FUNCTIONAL HYDROGELS IN DRUG DELIVERY

Key Features and Future Perspectives

FUNCTIONAL HYDROGELS IN DRUG DELIVERY

Key Features and Future Perspectives

Editors

Umile Gianfranco Spizzirri and Giuseppe Cirillo
Department of Pharmacy, Health and Nutritional Sciences
University of Calabria
Rende (CS)
Italy

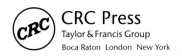

CRC Press
Taylor & Francis Group
Boca Raton London New York

CRC Press is an imprint of the
Taylor & Francis Group, an **informa** business
A SCIENCE PUBLISHERS BOOK

Cover illustration reproduced by permission of Drs. Derya Aydın, Mohammad Alipour and Seda Kizilel (authors of Chapter 1).

CRC Press
Taylor & Francis Group
6000 Broken Sound Parkway NW, Suite 300
Boca Raton, FL 33487-2742

First issued in paperback 2021

© 2017 by Taylor & Francis Group, LLC
CRC Press is an imprint of Taylor & Francis Group, an Informa business

No claim to original U.S. Government works

Version Date: 20170601

ISBN-13: 978-0-367-78202-3 (pbk)
ISBN-13: 978-1-4987-4901-5 (hbk)

Library of Congress Cataloging-in-Publication Data

Names: Spizzirri, Umile Gianfranco, editor. | Cirillo, Giuseppe, 1980- editor.
Title: Functional hydrogels in drug delivery : key features and future perspectives / editors, Umile Gianfranco Spizzirri and Giuseppe Cirillo, Department of Pharmacy, Health and Nutritional Sciences, University of Calabria, Rende (CS), Italy.
Description: Boca Raton, FL : CRC Press/ Taylor & Francis Group, 2017. | Includes bibliographical references and index.
Identifiers: LCCN 2017018991| ISBN 9781498749015 (hardback : alk. paper) | ISBN 9781498749022 (e-book)
Subjects: LCSH: Colloids in medicine. | Colloids--Biotechnology. | Pharmaceutical chemistry.
Classification: LCC R857.C66 F86 2017 | DDC 615.1/9--dc23
LC record available at https://lccn.loc.gov/2017018991

Visit the Taylor & Francis Web site at
http://www.taylorandfrancis.com

and the CRC Press Web site at
http://www.crcpress.com

Preface

Pharmaceutical application of hydrophilic materials has emerged as one of the most significant trends in the area of nanotechnology. "Intelligent" polymeric devices able to undergo morphological modifications in response to an internal or external stimulus, such as pH, redox balance, temperature, magnetic field, and light have been actively pursued. In an effort to further improve the performances of the drug delivery device, stimuli-responsive hydrogels responsive to a combination of two or more signals have recently been developed by incorporating different stimulus responsive elements into a network *via* polymerization processes. Notably, these combined responses take place either simultaneously at the pathological site, or sequentially from hydrogel preparation, hydrogel transporting pathways, to cellular compartments. These stimuli responsive polymeric materials lead to superior *in vitro* and/or *in vivo* therapeutic efficacy, with programmed site-specific feature and remarkable potential for targeted therapy. This book highlights the recent developments in the synthesis of stimuli-responsive hydrogels for applications in the pharmaceutical field, with a particular focus on the correlation between the hydrogel physical feature and the precision *situ*-controlled delivery of bioactive compounds. In this analysis, each chapter includes the last updates about the different materials employed and the improvement of their physico-chemical and biological properties to fabricate high performing carriers for specific use, including stimuli-responsive materials, molecularly imprinted polymers, carrier for the delivery of high MW drugs. Furthermore, the peculiar features of specific administration routes (e.g., oral, parenteral, vaginal, ocular and pulmonary) will be exploited with the aim to improve the efficiency of hydrogel devices.

Contents

Preface   **v**

1. **Design of Stimuli-Responsive Drug Delivery Hydrogels:**   **1**
   Synthesis and Applications
   Derya Aydın, Mohammad Alipour and *Seda Kizilel*

2. **Nanocomposite Hydrogels as Drug Delivery Systems**   **24**
   Teresa del Castillo Castro, María Mónica Castillo Ortega,
   Dora Evelia Rodríguez Félix and *José Carmelo Encinas Encinas*

3. **Vesicles, Micelles and Cyclodextrins Immobilized into**   **52**
   Hydrogel: Multi-component Devices for Controlled
   Drug Delivery
   Lorena Tavano and *Rita Muzzalupo*

4. **Molecularly Imprinted Hydrogels for the Selective Release**   **64**
   of Therapeutics
   Piotr Luliński and *Marcin Woźnica*

5. **Prodrugs and Bioconjugate Hydrogels: A Valuable Strategy**   **88**
   for the Prolonged-Delivery of Drugs
   Ankit Jain, Anamika Sahu, Aviral Jain and *Arvind Gulbake*

6. **Carbohydrate based Hydrogels for Controlled Release of**   **113**
   Cancer Therapeutics
   S. Eswaramma, K.S.V. Krishna Rao, Qian Zhong and
   K. Madhusudana Rao

7. **Porous Hydrogels as Carrier for Delivery of**   **154**
   Macromolecular Drugs
   Ecaterina Stela Dragan, Ana Irina Cocarta and *Maria Valentina Dinu*

8. **Biopolymer-based Interpenetrating Network Hydrogels for**   **197**
   Oral Drug Delivery
   Sabyasachi Maiti and *Sougata Jana*

9. **Stimuli-Responsive Hydrogels for Parenteral Drug Delivery**   **234**
   Gayatri C. Patel

10. Hydrogels for Vaginal Drug Delivery   259
    Željka Vanić and Nataša Škalko-Basnet

11. Advances in Composite Hydrogels for Ocular Drug   303
    Delivery and Biomedical Engineering Application
    Andreza Maria Ribeiro and Ivan Antonio Neumann

12. Hydrogels for Pulmonary Drug Delivery   327
    Ibrahim M. El-Sherbiny, Mohammed Sedki, Habiba Soliman and
    Magdi H. Yacoub

Index   353

1

Design of Stimuli-Responsive Drug Delivery Hydrogels

Synthesis and Applications

Derya Aydın, Mohammad Alipour and *Seda Kizilel**

ABSTRACT

Stimuli-responsive hydrogels have become popular in medicine and polymer science as useful 'smart' devices due to their various properties such as overall biocompatibility, high drug loading capacity, and controlled molecule delivery. By tuning the polymer side chains and degree of crosslinking, these gels may exhibit swelling/shrinking behaviour in response to environmental stimuli such as light, pH, chemicals, temperature, mechanical strain, and electrical field. Sensitivity of these hydrogels enables precise control over fundamental material properties such as physical structure, porosity, swelling behaviour, mechanical strength and drug permeability. Temperature and pH alterations are examples of physiological deviations that are commonly considered for the design of responsive hydrogels, specifically for site-specific controlled drug delivery. A class of hydrogels known as multi-responsive hydrogels can respond to more than one stimuli which make them tunable and controllable with improved biomimetic properties well-suited for controlled and site specific drug delivery. Despite all these attractive properties of stimuli-responsive hydrogels, slow response time may cause some limitations in practical applications. Reduced hydrogel thickness may decrease the response time of the gel to a stimulus; however, this

Department of Chemical and Biological Engineering, Koc University, Sariyer, Istanbul, Turkey, 34450.

* Corresponding author

may lead to mechanically fragile hydrogel structures. Therefore, practical applications need significant improvement in hydrogel design to improve response time considering mechanical properties, biocompatibility, and biodegradability. This chapter highlights recent progress in the field of stimuli-responsive hydrogels, focusing primarily on drug delivery vehicles.

Keywords: stimuli-responsive, hydrogel, drug delivery

1. Introduction

During the past decades, most of the pharmaceutical research has focused on controlled drug delivery systems. Novel drug delivery vehicles have been developed using systems that include micelles, liposomes, dendrimers, nanoparticles and lipo-protein drug carriers (Taghizadeh et al. 2015, des Rieux et al. 2006, Alamdarnejad et al. 2013, Fattal et al. 2002). Among many types of polymeric systems that are used as drug carriers, hydrogels have attracted considerable interest and have been reviewed from different perspectives (Peppas 1997, Hoare and Kohane 2008).

Hydrogels are a unique class of macromolecular networks that have a high water swelling ratio. Many advantages of hydrogels such as biocompatibility, water retention, external and internal stimulus in the hydrogels provide suitable platform for the diffusion of therapeutic substance (Hoffman 2012). Hydrophilic and hydrophobic properties of hydrogels and the degree of cross-linking and ionization are important parameters that control equilibrium swelling, dimensional alterations and release profiles of drugs through these carriers (Peppas 1987, Brannon-Peppas and Peppas 1991, Bal et al. 2014, Giray et al. 2012).

In recent years, stimuli-responsive hydrogels have attracted significant attention for the development of controlled-released drug delivery systems and their clinical applications. Increasing number of studies have been published about drug delivery through stimuli-responsive systems as is shown in Fig. 1. An ideal drug delivery system should be capable of synchronizing the drug release profile with the physiological condition (Gupta et al. 2002). Responsive properties of special hydrogels to environmental stimulus are especially desirable for clinical applications. In response to internal or external stimuli, hydrogels undergo significant change in their network structure, swelling behaviour, and permeability (Bajpai et al. 2008). External stimuli such as light and electric field have been applied with stimuli generating devices, whereas internal stimuli occur within the native environment of the body (Gupta et al. 2002). Commonly used external and internal stimuli to control drug release behaviour include pH, temperature, chemical, mechanical strain, light, electric field, and magnetic field which are illustrated in Fig. 2 (Popescu et al. 2011). In this chapter, we address opportunities and challenges related to the synthesis,

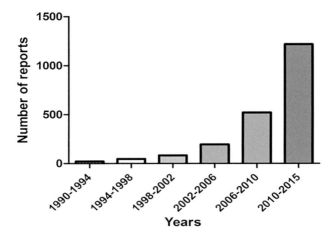

Fig. 1. Number of studies reported about stimuli-responsive hydrogels in drug delivery from 1990 to 2015.

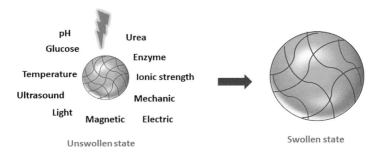

Fig. 2. Schematic representation of possible stimuli used to trigger structural alterations in hydrogel networks.

swelling and drug delivery through stimuli-responsive hydrogels and provide future directions on further requirements for clinical applications.

2. Thermo-responsive Hydrogels

Thermo-responsive hydrogels and polymers is the most commonly studied class of responsive polymeric systems in drug delivery research (Bawa et al. 2009, Bromberg and Ron 1998, Gil and Hudson 2004, Qiu and Park 2012). Temperature can act as an external or internal stimulus. Thermal stimulus is important due to universal physiological temperature of 37°C and development of several mechanisms to manipulate and control temperature *in vivo* (Klouda and Mikos 2008, Koetting et al. 2015). Drug delivery can be triggered by temperature changes due to increased body temperature in a disease state or due to modulated external temperature (Bawa et al. 2009).

2.1 Properties of temperature-sensitive hydrogels

Characteristic feature of thermoresponsive polymers is the presence of hydrophobic units such as methyl, ethyl and propyl groups (Qiu and Park 2012). Critical solution temperature is a key parameter in temperature-sensitive polymers. At a specific temperature the polymer phase changes according to its composition (Gil and Hudson 2004). If the polymer solution has a lower critical solution temperature (LCST), its solubility in water decreases upon heating. Otherwise, it is called an upper critical solution temperature (UCST) (Schmaljohann 2006).

For the case of hydrogels, the solubility decreases and hydrogels shrink as temperature increases above the LCST. This type of swelling behaviour is known as inverse temperature dependence (Chaterji et al. 2007). These hydrogels show this property due to the presence of polymer chains that have both hydrophobic and hydrophilic groups. The hydrophobic segments have strengthened high temperatures due to weakening of hydrogen bond and solubility which leads to the shrinking of the hydrogels (Qiu and Park 2012). Poly(N-isopropylacrylamide) (PNIPAAm) based hydrogels are used for this unique phase transition with reversible swelling-shrinkage abilities, which is very useful for the controlled release of encapsulated or loaded hydrophilic drugs. These hydrogels start shrinking when the temperature increases above LCST and leads to the release of drug from hydrogel network (Fig. 3). Many studies have focused on the design of thermo-responsive PNIPAM-based hydrogels for their use in controlled drug delivery systems (Liu et al. 2012, Gao et al. 2013, Zhang et al. 2009, Cheng et al. 2015).

2.2 Common monomers of thermo-responsive hydrogels

PNIPAAm is the most commonly used thermo-responsive polymer in drug delivery, as its phase transition occurs at approximately body temperature (Bawa et al. 2009, Qiu and Park 2012, Koetting et al. 2015, Schmaljohann 2006, Kamath and Park 1993). The LCST of PNIPAAm has been modified by a number of comonomers (Liu et al. 2009). The inclusion of hydrophilic monomers raises the LCST, while hydrophobic comonomers depress the critical point. However, there are limitations about the shift of the LCST due to the necessary amount of NIPAAm units (Liu et al. 2009). It has phase transition at 32°C in water and can be increased to a temperature of about 40°C with the addition of a hydrophilic co-monomer such as *N,N*-dimethylacrylamide (PDMAAm) (Gan et al. 2001). Poly(PDEAAm)

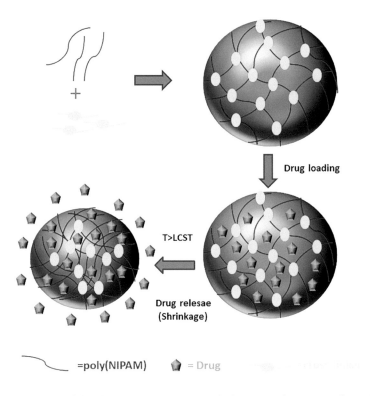

Fig. 3. Schematic of the thermo-responsive morphology transformation of crosslinked poly(NIPAM) hydrogels.

is also widely used because of its LCST within the range of 25–32°C. Copolymers of NIPAAm can also be synthesized using other monomers such as butylmethacrylate (BMA) in order to alter LCST (Qiu and Park 2012). Another novel thermo-responsive polymer that has also pH-responsive characteristics is poly(*N*-acryloyl-*N*-alkylpiperazine) (Gan et al. 2001). Polyethylene-glycol (PEG) also shows negative temperature response in aqueous environments. PEG methacrylate hydrogels decrease in swelling ratio as temperature increases and longer chains lead to lower solubility at lower temperatures (Koetting et al. 2015).

Besides swelling–shrinking transition, temperature-sensitive hydrogels that are not covalently crosslinked may demonstrate sol–gel phase transitions, instead of swelling–shrinking transitions. The thermally reversible gels with inverse temperature dependence become sol at higher temperatures. Some block copolymers made of poly(ethylene oxide) (PEO) and poly(propylene oxide) (PPO) demonstrate this inverse temperature response (Bawa et al. 2009, Qiu and Park 2012).

2.3 *Applications of temperature-responsive hydrogels in drug delivery*

Temperature-sensitive hydrogels have been studied most extensively and their unique applications have been reviewed in earlier reports (Bawa et al. 2009, Qiu and Park 2012, Klouda and Mikos 2008, Schmaljohann 2006, Aoyagi et al. 2000). These gels are basically classified as negatively thermo-sensitive, positively thermo-sensitive, and thermally reversible gels (Qiu and Park 2012). Negatively thermo-sensitive hydrogels have been used in on–off drug release systems in response to a stepwise temperature change (Bae et al. 1991a). Crosslinked P(NIPAAm–co-BMA) hydrogels (Chun and Kim 1996, Cevik et al. 2015, Ritger and Peppas 1987), and interpenetrating polymer networks (IPNs) of P(NIPAAm) and poly(tetramethyleneether glycol) (PTMEG) have been considered in these on–off drug release studies (Bae et al. 1991b). Hydrophobic comonomer BMA was introduced into NIPAAm gels to increase their mechanical strength. For example, on–off release of indomethacin through these gels was monitored at low temperature (on) and high temperature (off) because of shrinkage of the surface that leads to less permeable barrier. This shrinking of the surface was observed due to sudden differences in the hydrogel interior and surface temperatures. The shrinking of the surface was explained by the length of methacrylate alkyl side-chain and hydrophobicity of the comonomer (Yoshida et al. 1992).

Various forms of thermo-responsive hydrogels formed by IPNs demonstrate positive thermosensitivity which means swelling at high temperature and shrinking at low temperature. IPNs synthesized with poly(acrylic acid) and polyacrylamide (PAAm) or P(AAm–co-BMA) have this positive thermosensitivity (Katono et al. 1991). Increasing BMA content in this network shifts the transition temperature to higher temperature. The swelling of those hydrogels resulted in reversible changes in the release rate of ketoprofen, a model drug, in response to temperature alterations (Katono et al. 1991).

Different PEO-PPO thermoreversible gels have also been used in controlled drug delivery systems based on sol–gel transition at body temperature (Qiu and Park 2012). Some of these gels are commercially available under the names of Pluronics® and Tetronics, which have been approved by Food and Drug Administration and Environmental Protection Agency for applications in pharmaceutical ingredients and have many applications in drug delivery (Bromberg and Ron 1998).

Another application of thermo-responsive hydrogels is hyperthermia whose combination with chemo and radiotherapy is important for enhancing solid tumour cytotoxicity, permeability and drug delivery to tumours (Issels 1999). Hyperthermia treatment is usually performed at temperatures higher than body temperature, thus LCST of temperature-responsive delivery systems should be above the body temperature (Meyer et al. 2001). Polymeric micelles of block copolymers with thermo-responsive property have been studied as drug delivery systems for enhanced permeation and retention effect of tumour sites (Matsumura and Maeda 1986). Block copolymers with hydrophobic polymers, such as poly(butyl methacrylate) (PBMA), polystyrene or poly(lactic acid), were prepared with end-functionalized thermo-responsive polymer such as PNIPAAm (Chung et al. 1999, Chung et al. 2000). These micellar structures showed hydration in aqueous solution below transition temperature of PNIPAAm. Upon a temperature rise above 32°C, these chains become hydrophobic due to dehydration of polymer chains. Since dehydrated chains aggregate and precipitate, the core of micelles becomes a reservoir for a hydrophobic anticancer drug, Adriamycin (Fig. 4) (Bawa et al. 2009, Chung et al. 2000).

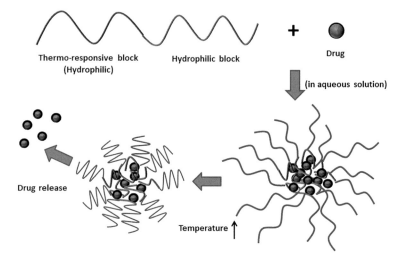

Fig. 4. Structure and drug release from a thermo-responsive polymeric micelle.

In a very recent study, dual stimuli-responsive hydrogel was synthesized by cross-linking copolymers of nisopropylacrylamide (NIPAM) and 2-hydroxyethyl acrylate (HEA) with a diselenide-bearing cross-linking agent (Cheng et al. 2015). This thermo and oxidant responsive poly(NIPAM-co-HEA) hydrogels have diselenide linkages, so they could degrade in the presence of oxidizing agents and become water soluble. Since these hydrogels have PNIPAM units, they demonstrate swelling–shrinkage behaviour in response to temperature alterations (Cheng et al. 2015).

2.3.1 Thermo-responsive hydrogels in particle based drug delivery

Majority of the applications related to thermal responsive hydrogel particle involve the design of composites for therapeutic and diagnostic objectives. These systems are usually composed of a traceable particle, such as iron oxide or gold, coated in a thermally responsive, drug loaded hydrogel. One application of these systems is the chemotherapeutic delivery where highly toxic drugs show improved effectiveness when localized and concentrated at the site of a tumour (Koetting et al. 2015). Temperature-sensitive hydrogel microparticles are also used by grafting them to the surface of rigid membranes. PNIPAAm hydrogel microparticles were dispersed into a crosslinked gelatin matrix and temperature dependent release of a model drug, 4-acetamidophen, from membranes was demonstrated (Chun and Kim 1996).

3. pH-responsive Hydrogels

pH-responsive hydrogels are of great importance since these systems could respond to the naturally dynamic variation of pH in several parts of the body such as gastrointestinal tract, vagina and blood vessels (Gupta et al. 2002). Principally, pH-responsive hydrogels sense the perturbation in the environment pH contributing to change in physical properties of the hydrogel such as shape and size (Cevik et al. 2015). In particular, two main strategies are used for the design of pH-responsive drug delivery systems: (1) the use of polymeric systems with ionizable pendant moieties on their backbone structure and, (2) the use of polymers bearing acid sensitive bonds where breaking of these bonds contribute to the release of drug molecules attached to the polymer backbone (Taghizadeh et al. 2015). Among various kinetic models developed for drug or protein release from swollen hydrogel structure, the following model proposed by Ritger and Peppas has been commonly used (Ritger and Peppas 1987):

$$\frac{Mt}{M\infty} = kt^{n} \tag{1}$$

where in Eq. (1) Mt/M_{∞} is the fractional release of drug in time t, 'k' is the characteristic constant of the hydrogel and 'n' is the diffusion exponent characteristic of the release mechanism.

3.1 Polymer composition and swelling behaviour

The presence of ionizable pendant groups in the polymer backbone, contribute to the pH-responsibility of hydrogel systems (Koetting et al. 2015). Ionization of the pendant group in the aqueous solution at appropriate pH and ionic strength will result in an accumulation of fixed charge along polymer network contributing to pH-dependent swelling or shrinking behaviour (Gupta et al. 2002). Swelling behaviour of hydrogels could be tuned with polymer properties such as cross-linking density, hydrophobicity/hydrophilicity, degree of polymerization and the charge, pKa, and concentration of the ionizable groups and also properties of swelling medium such as pH and ionic strength (Anderson and Quinn 1974). Increasing ionic strength of the swelling buffer will result in ion exchange between buffer and hydrogel. The ionic contribution to overall swelling is represented by osmotic pressure (π_{ion}) which is calculated by the following:

$$\pi_{ion} = RT \sum (C_i - C_i^*) \tag{2}$$

In Eq. (2) C_i and C_i^* are counterion concentration inside and outside of hydrogel, R is universal gas constant and T is absolute temperature respectively (Khare and Peppas 1995). The most common synthetic polymers investigated for pH-responsive behaviour include acrylic acid (AA), methacrylic acid (MAA), dimethylaminoethyl methacrylate (DMAEMA), diethylaminoethyl methacrylate (DEAEMA) and acrylamide (AAm). Natural hydrogels such as gelatin, albumin, alginate, and chitosan can exhibit pH-responsive behaviour as well (Koetting et al. 2015). Depending on the ionizable pendant group, pH-responsive hydrogels are categorized into two main groups as cationic and anionic hydrogels (Podual et al. 2000). As the external pH increases, the hydrogel network undergoes swelling if it contains anionic pendant groups or shrinks if it contains cationic pendant groups in its polymeric backbone (Bajpai et al. 2008). The pH-responsive behaviour of anionic and cationic hydrogels is depicted in Fig. 5.

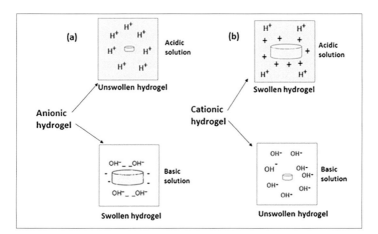

Fig. 5. Schematic representation of the pH-responsive swelling of (a) anionic and (b) cationic hydrogels.

3.1.1 Anionic hydrogel

Anionic hydrogels exhibit swelling behaviour when pH of the swelling buffer is above acid dissociation constant, pKa, due to a simultaneous effect of electrostatic repulsion and water absorption. The structure of these gels remains collapsed at low pH because of the tight physical interactions in the network (Gupta et al. 2002).

3.1.2 Cationic hydrogel

In cationic hydrogels, drug is mostly released at low pH conditions such as stomach (Risbud et al. 2000). In contrary to anionic hydrogels, cationic hydrogels swell at low pH condition (pH < pKa) and collapse when exposed to an environment with high pH (pH > pKa) (Koetting et al. 2015). The swelling behaviour of pH responsive anionic or cationic hydrogels is different in acidic and alkaline buffer solutions (Gupta et al. 2002).

3.2 Application of pH-responsive hydrogels in controlled drug delivery

Both anionic and cationic pH-responsive hydrogels have been investigated for controlled delivery of therapeutic drugs (Liu et al. 2006), genetic agents (Forbes and Peppas 2014), and proteins (Peppas et al. 2004). A wide variety of existing synthetic and natural pH-responsive polymers enable researchers to tune hydrogel swelling properties (Koetting et al. 2015). pH-responsive hydrogels are potentially useful for oral administration of the drug along the digestive tract due to the dramatic different pH conditions observed at different sites, or for targeted drug delivery into a tumour site due to alterations in the acidity of tumour tissue (Cevik et al. 2015). Singh and Sharma applied different kinetic models to study antibiotic drug release from tragacanth gum and poly(acrylic acid) based polymer networks (Singh and Sharma 2014). Liu et al. developed an amphiphilic hydrogel interpenetrating polymer network (IPN) as a carrier for controlled drug delivery, where hydrophilic network was important for swelling of IPN and hydrophobic network was useful to encapsulate drug molecules (Popescu et al. 2011). Popescu et al. investigated a novel drug delivery composite system consisting of a pH-sensitive nanostructured hydrogel (matrix) encapsulating PC/Chol liposomes as nano-carrier loaded with calcein as hydrophilic model drug (Liu et al. 2006).

Besides all advantages mentioned for pH-responsive hydrogels, non-biodegradable character of these gels limits their use for clinical applications, since hydrogels made up of non-degradable polymers should be removed from the body after their use (Qiu and Park 2012). Subsequently, synthesizing pH-responsive hydrogels based on polypeptides, proteins, and polysaccharides attracted significant attention (Markland et al. 1999, Chiu et al. 1999).

4. Photo-responsive Hydrogels

Photo responsive hydrogels are particularly interesting for drug delivery applications due to remote, temporary, and spatial control over particle release from these 3D structures. More importantly, the light irradiation does not interfere with most proteins activity (Peng et al. 2010). These type of responsive hydrogels are classified into two main groups: (1) photodegradable hydrogels which have degradable moieties (e.g., o-nitrobenzyl and azobenzene) in their backbone, (2) thermo-sensitive hydrogels (e.g., poly(N-isopropylacrylamine)) that contain near infrared (NIR)-absorbing nanostructures such as nanoshells and carbon nanotubes in the matrix (Wang et al. 2016).

4.1 Common photo-responsiveness mechanisms

Photo-sensitive molecules respond to light *via* three main mechanisms: isomerization or cyclization, degradation, and dimerization (Koetting et al. 2015). Azobenzenes, incorporated within hydrogel structure both as pendant groups or cross-linkers, are one of the most common structures that undergo isomerization as cis-trans shift and vice versa in response to 360 and 440 nm light, resulting in the dissolution of the hydrogel (Peng et al. 2010, Yager and Barrett 2006, Barrett et al. 2007). The other common form of isomerization mechanism is cyclization. The balanced cyclic structures of these functional groups such as spirobenzo-pyran, make these molecules prime targets for low energy photo-irradiation. Degradation is based on cleavage of covalent bonds. The most common monomer used as photo-degradable moieties is the o-methoxy nitro-benzene family (Kloxin et al. 2009). The last mechanism is dimerization, which involves combination of two units. The most common reaction type of this mechanism is cyclization of two double bonds to form acyclo-butyl ring, but due to high ring strain, they readily break up in response to 350 and 250 nm light respectively (Koetting et al. 2015).

4.2 Applications

Delivery systems with a pulsatile or triggered release pattern are receiving higher interest compared to continuous release systems. Since the release of particles from hydrogel networks can be controlled by alteration of network mesh size, photo-responsive hydrogel systems are potentially useful for drug delivery systems with a controlled release (Tomatsu et al. 2011). Peng et al. functionalized dextran with azobenzene (AB) or b-cyclodextrin (CD) moieties for a light controlled release of protein. The cis-trans configuration of azobenzene changes upon exposure to UV light (365 nm) resulting in the dissociation of hydrogel as illustrated in Fig. 6 (Peng et al. 2010). Griffin and Kasko synthesized and characterized release of a model therapeutic agent from a light induced polymeric release system using an ortho-nitrobenzyl (o-NB) ether linker as the photosensitive moiety. They investigated the effect of different parameters such as wavelength, light intensity, sample geometry, and exposure time on the release profile of therapeutic agent (Griffin and Kasko 2012). Despite wide applications of photo responsive hydrogels, they are not fully satisfactory for drug release systems due to slow reaction in response to light as an external stimuli. Furthermore, in some cases chromophores can leach out during swelling–deswelling cycles as they are covalently linked to polymer backbone (Qiu and Park 2012).

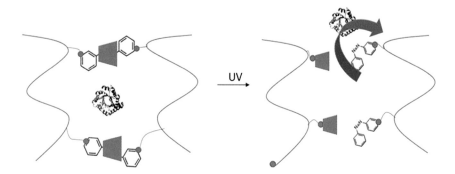

Fig. 6. Schematic representation of photo-responsive protein release from a network consisting of trans AB-Dex and CD-Dex. Azobenzene moieties isomerize from trans to cis configuration once exposed to UV light, resulting in protein release as crosslinking points disbanded.

5. Chemically Responsive Hydrogels

Another important class of stimuli-responsive hydrogels is chemically responsive hydrogels which shows swelling or degradation in response to certain target molecules. Even though there is wide range of chemicals which can act as stimuli for some useful functions, the most widely known are glucose-responsive, enzyme-responsive and molecularly imprinted polymers (Koetting et al. 2015).

5.1 Glucose-responsive hydrogels

Glucose-responsive hydrogel systems have the capability to provide self regulated insulin release in response to a specific concentration of glucose in the blood (Bawa et al. 2009). Regulation of insulin concentration is important because an overdose of insulin may cause a hypoglycemic coma or when insufficient insulin is injected, hyperglycemia may result. Regular glucose measurement is also critical in cell growth since glucose is the primary carbon source in most fermentation processes (Kabilan et al. 2004). Therefore, precisely engineered glucose-responsive delivery systems is required for maintaining appropriate glucose levels.

5.1.1 Properties, common monomers and applications of glucose-responsive hydrogels

Glucose-responsive hydrogels generally utilize immobilized enzymes or biocatalysts, more specifically glucose oxidase. These biocatalysts catalyze an enzymatic reaction in their soluble state and the products of this enzymatic reaction then triggers phase transition of gel network. Glucose-responsive hydrogels have mostly relied on two mechanisms for detecting glucose and responding in an appropriate way. In one of these mechanisms, glucose oxidase acts as a detecting enzyme and its reaction with glucose as a transduction pathway for stimulating response. For insulin delivery case, glucose oxidase utilizes the pH sensitivity of the polymer where the enzyme is immobilized. The glucose oxidase converts glucose to form gluconic acid which leads to pH change which results in volume transition in ph-sensitive hydrogel. Thus, the swelling ratio of the hydrogel is regulated by the glucose concentration of the environment (Bawa et al. 2009).

The second main pathway for glucose-responsiveness is based on concanavalin A which is a glucose-binding protein (Ballerstadt and Schultz 1998, Adams et al. 2006, Kim and Park 2001, Miyata et al. 2004). In this mechanism, Con A binds to glycosylated moieties in the hydrogel that consists of glycosylated polymer backbone resulting in the formation of a tight matrix that keeps insulin entrapped within the network. Since Con A has greater affinity for glucose than for glycosylated moieties, when glucose diffuses into the polymer matrix, the glucose displaces glycosylated polymer. This replacement promotes hydrogel swelling and results in insulin release by diffusion (Fig. 7). The mechanism has some limitations such as slow response time and leakage of Con A from the hydrogel. Various improvements were performed such as conjugation Con A with PEG chains (Kim and Park 2001a,b) or covalent binding of Con A (Miyata et al. 2004) to increase the stability and affinity of Con A to glucose for insulin delivery.

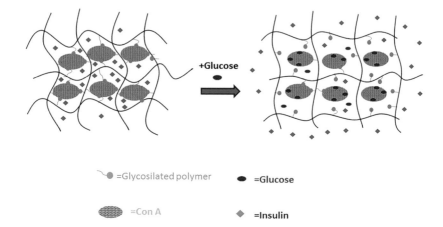

Fig. 7. Insulin release during Con A based sol–gel phase-transition of a glucose-sensitive hydrogel.

These improvements prevented leaching of Con A out of the polymer and resulted in repeatable swelling behaviour.

5.2 Enzyme-responsive hydrogels

Enzyme-responsive hydrogels are another important chemically sensitive hydrogels that are responsive only to specific enzymes. These enzymes have been utilized as signals of physiological changes and can be used in site-specific drug delivery (Bawa et al. 2009). The most common approach for the design of enzyme-responsive hydrogels involves incorporation of peptide chains into the gel network as linker or crosslinker to make the network biodegradable with specific enzymes. In a previous study, an effective approach was reported for creating tumour targeting nanocarriers for drug delivery. Magnetic iron oxide nanoparticles (MIONPs) were coated with integrin-targetted and matrix-metalloproteinase (MMP) sensitive PEG hydrogel scaffolds. The functional PEG hydrogel coating has been designed for active loading and triggered intra-cellular release of the cancer therapeutic agent doxorubicin (DOX). This study demonstrated that coated nanocarriers could be taken into cancer cells 11 times more efficiently than uncoated ones (Nazli et al. 2014). In another study, oligopeptide sequences such as GFLG, GFLGK was targetted for cathepsin B-based degradation for the delivery of plasmid DNA and antibodies (Koetting et al. 2015, Rejmanová et al. 1983). N-(2-hydroxypropyl) methacrylamide (HPMA) backbone with drugs attached *via* GFLG was synthesized and cleaved by cathepsin B for release of doxorubicin and ampicillin (Koetting et al. 2015). Peptides have also been used as cross-linkers in these drug delivery systems (Glangchai et al. 2008).

Enzyme-responsive hydrogels can be used in colon targetted drug delivery and can potentially be useful for the treatment of colon cancer or the systemic delivery of drugs in the upper gastro-intestinal tract (Yang et al. 2002). Since in the microenvironment of colon, reductive enzymes (e.g., azoreductase) or hydrolytic enzymes (e.g., glycosidases) degrade various types of polysaccharides such as pectin, chitosan, cyclodextrin and dextrin, design of hydrogels cross-linked with diisocyanate can be useful for targeting of colon (Sinha and Kumria 2001).

5.3 Molecularly imprinted polymers (MIP)

Molecular imprinting is used for the synthesis of artificial receptors for a given target molecule based on synthetic polymers. Hydrogels are synthesized using a template to produce binding sites that are capable of binding target molecules. MIPs act like antibodies due to their molecule recognition property (Ansell 2004, Tang et al. 2005, Haupt et al. 2011).

MIPs have been considered to develop controlled drug delivery systems (Alvarez-Lorenzo and Concheiro 2004, Sellergren and Allender 2005). MIPs have the advantage of specific binding to target molecules. Commercial use of MIPs in drug delivery can attract great interest, if this specific binding property of MIPs can be used for the development of highly controlled release systems over conventional responsive hydrogels.

6. Mechanical Strain-Responsive Hydrogels

Mechanical strain responsive hydrogels as subset of the stimuli-responsive hydrogels have been classified as pressure responsive and shear stress responsive hydrogels (Qiu and Park 2012, Koetting et al. 2015). Based on the experimental results and thermodynamic calculations, pressure responsive hydrogels undergo volume expansion under high pressure and collapse under low pressure (Lee et al. 1990, Zhong et al. 1996). Shear stress responsive hydrogels exhibit shear-thinning and shear-thickening behaviour upon exposure to shear stress as illustrated in Fig. 8 (Hoffman 2013). Mechanical responsive properties of hydrogels allow for the design of injectable materials which are becoming significant for tissue engineering and therapeutic drug delivery (Guvendiren et al. 2012).

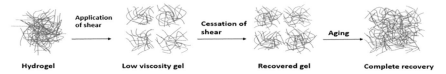

Fig. 8. Schematic representation of the network behaviour during shear-thinning and recovery or self-healing.

6.1 Common monomers

Injectable hydrogels can be classified into two major groups based on the nature of their *in situ* cross-linking mechanism (Guvendiren et al. 2012). *In situ* chemical cross-linking is based on photo-initiated, redox-initiated or Michael-type addition polymerization, while physically cross-linked hydrogels form as some peptides, proteins, or synthetic polymer microparticles which are self-assembling under external stimuli and do not rely on covalent bond formation (Kretlow et al. 2007). Poly(N-isopropylacrylamide) hydrogels are examples of sensitive hydrogels where they demonstrate swelling behaviour under hydrostatic pressure at temperature near to its LCST (Lee et al. 1990). Poly(N,N-propylacrylamide), poly(N,N-diethylacrylamide) and poly(N-isopropylacrylamide) are some other examples of pressure responsive hydrogels (Qiu and Park 2012). Shear stress responsive hydrogels could be derived both from natural proteins, engineered peptides, synthetic polymer species, or colloidal systems (Koetting et al. 2015). Naturally derived proteins such as silk fibroin self-assemble to a hydrogel that is composed of β-rich fibers (Matsumoto et al. 2006).

6.2 Applications of mechanical strain-responsive hydrogels

Mechanical strain responsive hydrogels have been investigated for a wide variety of applications in tissue engineering and drug delivery systems. Shear-thinning or shear-thickenings properties of these hydrogels make them capable of being injected by syringe very easily, undergoing a rapid sol–gel transition, then filling and adapting the shape of cavity or damaged tissues (Koetting et al. 2015, Guvendiren et al. 2012). Altunbas et al. developed a self-assembling peptide hydrogel system exhibiting shear thinning and immediate recovery properties that can form a solid physical hydrogel by *in vitro* assembly at physiological conditions allowing for three-dimensional and homogenous encapsulation of drug and other therapeutic molecules (Altunbas et al. 2011). Li et al. studied supramolecular structure of hydrogels formed by physical cross-linking induced by the supramolecular self-assembly of poly(ethylene oxide) (PEO) threaded with α-Cyclodextrin (α-CD). These gels were found as shear-thinning, reversible, and injectable through needles (Li et al. 2003). The release of labeled dextran was used as a model molecule through these gels. Furthermore, the drug release kinetics was found to be influenced by erosion of these hydrogels due to detaching of PEO chains from the cavities of CDs (Guvendiren et al. 2012, Li et al. 2003). Synthetic colloidal hydrogels developed by Wang et al. which consists of self-assembly of poly(D,L-lactic-co-glycolic acid) (PLGA) colloidal particles, exhibit shear-thinning behaviour due to the disruption of inter-particle interactions as the applied shear force was increased (Wang et al. 2008).

7. Electro-responsive Hydrogels

Electric signal can be used as an external stimulus which has various advantages. This stimuli can provide control over current magnitude and duration of electrical pulses (Bawa et al. 2009). Electric-responsive hydrogels demonstrate shrinking or swelling behaviour in response to applied electric field and this property allows for their application in drug delivery (Qiu and Park 2012). Delivery systems that utilize this property are designed with polyelectrolytes that have high concentration of ionizable groups on backbone (Bawa et al. 2009). Partially hydrolyzed polyacrylamide hydrogels in direct contact with both anode and cathode electrodes undergo a volume collapse if a minute change in electric potential is applied across the gel. On application of a potential, H+ ions migrate towards cathode, which results in a loss of water at anode side. Simultaneously, the electrostatic attraction that exists between the anode surface and the negatively charged acrylic acid groups creates a uniaxial stress along the gel axis. These two events lead to shrinking of the hydrogel on the anode side (Qiu and Park 2012, Tanaka et al. 1982, Gong et al. 1994).

7.1 Applications of electro-responsive hydrogels in drug delivery

Electro-responsive hydrogels have been used in controlled drug delivery (Sawahata et al. 1990, Kwon et al. 1991, Ramanathan and Block 2001, Yuk et al. 1992). One of the mechanism is based on chemomechanical shrinking and swelling of polymer gels under an electric field. The electric field-induced changes in the gel network results in on–off release profiles (Sawahata et al. 1990, Yuk et al. 1992). In one of these studies, electrically stimulated drug delivery systems using polyelectrolyte gel and microparticles have been reported. PAA hydrogel microparticles, which showed rapid shrinking with the applying electric current, are swollen back to their original size when the electric field was turned off. Pilocarpine hydrochloride, glucose and insulin could be released by switching the electric-field on and off. The electric field-induced volume changes of poly(dimethylaminopropylacrylamide) hydrogels were used for on–off release of insulin (Sawahata et al. 1990).

In another study, controlled release of edrophonium chloride was achieved from poly(2-acrylamido-2-methylpropane sulfonic acid-co-*n*-butylmethacrylate) poly(AMPS/BMA) monolithic device with electric stimulus (Kwon et al. 1991). The on–off drug release mechanism using electric stimulus was based on ion exchange between of the positively charged solute drug and hydrogen ion produced from electrolysis of water. The fast release pattern was also attributed to the electrostatic force, squeezing effect and the electro-osmosis of the gel (Kwon et al. 1991). Chitosan gels were also used as matrices for electrically modulated drug delivery.

8. Future Outlook

In this chapter, the synthesis and mechanisms, structural properties, release behaviours, and increasing applications of stimuli-responsive hydrogels in biomedical research, especially drug delivery systems, were reviewed. Significant progress has been achieved especially in the area of stimuli-responsive hydrogels allowing researchers to further investigate existing systems and develop new and smart responsive hydrogels based on detailed knowledge of the polymer-drug conjugates relationship.

Despite the possibility of responsive hydrogel design, temporal and spatial control delivery of particles to the desired site is still challenging which necessitates further investigation addressing all safety questions. Slow response time is one of the main obstacles for getting more efficient and desired drug release profile. However, making hydrogels with smaller size seems to be a good solution for decreasing response time but results in more fragile systems with insufficient mechanical strength.

Stimuli-responsive hydrogels provide many great advantages including controlled drug release, high specificity to tumour and intracellular drug delivery, and excellent therapeutic efficacy while minimizing drug and carrier associated side effects. However, further research is required to get smarter multi stimuli-responsive hydrogels providing less response-time, more biocompatibility and biodegradability, and sufficient mechanical strength.

Controlled drug delivery systems have attracted great interest of medical and industrial fields due to many desirable properties and functions of stimuli-responsive hydrogels. Since research is ongoing in an effort to find novel mechanisms, significant advances will occur in the near future both in healthcare and industry that arise directly from stimuli-responsive hydrogels.

References

Adams, G.G., Y. Cui, J.H. Mitchell and M.J. Taylor. 2006. Rheological and diffusion properties of a dextran-con A polymer in the presence of Insulin and Magnesium. Rheologica Acta. 45: 611–620.

Alamdarnejad, G., A. Sharif, S. Taranejoo, M. Janmaleki, M.R. Kalaee, M. Dadgar et al. 2013. Synthesis and characterization of thiolated carboxymethyl chitosan-graft-cyclodextrin nanoparticles as a drug delivery vehicle for albendazole. Journal of Materials Science-Materials in Medicine. 24: 1939–1949.

Altunbas, A., S.J. Lee, S.A. Rajasekaran, J.P. Schneider and D.J. Pochan. 2011. Encapsulation of curcumin in self-assembling peptide hydrogels as injectable drug delivery vehicles. Biomaterials. 32: 5906–5914.

Alvarez-Lorenzo, C. and A. Concheiro. 2004. Molecularly imprinted polymers for drug delivery. Journal of Chromatography B. 804: 231–245.

Anderson, J.L. and J.A. Quinn. 1974. Restricted transport in small pores. A model for steric exclusion and hindered particle motion. Biophys. J. 14: 130–150.

Ansell, R.J. 2004. Molecularly imprinted polymers in pseudoimmunoassay. Journal of Chromatography B. 804: 151–165.

Aoyagi, T., M. Ebara, K. Sakai, Y. Sakurai and T. Okano. 2000. Novel bifunctional polymer with reactivity and temperature sensitivity. Journal of Biomaterials Science, Polymer Edition. 11: 101–110.

Bae, Y.H., T. Okano and S.W. Kim. 1991a. "On–Off" thermocontrol of solute transport. I. Temperature dependence of swelling of N-isopropylacrylamide networks modified with hydrophobic components in water. Pharmaceutical Research. 8: 531–537.

Bae, Y.H., T. Okano and S.W. Kirn. 1991b. "On–Off" thermocontrol of solute transport. II. Solute release from thermosensitive hydrogels. Pharmaceutical Research. 8: 624–628.

Bajpai, A.K., S.K. Shukla, S. Bhanu and S. Kankane. 2008. Responsive polymers in controlled drug delivery. Progress in Polymer Science. 33: 1088–1118.

Bal, T., B. Kepsutlu and S. Kizilel. 2014. Characterization of protein release from poly(ethylene glycol) hydrogels with crosslink density gradients. Journal of Biomedical Materials Research Part A. 102: 487–495.

Ballerstadt, R. and J.S. Schultz. 1998. Kinetics of dissolution of Concanavalin A/Dextran sols in response to glucose measured by surface plasmon resonance. Sensors and Actuators B: Chemical. 46: 50–55.

Barrett, C.J., J.I. Mamiya, K.G. Yager and T. Ikeda. 2007. Photo-mechanical effects in azobenzene-containing soft materials. Soft Matter. 3: 1249–1261.

Bawa, P., V. Pillay, Y.E. Choonara and L.C. du Toit. 2009. Stimuli-responsive polymers and their applications in drug delivery. Biomedical Materials. 4: 022001.

Brannon-Peppas, L. and N.A. Peppas. 1991. Time-dependent response of ionic polymer networks to pH and ionic strength changes. International Journal of Pharmaceutics. 70: 53–57.

Bromberg, L.E. and E.S. Ron. 1998. Temperature-responsive gels and thermogelling polymer matrices for protein and peptide delivery. Advanced Drug Delivery Reviews. 31: 197–221.

Cevik, O., D. Gidon and S. Kizilel. 2015. Visible-light-induced synthesis of pH-responsive composite hydrogels for controlled delivery of the anticonvulsant drug pregabalin. Acta Biomaterialia. 11: 151–161.

Chaterji, S., I.K. Kwon and K. Park. 2007. Smart polymeric gels: redefining the limits of biomedical devices. Progress in Polymer Science. 32: 1083–1122.

Cheng, X., Y. Jin, T. Sun, R. Qi, B. Fan and H. Li. 2015. Oxidation-and thermo-responsive poly(N-isopropylacrylamide-co-2-hydroxyethyl acrylate) hydrogels cross-linked via diselenides for controlled drug delivery. RSC Advances. 5: 4162–4170.

Chiu, H.C., G.H. Hsiue, Y.P. Lee and L.W. Huang. 1999. Synthesis and characterization of pH-sensitive dextran hydrogels as a potential colon-specific drug delivery system. J. Biomater. Sci. Polym. Ed. 10: 591–608.

Chun, S.-W. and J.-D. Kim. 1996. A novel hydrogel-dispersed composite membrane of poly(N-isopropylacrylamide) in a gelatin matrix and its thermally actuated permeation of 4-acetamidophen. Journal of Controlled Release. 38: 39–47.

Chung, J., M. Yokoyama, M. Yamato, T. Aoyagi, Y. Sakurai and T. Okano. 1999. Thermo-responsive drug delivery from polymeric micelles constructed using block copolymers of poly(N-isopropylacrylamide) and poly(butylmethacrylate). Journal of Controlled Release. 62: 115–127.

Chung, J.E., M. Yokoyama and T. Okano. 2000. Inner core segment design for drug delivery control of thermo-responsive polymeric micelles. Journal of Controlled Release. 65: 93–103.

des Rieux, A., V. Fievez, M. Garinot, Y.-J. Schneider and V. Preat. 2006. Nanoparticles as potential oral delivery systems of proteins and vaccines: A mechanistic approach. Journal of Controlled Release. 116: 1–27.

Fattal, E., S. Pecquet, P. Couvreur and A. Andremont. 2002. Biodegradable microparticles for the mucosal delivery of antibacterial and dietary antigens. International Journal of Pharmaceutics. 242: 15–24.

Forbes, D.C. and N.A. Peppas. 2014. Polymeric nanocarriers for siRNA delivery to murine macrophages. Macromolecular Bioscience. 14: 1096–1105.

Gan, L., G.R. Deen, X. Loh and Y. Gan. 2001. New stimuli-responsive copolymers of N-acryloyl-N'-alkyl piperazine and methyl methacrylate and their hydrogels. Polymer. 42: 65–69.

Gao, X., Y. Cao, X. Song, Z. Zhang, C. Xiao, C. He and X. Chen. 2013. pH- and thermo-responsive poly(N-isopropylacrylamide-co-acrylic acid derivative) copolymers and hydrogels with LCST dependent on pH and alkyl side groups. Journal of Materials Chemistry B. 1: 5578–5587.

Gil, E.S. and S.M. Hudson. 2004. Stimuli-responsive polymers and their bioconjugates. Progress in Polymer Science. 29: 1173–1222.

Giray, S., T. Bal, A.M. Kartal and S. Kızılel. 2012. Controlled drug delivery through a novel PEG hydrogel encapsulated silica aerogel system. Journal of Biomedical Materials Research Part A. 100: 1307–1315.

Glangchai, L.C., M. Caldorera-Moore, L. Shi and K. Roy. 2008. Nanoimprint lithography based fabrication of shape-specific, enzymatically-triggered smart nanoparticles. Journal of Controlled Release. 125: 263–272.

Gong, J., T. Nitta and Y. Osada. 1994. Electrokinetic modeling of the contractile phenomena of polyelectrolyte gels. One-dimensional capillary model. The Journal of Physical Chemistry. 98: 9583–9587.

Griffin, D.R. and A.M. Kasko. 2012. Photoselective Delivery of Model Therapeutics from Hydrogels. Acs Macro Letters. 1: 1330–1334.

Gupta, P., K. Vermani and S. Garg. 2002. Hydrogels: from controlled release to pH-responsive drug delivery. Drug Discov. Today. 7: 569–579.

Guvendiren, M., H.D. Lu and J.A. Burdick. 2012. Shear-thinning hydrogels for biomedical applications. Soft Matter. 8: 260–272.

Haupt, K., A.V. Linares, M. Bompart and B.T.S. Bui. 2011. Molecularly imprinted polymers. pp. 1–28. *In*: K. Haupt (ed.). Molecular Imprinting. Springer, Berlin Heidelberg.

Hoare, T.R. and D.S. Kohane. 2008. Hydrogels in drug delivery: progress and challenges. Polymer. 49: 1993–2007.

Hoffman, A.S. 2012. Hydrogels for biomedical applications. Advanced Drug Delivery Reviews. 64: 18–23.

Hoffman, A.S. 2013. Stimuli-responsive polymers: Biomedical applications and challenges for clinical translation. Advanced Drug Delivery Reviews. 65: 10–16.

Issels, R. 1999. Hyperthermia combined with chemotherapy–biological rationale, clinical application and treatment results. Oncology Research and Treatment. 22: 374–381.

Kabilan, S., J. Blyth, M. Lee, A. Marshall, A. Hussain, X.P. Yang et al. 2004. Glucose-sensitive holographic sensors. Journal of Molecular Recognition. 17: 162–166.

Kamath, K.R. and K. Park. 1993. Biodegradable hydrogels in drug delivery. Advanced Drug Delivery Reviews. 11: 59–84.

Katono, H., A. Maruyama, K. Sanui, N. Ogata, T. Okano and Y. Sakurai. 1991. Thermoresponsive swelling and drug release switching of interpenetrating polymer networks composed of poly(acrylamide-co-butyl methacrylate) and poly(acrylic acid). Journal of Controlled Release. 16: 215–227.

Khare, A.R. and N.A. Peppas. 1995. Swelling deswelling of anionic copolymer gels. Biomaterials. 16: 559–567.

Kim, J.J. and K. Park. 2001a. Glucose-binding property of pegylated concanavalin A. Pharmaceutical Research. 18: 794–799.

Kim, J.J. and K. Park. 2001b. Modulated insulin delivery from glucose-sensitive hydrogel dosage forms. Journal of Controlled Release. 77: 39–47.

Klouda, L. and A.G. Mikos. 2008. Thermoresponsive hydrogels in biomedical applications. European Journal of Pharmaceutics and Biopharmaceutics. 68: 34–45.

Kloxin, A.M., A.M. Kasko, C.N. Salinas and K.S. Anseth. 2009. Photodegradable Hydrogels for Dynamic Tuning of Physical and Chemical Properties. Science. 324: 59–63.

Koetting, M.C., J.T. Peters, S.D. Steichen and N.A. Peppas. 2015. Stimulus-responsive hydrogels: Theory, modern advances, and applications. Materials Science and Engineering: R: Reports. 93: 1–49.

Kretlow, J.D., L. Klouda and A.G. Mikos. 2007. Injectable matrices and scaffolds for drug delivery in tissue engineering. Adv. Drug Deliv. Rev. 59: 263–273.

Kwon, I.C., Y.H. Bae, T. Okano and S.W. Kim. 1991. Drug release from electric current sensitive polymers. Journal of Controlled Release. 17: 149156–149153.

Lee, K.K., E.L. Cussler, M. Marchetti and M.A. McHugh. 1990. Pressure-dependent phase-transitions in hydrogels. Chemical Engineering Science. 45: 766–767.

Li, J., X. Ni and K.W. Leong. 2003. Injectable drug-delivery systems based on supramolecular hydrogels formed by poly(ethylene oxide)s and alpha-cyclodextrin. J. Biomed. Mater. Res. A. 65: 196–202.

Liu, R., M. Fraylich and B.R. Saunders. 2009. Thermoresponsive copolymers: from fundamental studies to applications. Colloid and Polymer Science. 287: 627–643.

Liu, Y., Z. Li and D. Liang. 2012. Behaviors of liposomes in a thermo-responsive poly(N-isopropylacrylamide) hydrogel. Soft Matter. 8: 4517–4523.

Liu, Y.Y., X.D. Fan, X.B. Wei, Q.F. Si, W.X. Chen and L. Sun. 2006. pH-responsive amphiphilic hydrogel networks with IPN structure: A strategy for controlled drug. International Journal of Pharmaceutics. 308: 205–209.

Markland, P., Y. Zhang, G.L. Amidon and V.C. Yang. 1999. A pH- and ionic strength-responsive polypeptide hydrogel: synthesis, characterization, and preliminary protein release studies. J. Biomed. Mater. Res. 47: 595–602.

Matsumoto, A., J. Chen, A.L. Collette, U.-J. Kim, G.H. Altman, P. Cebe et al. 2006. Mechanisms of silk fibroin sol-gel transitions. Journal of Physical Chemistry B. 110: 21630–21638.

Matsumura, Y. and H. Maeda. 1986. A new concept for macromolecular therapeutics in cancer chemotherapy: mechanism of tumoritropic accumulation of proteins and the antitumor agent smancs. Cancer Research. 46: 6387–6392.

Meyer, D.E., B. Shin, G. Kong, M. Dewhirst and A. Chilkoti. 2001. Drug targeting using thermally responsive polymers and local hyperthermia. Journal of Controlled Release. 74: 213–224.

Miyata, T., A. Jikihara, K. Nakamae and A.S. Hoffman. 2004. Preparation of reversibly glucose-responsive hydrogels by covalent immobilization of lectin in polymer networks having pendant glucose. Journal of Biomaterials Science, Polymer Edition. 15: 1085–1098.

Nazli, C., G.S. Demirer, Y. Yar, H.Y. Acar and S. Kizilel. 2014. Targeted delivery of doxorubicin into tumor cells *via* MMP-sensitive PEG hydrogel-coated magnetic iron oxide nanoparticles (MIONPs). Colloids and Surfaces B: Biointerfaces. 122: 674–683.

Peng, K., I. Tomatsu and A. Kros. 2010. Light controlled protein release from a supramolecular hydrogel. Chem. Commun. (Camb). 46: 4094–4096.

Peppas, N.A. 1987. Hydrogels in Medicine and Pharmacy, Vol. 3. CRC Press, Boca Raton, FL.

Peppas, N.A. 1997. Hydrogels and drug delivery. Current Opinion in Colloid & Interface Science. 2: 531–537.

Peppas, N.A., K.M. Wood and J.O. Blanchette. 2004. Hydrogels for oral delivery of therapeutic proteins. Expert Opinion on Biological Therapy. 4: 881–887.

Podual, K., F.J. Doyle and N.A. Peppas. 2000. Preparation and dynamic response of cationic copolymer hydrogels containing glucose oxidase. Polymer. 41: 3975–3983.

Popescu, M.T., S. Mourtas, G. Pampalakis, S.G. Antimisiaris and C. Tsitsilianis. 2011. pH-responsive hydrogel/liposome soft nanocomposites for tuning drug release. Biomacromolecules. 12: 3023–3030.

Qiu, Y. and K. Park. 2012. Environment-sensitive hydrogels for drug delivery. Advanced Drug Delivery Reviews. 64: 49–60.

Ramanathan, S. and L.H. Block. 2001. The use of chitosan gels as matrices for electrically-modulated drug delivery. Journal of Controlled Release. 70: 109–123.

Rejmanová, P., J. Kopeček, J. Pohl, M. Baudyš and V. Kostka. 1983. Polymers containing enzymatically degradable bonds, 8. Degradation of oligopeptide sequences in N-(2-hydroxypropyl) methacrylamide copolymers by bovine spleen cathepsin B. Die Makromolekulare Chemie. 184: 2009–2020.

Risbud, M.V., A.A. Hardikar, S.V. Bhat and R.R. Bhonde. 2000. pH-sensitive freeze-dried chitosan-polyvinyl pyrrolidone hydrogels as controlled release system for antibiotic delivery. Journal of Controlled Release. 68: 23–30.

Ritger, P.L. and N.A. Peppas. 1987. A simple equation for description of solute release II. Fickian and anomalous release from swellable devices. Journal of Controlled Release. 5: 37–42.

Sawahata, K., M. Hara, H. Yasunaga and Y. Osada. 1990. Electrically controlled drug delivery system using polyelectrolyte gels. Journal of Controlled Release. 14: 253–262.

Schmaljohann, D. 2006. Thermo- and pH-responsive polymers in drug delivery. Advanced Drug Delivery Reviews. 58: 1655–1670.

Sellergren, B. and C.J. Allender. 2005. Molecularly imprinted polymers: A bridge to advanced drug delivery. Advanced Drug Delivery Reviews. 57: 1733–1741.

Singh, B. and V. Sharma. 2014. Influence of polymer network parameters of tragacanth gum-based pH responsive hydrogels on drug delivery. Carbohydr. Polym. 101: 928–940.

Sinha, V. and R. Kumria. 2001. Polysaccharides in colon-specific drug delivery. International Journal of Pharmaceutics. 224: 19–38.

Taghizadeh, B., S. Taranejoo, S.A. Monemian, Z.S. Moghaddam, K. Daliri, H. Derakhshankhah et al. 2015. Classification of stimuli-responsive polymers as anticancer drug delivery systems. Drug Delivery. 22: 145–155.

Tanaka, T., I. Nishio, S.-T. Sun and S. Ueno-Nishio. 1982. Collapse of gels in an electric field. Science. 218: 467–469.

Tang, Y., Z. Huang, T. Yang, X. Hu and X. Jiang. 2005. The characteristic and application of molecularly imprinted polymer: efficient sample preconcentration of antibiotic cefathiamidine from human plasma and serum by solid phase extraction. Analytical Letters. 38: 219–226.

Tomatsu, I., K. Peng and A. Kros. 2011. Photoresponsive hydrogels for biomedical applications. Advanced Drug Delivery Reviews. 63: 1257–1266.

Wang, Q., L. Wang, M.S. Detamore and C. Berkland. 2008. Biodegradable colloidal gels as moldable tissue engineering scaffolds. Advanced Materials. 20: 236–+.

Wang, X.Y., C.P. Wang, Q. Zhang and Y.Y. Cheng. 2016. Near infrared light-responsive and injectable supramolecular hydrogels for on-demand drug delivery. Chemical Communications. 52: 978–981.

Yager, K.G. and C.J. Barrett. 2006. Novel photo-switching using azobenzene functional materials. Journal of Photochemistry and Photobiology a-Chemistry. 182: 250–261.

Yang, L., J.S. Chu and J.A. Fix. 2002. Colon-specific drug delivery: new approaches and *in vitro/in vivo* evaluation. International Journal of Pharmaceutics. 235: 1–15.

Yoshida, R., K. Sakai, T. Okano, Y. Sakurai, Y.H. Bae and S.W. Kim. 1992. Surface-modulated skin layers of thermal responsive hydrogels as on-off switches: I. Drug release. Journal of Biomaterials Science, Polymer Edition. 3: 155–162.

Yuk, S.H., S.H. Cho and H.B. Lee. 1992. Electric current-sensitive drug delivery systems using sodium alginate/polyacrylic acid composites. Pharmaceutical Research. 9: 955–957.

Zhang, J., R. Xie, S.-B. Zhang, C.-J. Cheng, X.-J. Ju and L.-Y. Chu. 2009. Rapid pH/temperature-responsive cationic hydrogels with dual stimuli-sensitive grafted side chains. Polymer. 50: 2516–2525.

Zhong, X., Y.-X. Wang and S.-C. Wang. 1996. Pressure dependence of the volume phase-transition of temperature-sensitive gels. Chemical Engineering Science. 51: 3235–3239.

2

Nanocomposite Hydrogels as Drug Delivery Systems

Teresa del Castillo Castro,* María Mónica Castillo Ortega,
Dora Evelia Rodríguez Félix and *José Carmelo Encinas Encinas*

Abstract

Current requirements of the novel therapeutic treatments have led to the designing of composite materials with superior clinical properties compared with their individual counterparts. The inclusion of nanostructures of different nature into cross-linked polymer networks allows obtaining nanocomposite hydrogels with suitable multifuncionalities for drug delivery applications. This chapter reviews the main contributions and general limitations of the recent researches regarding the use of nanocomposite hydrogels of different compositions in drug delivery field.

Keywords: nanocomposite hydrogel, drug delivery, stimuli-responsive systems

1. Introduction

Hydrogels have been extensively used as drug carriers in drug controlled delivery devices (Hamidi et al. 2008, Hoare and Kohane 2008, Salatin et al. 2016, Y. Zhang et al. 2016). Optimization studies of chemical, biological and physical properties of these hydrophilic polymeric networks have been developed as a typical strategy to achieve a suitable control of release

Departamento de Investigación en Polímeros y Materiales, Universidad de Sonora, CP 83000, Hermosillo, Sonora, Mexico.
* Corresponding author: terecat@polimeros.uson.mx; terecat@hotmail.com

mechanism, biocompatibility requirements, loading and releasing capacity of therapeutic levels of the bioactive specie, mechanical consistency to mimic the tissue environments, and some other desirable features for the application.

Alternatively, recent research in nanotechnology area suggests that nanostructures might solve challenges in the controlled release of drugs, specifically those related with the transportation of therapeutic compounds to the target sites (Brannon-Peppas and Blanchette 2004, Cheng et al. 2007, Cho et al. 2008, Manzoor et al. 2012, Karimi et al. 2016, Luque-Michel et al. 2016). The nanostructures exhibit unique physicochemical properties such as the small size, surface charge, large surface to mass ratio, functional surfaces and the ability to bind, adsorb and carry other compounds. However, in some cases, the high instability and the low biocompatibility of nanostructures still remain a significant problem to their clinical use (Donaldson et al. 2002, Duncan and Izzo 2005, Chang et al. 2007, Warheit et al. 2004).

The development of nanocomposite hydrogels (NCHs) is an emerging approach to obtain tailored functionality and superior properties compared to their individual counterparts for various biomedical applications, including drug delivery. The NCHs, also known as hybrid hydrogels, can be defined as a composite material that physically or covalently incorporates nanosized particles or nanostructures into a cross-linked polymer network (Zhao et al. 2015). Nanostructures of different nature such as polymeric, ceramic, metallic and carbonaceous materials have been embedded within bulk hydrogel frameworks to obtain hybrid hydrogels. In the drug delivery area, the innovative combination of these two different materials has been focused on the generation of synergistic property enhancements for the application and the avoidance of nanomaterial aggregation. It is also considered that the confinement of nanostructures in the water-rich environment of biocompatible hydrogels can change the interaction of the nanostructure with cells/tissues and thus prevent the risks of toxic nanostructured drug carriers to the human health (Fig. 1).

Moreover, these multifunctional systems are particularly useful as stimuli-responsive release systems (SRSs). The SRSs are engineering devices designed for producing a programmed drug release profile by the application of a specific internal or external stimuli. The fabrication of SRSs has become one of the promising advanced technology in the field of polymers as well as in modern-day medical and pharmaceutical science. Unlike controlled drug delivery systems that involve spontaneous release patterns, the SRSs offer the promise of new treatments that require accurate and on-demand doses of medication for particular patient's physiological conditions.

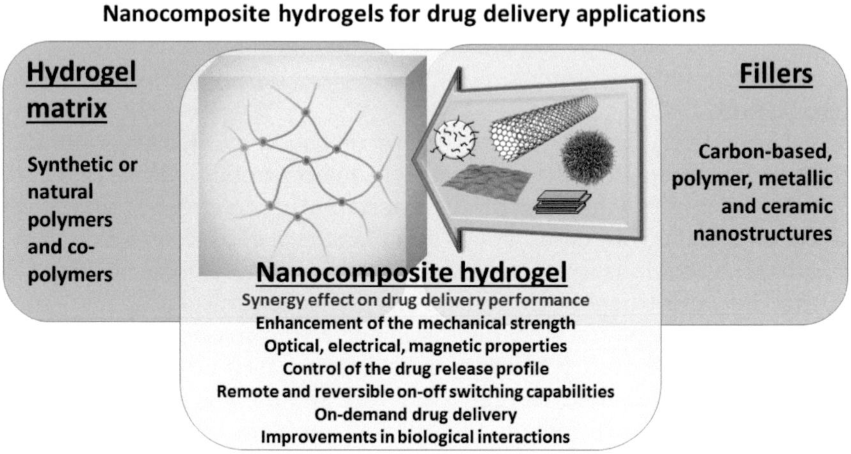

Nanocomposite hydrogels for drug delivery applications

Fig. 1. Nanocomposite hydrogels for drug delivery applications. Carbon-based, polymer, metallic and ceramic nanostructures are embedded within bulk hydrogel networks to obtain nanocomposite hydrogels. Tunable kinetics of drug release satisfy the requirements of advanced clinical treatments.

The physicochemical understanding of NCHs under the conditions of application is neither simple nor well developed. It is evident that the analysis and prediction of their swelling and response behavior is rather complex (Kryscio and Peppas 2012, Peppas and Van Blarcom 2015). The drug release kinetic from such hydrogels may follow a complex mechanism. Each individual component of the material has a particular behavior under the specific condition of the release medium and/or the applied stimulation. Accordingly, the mass transport from the NCHs may be controlled by spontaneous diffusion mechanisms or through the independent response of the hydrogel matrix, the nanostructured filler and the drug, plus the combined contribution of all components. Additionally, the combination of the individual responses depends on the material structure and composition as well as on the thermodynamically non-ideal interactions between its components. Essentially, the preparation method and the composition of the NCH influence its structure at nano-scale and molecular level, which determine the final behavior of the material in drug delivery.

Several methods have been reported for the preparation of nanoparticle-hydrogel composites (Thoniyot et al. 2015); the main approaches include the hydrogel formation in a nanoparticle suspension (Pérez-Martínez et al. 2016, Sershen et al. 2002, Ravi et al. 2005), the physically embedding the nanoparticles into hydrogel matrix after gelation (Hu et al. 2003), the reactive nanoparticle formation within a preformed gel (Wang et al. 2004, Saravanan et al. 2007), and the crosslinking using nanoparticles to form hydrogels (Castaneda et al. 2008, Skardal et al. 2010). The selection of the appropriate procedure should render the desired properties of the nanoparticle-hydrogel composite.

This chapter focuses on the most recent developments in the field of NCHs with emphasis on drug delivery applications. In particular, we examine the preparation, properties and behavior of the NCHs with different composition as drug release systems, and discuss some current examples of their performance as stimuli-responsive materials for drug delivery.

2. Carbonaceous Nanostructures-hydrogel Composites

In the past decade, carbon-based nanomaterials such as fullerene, carbon nanotubes (CNTs), graphene and graphene oxide (GO) have been intensively investigated for potential applications in biomedicine (Steinmetz et al. 2009, Goenka et al. 2014, Hong et al. 2015). These nanostructures are advantageous primarily owing to their small size, unique optical, electrical and mechanical properties, and large surface area. The favorable sizes of carbon nanomaterials have made them ideal nanocapsules and nanocarriers to load and deliver drugs and genes to specific targets *in vivo* (Li et al. 2015, Tian et al. 2016, Singh et al. 2016).

Significant efforts are being developed in designing hybrid hydrogels containing carbonaceous nanomaterials, particularly CNTs and GO, for drug delivery applications.

Carbonaceous nanomaterials provide to polymer networks, suitable mechanical properties for *in vivo* applications, and some electrical and optical functions needed, for example, in SRSs. These NCHs combine multiple functionalities, which is otherwise not possible by using conventional polymeric hydrogels.

2.1 CNTs–hydrogel composites

The CNTs have received much attention as suitable material to enhance the electrical and mechanical properties of hydrogels. The key problem for the nanotube incorporation to the hydrogel structure is their hydrophobic nature. To overcome this drawback, several techniques have been developed to enhance the dispersion of the CNTs within the nanocomposite network. The pretreatments with strong acids and modification with various polar groups are commonly used to facilitate the dispersion of the CNTs in the hydrophilic polymers.

For example, carboxylic acid functionalized CNTs were used to prepare nanohydrogels based on tragacanth gum carbohydrate in the presence of glycerol diglycidyl ether (Badakhshanian et al. 2016). The general toughening effect of CNT nanoparticles reflects itself in a significantly larger roughness of the fractured surface. Interestingly, CNT-containing hydrogel exhibited a higher release rate of indomethacin at pH 9 as compared with the hydrogel without nanotubes. This behavior was explained based on the ionization of carboxylic acid groups of the CNT at basic medium; the repulsion force between these carboxylic anions expand nanohydrogels particles leading to more space among the polymer chains which facilitates migration of drug out of the networks.

In another contribution, the oxyfluorination of CNTs was efficiently used to achieve a suitable dispersion of the nanotubes in poly(vinyl alcohol)/poly(acrylic acid) matrix (Yun et al. 2011). The surface modification of CNTs was crucial in the electro-responsive swelling and drug releasing behavior of this composite material.

Other strategies to improve the solubility of the CNTs in aqueous solutions involve the surface modification of nanotubes with surfactants, polymers and proteins. In an example of this approach, carboxymethyl guar gum-chemically modified CNT hybrid hydrogels were synthesized as a potential device for sustained trans-dermal release of diclofenac sodium (Giri et al. 2011). The non-covalent functionalization can also be achieved by Van der Waals forces, electrostatic interaction, hydrogen bonding, coordination bonds and π–π stacking interactions (Apartsin et al. 2013, Gheorghiu et al. 2014).

The CNTs were also used to improve the loading amount of hydrophobic drugs into the hydrophilic hydrogel matrix. Regarding this approach, carboxylated CNTs were modified with polyethylene glycol monomethyl ether to fabricate a hybrid supramolecular hydrogel by inclusion interactions with α-cyclodextrin, for the controlled and sustained release of hydrophobic camptothecin (Mu et al. 2015). Recently, Giri et al. reported the preparation of sustainable hydrophobic membranes containing carboxy functionalized CNTs in poly(diethylene glycol dimethacrylate) grafted carboxymethyl guargum (Giri et al. 2016). The composite membranes of "honey comb" morphology were applied for transdermal delivery of hydrophobic diclofenac sodium. At higher CNT loading, the membranes were less hydrophobic and faster drug eluting because of the relatively poor matrix–filler interaction and copolymer wrapping.

2.2 GO–hydrogel composites

Among graphene family nanomaterials, the GO has been extensively explored as filler of hydrogels for biomedical applications owing to its outstanding properties, such as large surface area, high aspect ratio, high intrinsic mechanical strength, excellent thermal and electrical conductivity as well as its amphiphilic nature that facilitates its dispersion in aqueous or alcoholic solutions of polymers (Memic et al. 2015, Patel et al. 2016, Kim et al. 2016, Peng et al. 2016). The surface modification of GO by covalent bonding is possible due to the presence of carboxylic acid, epoxide and hydroxyl groups in the graphene lattice as sites for reactivity.

Recently, Paul et al. reported the incorporation of polyethylenimine functionalized GO nanosheets, complexed with vascular endothelial growth factor plasmid DNA, in methacrlylated gelatin hydrogel (Paul et al. 2014). The NCH was used to promote the controlled and localized gene therapy in damaged cardiac tissues.

The formation of stable aqueous polymer-GO solutions can also be achieved by noncovalent interaction between hydrophobic segments of block copolymers and the hydrophobic domains of GO surface. Zu and Han formed a supramolecular hybrid hydrogel based on GO-Pluronic copolymer complex and α-cyclodextrin with potential as controlled release system (Zu and Han 2009). In another work, Byun and Lee reported that the inclusion of GO in hyaluronic acid (HA) hydrogel improves the loading efficiency in nearly 90% of small, hydrophobic drugs (e.g., doxorubicin, DOX) (Byun and Lee 2014). The HA/GO composite hydrogel not only enhanced the loading amount but also exhibited long-lasting anticancer activity over 10 days.

The pH-dependent drug binding and releasing behaviors have been observed in GO-based nanocomposite hydrogels. A series of pH sensitive konjac glucomannan/sodium alginate/GO hydrogels were used for the controlled delivery of 5-fluorouracil (Wang et al. 2014). The authors highlighted the drug-binding effect of the GO during the anticancer drug loading and releasing. Piao and Chen prepared a physically crosslinked GO-gelatin hydrogels with potential in pH-sensitive drug delivery (Piao and Chen 2015). Physically crosslinked hydrogels are considered an attractive alternative in biomedical applications over chemically crosslinked hydrogels mainly due to the absence of toxic crosslinking agents. The storage modulus of the swollen GO-gelatin hydrogels reached 114.5 kPa, owing to the relatively strong physical bonding (i.e., hydrogen bonding and electrostatic forces) between GO and gelatin (Piao and Chen 2015).

2.3 Carbonaceous nanomaterials–hydrogel composites as stimuli-responsive materials

As mentioned earlier, particular attention has been focused on materials that exhibit stimuli-responsive properties for controlled drug delivery, among other biomedical applications. Carbon-based NCHs have shown excellent capabilities as SRSs; the carbonaceous nanomaterials embedded in the hydrogel framework are able to sense a specific stimuli (e.g., light, electric potential) and generate a local heating. The heating effect and the ensuing structural changes can be produced by remote control.

Light is a particularly attractive stimulus for controlling SRSs' behavior because its intensity and wavelength can be easily controlled. Specially, light from a near-infrared (NIR) laser penetrates human tissue on the order of hundreds of micrometers to centimeters without harm because of its minimal absorbance by skin and tissue. Thus, it is defined as an NIR window between ca. 650 and 1000 nm (Cheng et al. 2013).

Smart hydrogels containing carbonaceous nanomaterials have shown remarkable phase transitions upon NIR laser irradiation. For example, Wang et al. prepared a NIR triggered drug delivery platform based on the chitosan-modified chemically reduced GO incorporated into a thermosensitive nanogel (Wang et al. 2013). The nanogel exhibited a reversible thermo-responsive characteristics at 37–42°C and high DOX hydrochloride loading capacity (48 wt%). The irradiation with NIR light produced a repetitive and rapid drug release. Furthermore, the cancer cells incubated with the drug-loaded hydrogel and irradiated with NIR light displayed a greater cytotoxicity than those without irradiation.

The local high temperature produced by the light absorption in the carbonaceous nanomaterials can be directly used to kill cancer cells. In this sense, there has been demonstrated the promising prospect of CNT-based thermo-sensitive hydrogel as injectable *in situ* drug delivery system as well as hyperthermia therapy media. Zhou et al. prepared a NCH based on poly(n-isopropyl acrylamide) and CNTs to deliver DOX for the treatment of gastric cancer mice in a chemo-combined photothermal therapy (Zhou et al. 2015). The drug was directly delivered in the tumour site for enabling its anticancer effect and meanwhile, NIR was applied to stimulate the CNTs located in tumour site.

Furthermore, the hydrogels containing carbonaceous nanomaterials can be used as a pulsatile drug release system by a NIR laser remotely controlled mode. The carbon additives effectively rise the local temperature of the gel, which leads to the shrinking of the network and the promotion of the water expulsion. In a novel approach, Cheng et al. studied the photothermal conversion effect of a thermosensitive poly(N-isopropylacrylamide-*co*-acrylamide) composite hydrogel with structural hierarchy: $NaYF_4:Yb^{3+}/Er^{3+}$ nanocrystals were integrated into a one-layer gel for the action of up-conversion luminescence tagging, and CNTs were introduced into the other layer as the molecular antenna of NIR light (Cheng et al. 2013). The lysozyme-loaded hydrogel was allowed a triggered release *in vitro* by NIR laser irradiation depending on the swelling and de-swelling process of the polymer network (Fig. 2).

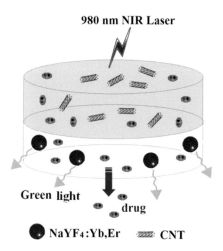

Fig. 2. Functional materials of $NaYF_4:Yb^{3+}/Er^{3+}$ nanoparticles and CNTs were incorporated into different layers of the poly(N-isopropylacrylamide-co-acrylamide) hydrogel for the purpose of up-conversion luminescence labelling and the NIR light antenna effect, respectively. Improved drug release from composite hydrogels was achieved in response to 980 nm NIR light irradiation by using lysozyme as a macromolecular drug. Reprinted with permission from Cheng et al. Langmuir 29 (2013) 9573–80. Copyright (2016) American Chemical Society.

On the other hand, the use of an electric field as an external stimulus is an efficient method that has been successfully employed to enhance the amount of released drug by simply controlling the applied voltage. Besides, the electrical signals are easy to generate and control. NCHs based on carbonaceous nanomaterials have been evaluated as electro-sensitive hydrogels in transdermal drug delivery systems and implantable electronic delivery devices (Yun et al. 2012, Choi et al. 2015). The carbon additives have played an important role for maximizing the effect of the applied electric voltage.

In an example of this approach, Im et al. prepared a NCH of polyethylene oxide/pentaerythritol triacrylate/CNT by using the electrospinning method (Im et al. 2010). Drug release was effectively increased with increasing applied electric voltage, due to the excellent conductivity of the CNTs. The suggested mechanism of drug release involves polyethylene oxide of the semi-interpenetrating polymer network being dissolved under the effects of CNTs.

Other reports have suggested that the mechanism of drug release from such NCHs involved a compressing effect and intensified stress on the polymeric network as result of the electrical properties of nanotubes. For example, Servant et al. reported that when CNTs were incorporated into a polymethacrylic acid-based hydrogel, radio-labelled sucrose release from the gels was significantly enhanced after two short electrical stimulations

(Servant et al. 2013). Damage to the hybrid gel surfaces and the loss of the pulsatile release profile were detected as a result of the DC electrical stimulation.

Despite studies having confirmed the potential of the carbon-based NCHs as stimuli-responsive materials, these systems have limited use as drug delivery platforms nowadays. Major limitations need to be overcome. The limitations include the passive loss of loaded drug molecules by diffusion (particularly in the case of hydrophilic drugs) and poor control of the release kinetics by the stimulation. The pulsatile controlled release of drugs at therapeutic levels still remains a challenge. Moreover, more detailed and mechanistic studies are required to investigate the biological properties of carbon-based NCHs under *in vitro* and *in vivo* conditions.

3. Polymeric Nanostructures–hydrogel Composites

The inclusion of polymeric nanostructures into a hydrogel system has been carried out to improve the performance of their individual counterparts. A wide variety of polymeric nanostructures have been developed and gained great attention in biomedical and pharmaceutical applications. In this sense, synthetic polymeric nanostructures, such as nanospheres, nanofibers, dendrimers and micelles, which are widely utilized as drug delivery systems, have been incorporated into hydrogels to utilize their drug releasing capabilities, as well as enhance their mechanical properties. This section includes information about different NCHs containing polymeric nanostructures with interesting properties as drug carriers.

3.1 Micro/nanospheres–hydrogel composites

The polymeric micro/nanospheres can act as matrix systems in which the drug is uniformly dispersed. The nanospheres are colloidal particles consisting of macromolecular substances that vary in size from 10 nm to 1000 nm (Singh and Lillard 2009). Typically, the drug of interest is dissolved, entrapped, adsorbed, attached and/or encapsulated into or onto a nano-matrix for drug delivery applications.

NCHs containing micro/nanospheres of polymer/drug complexes have been studied for controlled drug delivery applications. The complexing of drugs with polymers prior to microencapsulation, successfully preserved the drug bioactivity and reduced the burst release. Burst release was suggested to be due to the immediate discharge of drugs associated with the peripheral surface of the particles that were not fully encapsulated in the manufacturing process (O'Donnell and McGinity 1997). High initial burst release is one of the major challenges in drug-encapsulated micro/nanosphere systems.

Regarding this, Kastellorizios et al. prepared a composite hydrogel containing poly(lactic-*co*-glycolic acid) microspheres loaded with dexamethasone, vascular endothelial growth factor (VEGF) and platelet derived growth factor (PDGF) into polyvinyl alcohol matrix (Kastellorizios et al. 2015). The release of these three components seeks to reduce foreign body reaction (FBR). The authors found that the three tissue response modifiers were required for maximum promotion of angiogenesis, blood vessel maturation and prevention of the FBR, the VEGF had to be administered at higher doses than PDGF, and an increase in dexamethasone dosing must be accompanied by a proportional increase in growth factor dosing. The authors highlighted that the osmosis-driven process used for the encapsulation of proteins in microspheres contributed to a low burst release of the drugs.

In a similar contribution, Rhamani et al. investigated the local controlled release of stratifin from an NCH for the prevention of fibrosis (Rahmani-Neishaboor et al. 2012). In this study, complexing the drug with chitosan particles, then encapsulating into poly(lactic-*co*-glycolic acid) microspheres followed by embedding in poly(vinyl alcohol) hydrogels reduced the burst release to 8% in 24 h. The controlled release of the anti-fibrogenic factor minimized the collagen deposition (the main criterion of fibrosis) as well as decreased the total tissue cellularity and T cell-associated inflammation. The very low burst release of stratifin decreased the probability of adversely impacting the initial phase of wound healing. The authors suggested the suitability of the composite to reduce the fibrosis particularly around breast implants and vascular stents.

The potential of the composite hydrogels containing intrinsically electroconductive polymeric nanospheres as electric field responsive drug delivery system has been recently demonstrated. These systems have shown excellent spatial and temporal control. Regarding this, Ge et al. developed an SRS by the combination of a temperature-sensitive hydrogel of poly[(D,L-lactic acid)-*co*-(glycolic acid)]-*b*-poly(ethylene oxide)-*b*-poly[(D,L-lactic acid)-*co* (glycolic acid)] and nanoparticles of polypyrrole loaded with fluorescein or daunorubicin (Ge et al. 2012). The electroactive properties of polypyrrole allowed the drug release from nanoparticles by electrochemical oxidation/reduction of this polymer. After that, the electric-field-driven migration triggered the movement of charged entities toward the electrode of opposite charge, which resulted in the escape of drugs from the hydrogel.

3.2 Nanofibers–hydrogel composites

When the diameters of polymer fiber materials are on the micro- to nanometer scale, these materials have a very large surface area to volume ratio (this ratio for a nanofiber can be as large as 103 times of that of a microfiber), flexibility in surface functionalities, and superior mechanical performance (e.g., stiffness and tensile strength) compared to any other geometry of the material. These outstanding properties make the polymer nanofibers optimal candidates for a controlled drug release (Huang et al. 2003, Castro-Enríquez et al. 2012). The large surface area of nanofibers ensures a high drug take-up and reduces the constraint to drug diffusion, leading to an increase in the amount of drug that can be released from fibers. Other properties of polymeric fibers such as porosity and drug binding capabilities, are highly customizable through material choice, therefore, the rate of drug release can be tailored according to the therapeutic requirements.

Studies have shown that the inclusion of drug-loaded fibers into hydrogel matrix can enhance the capability for sustained release and preservation of biomolecules (Cutiongco et al. 2015). Typically, the drug release kinetics from polymeric nanofibers show a high degree of initial burst. The incorporation of drug-loaded fibers into a polymer network induces changes in the release kinetics, which is mostly altered by the barrier function of the hydrogel (Xu et al. 2016, Lee et al. 2013, Han et al. 2012).

Despite the large numbers of reports about the evaluation of hydrogel/polymeric nanofiber composites for tissue engineering applications, there are few articles specializing on such materials for drug delivery. Heterogeneous transport properties within a composite matrix pose significant optimization challenges in their applications as drug carriers.

Recently, an interesting work was published related to an electric stimuli-responsive material for the pulsatile delivery of amoxicillin (Pérez-Martínez et al. 2016). The drug-delivery platform was prepared by the encapsulation of amoxicillin-loaded polyaniline nanofibers of large-aspect-ratio into a polyacrylamide hydrogel. Transmission electron microscopy images of cross sections of the NCH revealed a continuous 3D nanofiber network of polyaniline supported by the hydrogel matrix. Drug release profile from composite hydrogel showed an "ON-OFF" release pattern in cycles of application/removal of cathodic electrical stimulation, in response to activation/deactivation of the electrochemical reduction of polyaniline (Fig. 3).

3.3 Dendrimers–hydrogel composites

Dendrimers are a new class of polymeric materials which are typically symmetrical around the core and often adopt a spherical three dimensional architecture. This particular geometry provides a high degree of surface functionality and versatility in comparison with conventional macromolecules, which promotes the application of dendrimers to enhance the solubility of many drugs (Tomalia et al. 1990, Milhem et al. 2000, Cheng et al. 2008). In addition, dendrimers possess empty internal cavities and

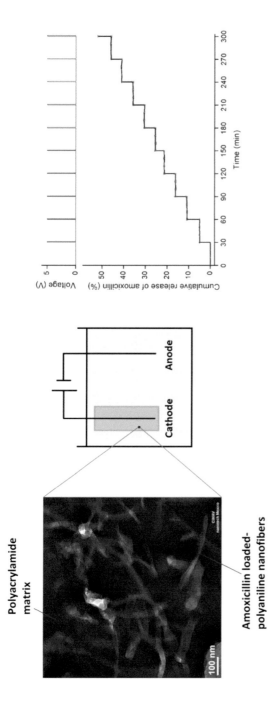

Fig. 3. Drug-delivery platform prepared by the encapsulation of amoxicillin-loaded polyaniline nanofibers of large-aspect-ratio into a polyacrylamide hydrogel. Drug release profile from composite hydrogel showed an "ON-OFF" release pattern in cycles of application/removal of cathodic electrical stimulation, in response to activation/deactivation of the electrochemical reduction of polyaniline. Reprinted with permission from Pérez-Martínez et al. React. Funct. Polym. 100 (2016) 12–1. Copyright (2016) American Chemical Society.

open conformations (for low-generation dendrimers), which make it possible to encapsulate hydrophobic drug molecules (Jansen et al. 1994). Based on previous considerations, dendrimers have a significant potential as controlled drug release systems.

The inclusion of dendrimers into hydrogel matrix affects the structure, swelling properties and drug release characteristics of the original networks. The drug release rate could either be increased, due to formation of hydrophilic channels, or reduced, because of decreased swelling, depending on the properties of the polymer system and model drug. For example, Sara Bekhradnia and coworkers synthesized temperature responsive IPN–hydrogels by the introduction of the dendrimer polyamidoamine (PAMAM) into a chemically cross-linked poly(N-isopropylacrylamide) (Bekhradnia et al. 2014). The retention of a significant portion of the loaded drug (paracetamol) at specific conditions was attributed to the hydrogen bonding ability of the dendrimer. Moreover, improved conditions for drug delivery were achieved due to the incorporation of dendrimer molecules within the hydrogel. The authors suggested that the PAMAM entities expanded the hydrogel networks and that the gel became more homogeneous.

On the other hand, dendrimers might enhance the solubility of lipophilic drugs due to hydrophobic interactions, hydrogen bonding or electrostatic interaction between surface functional groups of the dendrimer and drug. Moreover, some of the dendrimers show antibacterial and antifungal activity (Iqbal et al. 2009, Janiszewska et al. 2012) and provide the opportunity for complex therapy in which the dendrimers are not only the drug carrier but also an adjunctive component of the dosage form. In an example of this approach, Carbopol hydrogel containing PAMAM dendrimer and ketoconazole (KET) was prepared (Winnicka et al. 2012). The KET, an imidazole derivative with well-known antifungal properties, is lipophilic and practically insoluble in water. It was shown that using PAMAM dendrimers not only improved the solubility and the *in vitro* release of KET, but also enhanced the antifungal activity of the material.

3.4 Micelles–hydrogel composites

Polymeric micelles are generally formed by self-assembled nanoparticles from amphiphilic block copolymers. This system provides a unique core-shell architecture wherein the hydrophobic core serves as a natural carrier environment for hydrophobic drugs and the hydrophilic shell allows particle stabilization in aqueous solution (Kwon 2003, Otsuka et al. 2003, Torchilin 2001). Moreover, they offer attractive characteristics such as a generally small size (100 nm) and a tendency to evade scavenging by the mononuclear phagocyte system (Kwon and Okano 1996).

When environmentally sensitive (pH, temperature, etc.) functional groups are introduced into these amphiphilic copolymers, "smart" micelles are formed, and they can be used as environmentally controlled drug release systems. For example, Wei and coworkers reported a dual-drug delivery system for the independent controlled release of aspirin (Asp) and DOX (Wei et al. 2009). The system was constructed from Asp dispersed poly(vinyl alcohol) or chitosan/poly(vinyl alcohol) hydrogel and DOX-loaded poly(L-glutamic acid)-b-poly(propylene oxide)-b-poly(L-glutamic acid) (GPG) micelles. Asp showed a short-term release while DOX had a long-term and sustained release behavior. The release of DOX was environmentally controlled due to the pH and temperature sensitivity of the micelle, though the Asp showed the pH controlled release behavior due to the pH sensitivity of the hydrogel.

On the other hand, a thermo-responsive poly(N-isopropylacrylamide) gel containing the polymer surfactant, the poly(2-(methacryloyloxy) decylphosphate) was reported as a potential ascorbic acid carrier (Yan and Tsujii 2005). In this system, the micelles of polymer surfactant were trapped by the entanglement of polymer chains inside the gel networks. The composite system showed a completely different release behavior as compared to the conventional hydrogel. The micelle-containing system seemed to be suitable for the rapid release of hydrophobic drugs by an external stimuli such as the infrared laser.

Novel strategies have been developed in order to minimize the use of toxic surfactant and additives during the encapsulation of drug in the micelles. For example, Gong and coworkers proposed the curcumin encapsulation into polymeric micelles using a one-step solid dispersion method without any surfactant and additive (Gong et al. 2013). During the solid dispersion process, curcumin was distributed in poly(ethylene glycol)-poly(e-caprolactone) copolymer as amorphous substance, and then, the co-evaporation self-assembled into micelles with curcumin encapsulated in. The drug-loaded polymeric micelles were trapped into a thermosensitive hydrogel of poly(ethylene glycol)-poly(e-caprolactone)-poly(ethylene glycol). This composite hydrogel enhanced the cutaneous wound healing process.

3.5 Liposomes–hydrogel composites

Liposomes are small vesicles of spherical shape that consist of either many, few or just one phospholipid bilayers with particle sizes ranging from 30 nm to several micrometers (Akbarzadeh et al. 2013). These vesicles have the distinctive advantage of being both nontoxic and biodegradable because they are composed of naturally occurring substances. The unique ability of liposomes to entrap drugs both in an aqueous and a lipid phase makes such delivery systems attractive for hydrophilic and hydrophobic drugs (Zhang et al. 2015, Peng et al. 2015).

In a novel strategy to obtain a sustained release of low-molecular-weight hydrophilic drugs, the bioactive compounds are loaded to liposomes and then, the resulting complex is incorporated into a hydrogel matrix. For example, an injectable *in situ* gelling thermosensitive chitosan–β glycerophosphate system containing liposomes was evaluated for the delivery of encapsulated carboxyfluorescein (Ruel-Gariépy et al. 2002). The gelation rate and gel strength were slightly increased by the presence of the liposomes. The results presented in this study indicated that the liposome-hydrogel system rapidly gels at body temperature and it could be used for the sustained delivery of small-molecular-weight hydrophilic compounds.

Other interesting work related with liposomes-hydrogel composites reported a pH-responsive triblock terpolymer, the poly(2-vinyl pyridine)-b-poly(acrylic acid)-b-poly(n-butylmethacrylate), entrapping phosphatidyl-choline/cholesterol liposomes loaded with calcein as hydrophilic model drug (Popescu et al. 2011). Excellent control of the calcein release was achieved by adjusting the gelator concentration; that is, from 1 to 1.5 wt% the drug release period was significantly prolonged from 14 to 32 days.

4. Metal Nanostructures–hydrogel Composites

The growing interest in designing NCHs with magnetic, electrical and optical properties has led to the inclusion of metal nanostructures to polymeric networks. Metal nanostructures have great potential as reinforcing elements of hydrogels. Consequently, the suitable combination of both materials allows to obtain NCHs with unique characteristics and tunable properties.

The metal nanostructures have been integrated into polymer hydrogels through covalent (Grubjesic et al. 2016, Mandal et al. 2014) or non-covalent methods (Bhat and Maitra 2006); the nature of the hydrogel-metal interaction significantly influences the physical, chemical and biological properties of the NCHs. For example, a significant increase in the stiffness has been observed when surface-functionalized metallic nanoparticles have covalently bonded to the polymer chains and crosslinked with the polymeric networks (Yu et al. 2014, Zhao et al. 2013).

Various types of metallic nanoparticles have been used to fabricate NCHs for drug delivery applications including gold (Au), silver (Ag), and other noble metal nanoparticles. It has been reported that the introduction of metal nanoparticles into hydrogels can reduce the burst drug release effect, increase the stability of biomolecules and provide a slower and more continuous release kinetics of drugs (Yadollahi et al. 2015, Satarkar and Hilt 2008).

4.1 Ag nanoparticles–hydrogel composites

Especially, Ag nanoparticles are known for their antimicrobial properties. These nanoparticles have been widely used in dental fillings and, more recently in wound and burn dressings to prevent infections (Anirudhan and Deepa 2016, Ito et al. 2016, Richter et al. 2015). During the last few years, there has been an increased interest in silver-based NCHs as antimicrobial platforms for the medical field. In this context, Ag-based NCHs have been studied as suitable systems for the efficient release of Ag nanoparticles and/or ions in wound treatment and soft tissue implants. Stojkovska et al. reported a comprehensive approach to evaluate the cytotoxicity, antibacterial activity, and Ag release kinetics of alginate microbeads comprising Ag nanoparticles at the concentration range of 0.3–5 mM (Stojkovska et al. 2014). In this study was found that bovine calf chondrocytes in monolayer cultures were more sensitive to released Ag nanoparticles and/or ions as compared to chondrocytes immobilized in alginate microbeads and cultured in perfusion bioreactors.

In another approach, hybrid hydrogels have been designed to combine the antimicrobial properties of Ag nanostructures with the controlled drug release of some other bioactive compound. For example, a novel chitosan/Ag NCH was prepared by *in situ* formation of Ag nanoparticles in the chitosan hydrogel matrix (Yadollahi et al. 2015). Ag nanoparticles caused an increase in the swelling capacity of composite beads. The chitosan/Ag NCH showed good antibacterial activity against gram-positive and gram-negative bactericides. Drug release studies of ibuprofen from chitosan/Ag NCHs revealed that Ag nanoparticles prolonged the release of drug from chitosan beads. The authors hypothesized that the release time of drug molecules from the NCH was extended due to a longer path for drugs to migrate from nanocomposite bead to the media.

In another study, a NCH was prepared by embedding curcumin-loaded Ag nanoparticles into a polyacrylamide hydrogel (Ravindra et al. 2012). The curcumin-loaded nanocomposites showed a higher bacterial inhibition as compared with the hydrogels without the drug. The authors mentioned that curcumin suppressed the growth of the bacteria and the release of Ag nanoparticles from the hydrogel networks, and in this way, the antimicrobial properties of the metallic nanoparticles were preserved.

In a similar effort, Bardajee and coworkers prepared NCHs containing Ag nanoparticles into an hydrogel of poly(acrylic acid)-grafted salep, a water soluble polysaccharide (Bardajee et al. 2012). The potential of the

NCHs in drug delivery applications was examined using tetracycline hydrochloride in simulated colon conditions.

4.2 Au nanoparticles–hydrogel composites

Au nanoparticles are considered the most stable metal nanoparticles and present many fascinating properties, such as size-related electronic and optical properties (Daniel and Astruc 2004). Considering this, SRSs based on NCHs containing Au nanoparticles have been developed by several groups (Yu et al. 2014, Zhang et al. 2016, Li et al. 2016, Das et al. 2015, Lu et al. 2013, Zhao et al. 2013, Jayaramudu et al. 2013, Salgueiro et al. 2013, Daniel-da-Silva et al. 2013, Chen et al. 2012, Bikram et al. 2007). An external stimuli such as temperature or pH might cause a change in the conductivity of the hydrogel due to the change in the interparticle distance. Moreover, when these NCHs are subjected to irradiation of light at the Au plasmonic peak, the Au nanoparticles induce a localized heating within the hydrogel matrix with the concomitant changes in its swelling behavior. This phenomenon can be used for remote-controlled drug delivery. The increase in the temperature of surrounding hydrogel above the lower critical solution temperature of the polymer can result in a coil-to-globule transition of the polymer chains. Such effect can be used to release therapeutic agents from the NCHs. However, the rise in temperature can also collapse the gel structure resulting in an on demand burst release of drugs as opposed to a diffusion-controlled kinetics (Thoniyot et al. 2015).

The development of photothermal–chemotherapy combinative treatments is an interesting approach for enhancing antitumour efficacy and inhibiting tumour recurrence, which supports selective and dose-controlled delivery of heat and anticancer drugs to tumour. Recently, an injectable NCH incorporating PEGylated Au nanorods and paclitaxel-loaded chitosan polymeric micelles in a triblock copolymer hydrogel was designed for cancer treatment (Zhang et al. 2016). After intratumoural injection, the Au nanostructures and the micelles can be simultaneously delivered and immobilized in the tumour tissue by the thermo-sensitive hydrogel matrix. Exposure to laser irradiation induces the photothermal damage confined to the tumour, sparing the surrounding normal tissue. The authors highlighted that this combination photothermal–chemotherapy presented superior effects on suppressing the tumour recurrence and prolonging the survival in the Heps-bearing mice, compared to the photothermal therapy alone.

In a novel approach, Wu and coworkers developed a class of core–shell structured multifunctional hybrid nanogels to combine targeting, optical sensing of environmental temperature change, fluorescence imaging of cancer cell, adequate drug loading, and controllable drug release into a single system (Wu et al. 2010). The hybrid hydrogel was comprised of Ag–Au bimetallic nanoparticle as core, thermo-responsive nonlinear poly(ethylene glycol)-based hydrogel as shell, and surface hyaluronic acid chains as targeting ligands. The release of the anticancer drug temozolomide was induced by both the heat generated by external NIR irradiation and the temperature increase of local environmental media. The ability of the hybrid nanogels to combine the local specific chemotherapy with external NIR photothermal treatment significantly improves the therapeutic efficacy due to a synergistic effect.

Recently, a thermosensitive hydrogel was used as a novel chemoradiotherapy strategy for the treatment of cancer. The thermosensitive hydrogel of Pluronic F127 comprised Au nanoparticles and DOX for the sustained release of metallic nanoparticles and the antitumoural drug (Li et al. 2016). When the tumour was irradiated by X-ray, the DOX acted as chemotherapeutics while Au nanoparticles killed tumour cells by enhancing the radiation dose. The superior radiosensitization and anti-tumour effects were verified *in vitro* and *in vivo*.

4.3 Transition metal/oxide compound nanoparticles–hydrogel composites

Despite Ag and Au noble metal nanoparticles, some nanostructures of transitional metals such as iron (Fe), cobalt (Co) and nickel (Ni) and their oxide compounds, have been integrated to hydrogel matrix for drug delivery applications (Giammanco et al. 2015, Ahmad 2016, Babić et al. 2016, Işıklan 2007, Kim et al. 2012, Perez et al. 2015). The incorporation of these magnetic nanoparticles to the polymer networks offers a high potential for several biomedical applications including drug delivery uses. The superior magnetic properties of such nanoparticles can cause a temperature rise under alternating magnetic fields. In this way, NCHs based on thermo-sensitive hydrogel matrix containing magnetic nanoparticles can exhibit a remotely-controlled thermal-responsive swelling behaviours by using magnetic fields. This effect was used to control the diffusion of encapsulated drugs to the target site.

The drug release from NCHs containing magnetic particles can be combined with the hyperthermia effect for killing cancer cells. Regarding this, Liu and coworkers fabricated an intelligent magnetic hydrogel by mixing poly(vinyl alcohol) hydrogel and Fe_3O_4 magnetic particles through freezing-thawing cycles (Liu et al. 2006). When an external magnetic field was applied to the ferrogel, the drug (vitamin B12) was accumulated in the NCH and the accumulated drug was instantanously released when the magnetic field was switched "off". The pulsatile release of vitamin B_{12} was achieved by the ON-OFF switching of the remote magnetic field (Fig. 4).

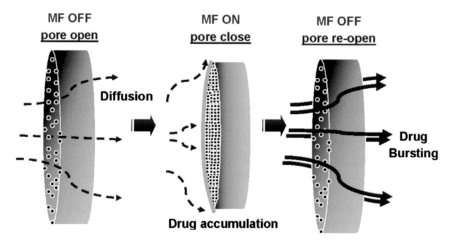

Fig. 4. Composite hydrogel fabricated by mixing poly(vinyl alcohol) hydrogel and Fe_3O_4 magnetic particles through freezing-thawing cycles. When magnetic field was applied to the ferrogel, the drug was accumulated around it, but the accumulated drug was spurt to the environment instantly when the magnetic fields instantly switched "off". Rapid to slow drug release can be tunable while the magnetic field was switched from "off" to "on" mode. Reprinted with permission from Liu et al. Langmuir. 22 (2006) 5974–8. Copyright (2016) American Chemical Society.

Overall, various types of metallic and metal-oxide nanostructures have been incorporated within polymer networks in order to generate NCHs with unique optical, electrical or magnetic properties. The resultant NCHs are mostly used as SRSs with highly suitable behavior for controlled drug delivery applications.

5. Ceramic Nanostructures–hydrogel Composites

Ceramic nanostructures have been widely used as fillers to produce polymer-based composites with improved mechanical properties (Depan et al. 2009, Ryu et al. 2016, Wang et al. 2007). Nanoceramic materials exhibit advantageous properties such as mechanical strength, toughness, bioactivity, controllable crystallinity, abundant grain boundaries, high thermal stability and chemical inertia.

Some ceramic nanostructures have played an important role in biomedical applications owing to their excellent biocompatible, osteoconductive and bioactivity properties, as well as their chemical and physical similarity to mineral component of bone tissues (Pastorino et al. 2015, Saif and Asif 2015, Ramiro-Gutiérrez et al. 2014). Thus, the inclusion of ceramic nanostructures within hydrogels can provide these bioactive properties to the polymeric network. The NCHs based on nanoceramics can combine the bioactive characteristics of nanofillers with the capability for *in situ* deliver antibiotics and growth factors, which can be an effective alternative in the bone regeneration treatments.

For example, a novel pH-sensitive ceramic-hydrogel of polyvinyl-alcohol, polyacrylic acid and synthetic hydroxyapatite was studied for bone healing and drug delivery applications (de Lima et al. 2015). The authors found that samples with lower concentration of the ceramic component released quicker theophylline than samples with higher concentration. Furthermore, the inclusion of hydroxyapatite promoted the ability of the scaffold to form an apatite layer when it was placed in simulated body fluid.

Nanoclays such as montmorillonite, attapulgite, palygorskite and halloysite have been incorporated into hydrogels for drug delivery applications. Clays can be exfoliated to produce layers or fibers with one or two dimensions in nanometric scale, which facilitates its dispersion within the polymer matrix. This nanoceramic has been traditionally used as carriers of drugs in pills and capsules, also known as excipients. Moreover, some clays have been recognized by the ability to retain drugs and slowly deliver them, which is a desirable feature of sustained drug release systems.

Particularly, montmorillonite clay is formed of thin silicate layers parallel to that stacked by rather weak interactions. Montmorillonite has been used as additive in NCHs for drug delivery applications. For example, novel hybrids of chitosan-g-lactic acid and sodium montmorillonite have been studied for the sustained delivery of ibuprofen and tissue engineering applications (Depan et al. 2009). A significant difference was observed in drug release kinetics from the material in form of smooth film and porous scaffold. The porous scaffolds have shown higher and faster drug release. Nanohybrids films increased the water absorption and took longer time for drying up indicating that the films can hold the moisture for longer time. The incorporation of montmorillonite allowed controlling the initial release of drug.

On the other hand, Wang and coworkers prepared pH-sensitive composite hydrogel beads of chitosan-g-poly (acrylic acid)/attapulgite/sodium alginate loaded with diclofenac sodium (Wang et al. 2009). They suggested that the inclusion of the attapulgite into the polymeric network generated longer paths for the drug migration from composite hydrogel to the media, and as a result, the release time was prolonged.

In another approach using clay-containing materials, microspheres based on chitosan and palygorskite, a one-dimensional clay, were evaluated as carrier of diclofenac sodium (Wu et al. 2014). As a natural cationic exchanger, palygorskite strongly interacts with cationic drugs in solution *via* electrostatic interaction. The microspheres were prepared by emulsion crosslinking technology with glutaraldehyde and the palygorskite was modified with hexadecyl betaine to enhance the compatibility with chitosan matrix. The microspheres containing 10–20% of the nanoceramic exhibited higher swelling ratio than those of pure chitosan, which was attributed to the hydrophilic nature of the palygorskite. Consequently, it was found that the nanoceramic addition modified the drug release behavior.

Halloysite is an aluminosilicate clay of predominantly cylindrical geometry with a diameter of 50 nm, an inner lumen of 15 nm and length of 600–900 nm. The inner lumen can be loaded with bioactive molecules for drug delivery applications. Typically, a successful drug loading reached 5–10 wt% of the tube weight. Clogging the tube ends in polymeric composites allows further extension of release time (Lvov et al. 2016). Both luminal and surface modifications of halloysite have been proposed to increase the loading efficiency of the nanostructure or to modify the drug release patterns.

In an example of this approach, a nanotubes-in-microgel oral system was designed for protein delivery (De Kruif et al. 2016). The halloysite nanotubes were selected as orally acceptable clay nanostructure and their lumen was chemically etched to increase drug loading capacity and to allow protection from enzymatic protein degradation. The ceramic nanotubes were combined with mono-N-carboxymethyl chitosan to form microgels. The combination of nanotubes and microgels had a synergic effect that prevented the digestion of albumin, the model protein used in the study.

Overall, the selection of the hydrogel matrix and the ceramic nanostructure allows the tuning of the bioactive capabilities and drug release profiles of the resulting NCHs. These multicomponent systems can be further used to create combined dosage forms with tailored release profiles and optimal protection of the drug in the gastrointestinal environment.

6. Conclusions and Perspectives

During the last decade, significant efforts have been developed to design, fabricate and implement nanocomposite hydrogels in drug delivery applications. These composite systems combine multiple functionalities, which is otherwise not possible by using conventional polymeric hydrogels. Nanostructures provide polymer networks with a prolonged release time of drugs, high loading efficiency, as well as suitable mechanical, electrical, optical and magnetic properties for the drug delivery applications. Moreover, nanostructures might show some bioactive properties and provide the opportunity for complex therapy in which nanomaterials are not only the drug carriers but also adjunctive components of the clinical treatment. On the other hand, hydrogel matrix acts as container of nanostructures, which prevents their agglomeration and decreases the toxicity risk of some non-biodegradable nanomaterials. A tunable kinetics of drug release has been achieved to satisfy the requirements of some advanced clinical treatments.

Recent trends in fabrication nanocomposite hydrogels for drug delivery are shifted toward designing stimuli-responsive release systems. However, despite the huge potential of these systems in drug delivery applications, the stimuli-responsive release systems have limited use as drug delivery platforms today. Major limitations, including the passive loss of loaded molecules by diffusion and poor control of the release kinetics by stimulus activation, need to be overcome to improve its efficacy in clinical treatments.

In order to achieve a more consistent prediction of drug release patterns, a fuller understanding of the underlying mechanism of drug delivery is required in each particular stimuli-responsive material and experimental condition. It is evident that the drug release kinetic from such multicomponent hydrogels follows complex mechanisms. It should be considered that each individual component of the material has a particular behaviour under the specific condition of the release medium and/or the applied stimulation. Consequently, mass transport from the nanocomposite system may be controlled by spontaneous diffusion mechanisms or through the independent response of the hydrogel matrix, the nanostructured filler and the drug, plus the combined contribution of all components.

Alongside further studies on the mechanistic aspects of drug delivery in nanocomposite hydrogels, more detailed studies are required to investigate the biological properties of such systems under *in vitro* and *in vivo* conditions.

Continuing work in this field will promote refinements and improvements in nanocomposite hydrogel performance for drug delivery applications, which may open up perspectives for their current application and future design of new advanced clinical treatments.

References

Ahmad, H. 2016. Evaluating a simple blending approach to prepare magnetic and stimuli-responsive composite hydrogel particles for application in biomedical field. Express Polym. Lett. 10: 661–78.

Akbarzadeh, A., R. Rezaei-Sadabady, S. Davaran, S.W. Joo, N. Zarghami, Y. Hanifehpour et al. 2013. Liposome: classification, preparation, and applications. Nanoscale Res. Lett. 8: 102.

Anirudhan, T.S. and B.J.R. Deepa. 2016. Functionalized polymeric silver nanoparticle hybrid network as a dual antimicrobe: synthesis, characterization, and antibacterial application. J. Appl. Polym. Sci. 133: 43479.

Apartsin, E.K., M.Y. Buyanova, D.S. Novopashina, E.I. Ryabchikova and A.G. Venyaminova. 2013. Nanomaterials imaging techniques, surface studies, and applications. Vol. 146. Springer Proceed. Phys. USA. 146: 291–307.

Babić, M.M., B.Đ. Božić, B.Đ. Božić, J.M. Filipović, G.S. Ušćumlić and S.L. Tomić. 2016. Evaluation of novel antiproliferative controlled drug delivery system based on poly(2-hydroxypropyl acrylate/itaconic acid) hydrogels and nickel complex with oxaprozin. Mater. Lett. 163: 214–217.

Badakhshanian, E., K. Hemmati and M. Ghaemy. 2016. Enhancement of mechanical properties of nanohydrogels based on natural gum with functionalized multiwall carbon nanotube: study of swelling and drug release. Polymer. 90: 282–289.

Bardajee, G.R., Z. Hooshyar and H. Rezanezhad. 2012. A novel and green biomaterial based silver nanocomposite hydrogel: synthesis, characterization and antibacterial effect. J. Inorg. Biochem. 117: 367–73.

Bekhradnia, S., K. Zhu, K.D. Knudsen, S.A. Sande and B. Nyström. 2014. Structure, swelling, and drug release of thermoresponsive poly(amidoamine) dendrimer–poly(n-isopropylacrylamide) hydrogels. J. Mater. Sci. 49: 6102–6110.

Bhat, S. and U. Maitra. 2006. Nanoparticle–gel hybrid material designed with bile acid analogues. Chem. Mater. 18: 4224–4226.

Bikram, M., A.M. Gobin, R.E. Whitmire and J.L. West. 2007. Temperature-sensitive hydrogels with sio2-au nanoshells for controlled drug delivery. J. Control. Release. 123: 219–227.

Brannon-Peppas, L. and J.O. Blanchette. 2004. Nanoparticle and targeted systems for cancer therapy. Adv. Drug Deliv. Rev. 56: 1649–1659.

Byun, E. and H. Lee. 2014. Enhanced loading efficiency and sustained release of doxorubicin from hyaluronic acid/graphene oxide composite hydrogels by a mussel-inspired catecholamine. J. Nanosci. Nanotechnol. 14: 7395–7401.

Castaneda, L., J. Valle, N. Yang, S. Pluskat and K. Slowinska. 2008. Collagen cross-linking with Au nanoparticles. Biomacromolecules. 9: 3383–3388.

Castro-Enríquez, D., F. Rodríguez-Félix, B. Ramírez-Wong, P. Torres-Chávez, M.M. Castillo-Ortega, D. Rodríguez-Félix et al. 2012. Preparation, characterization and release of urea from wheat gluten electrospun membranes. Materials. 5: 2903–2916.

Chang, J.-S., K.L.B. Chang, D.-F. Hwang and Z.-L. Kong. 2007. *In vitro* cytotoxicity of silica nanoparticles at high concentrations strongly depends on the metabolic activity type of the cell line. Environ. Sci. Technol. 41: 2064–2068.

Chen, R., Q. Chen, D. Huo, Y. Ding, Y. Hu and X. Jiang. 2012. *In situ* formation of chitosan-gold hybrid hydrogel and its application for drug delivery. Colloids and Surfaces. B, Biointerfaces. 97: 132–137.

Cheng, J., B.A. Teply, I. Sherifi, J. Sung, G. Luther, F.X. Gu et al. 2007. Formulation of functionalized PLGA-PEG nanoparticles for *in vivo* targeted drug delivery. Biomaterials. 28: 869–876.

Cheng, Y., Z. Xu, M. Ma and T. Xu. 2008. Dendrimers as drug carriers: applications in different routes of drug administration. J. Pharm. Sci. 97: 123–143.

Cheng, Z., R. Chai, P. Ma, Y. Dai, X. Kang, H. Lian et al. 2013. Multiwalled carbon nanotubes and NAYF4:Yb3+/Er3+ nanoparticle-doped bilayer hydrogel for concurrent nir-triggered drug release and up-conversion luminescence tagging. Langmuir. 29: 9573–9580.

Cho, K., X. Wang, S. Nie, Z.G. Chen and D.M. Shin. 2008. Therapeutic nanoparticles for drug delivery in cancer. Clin. Cancer Res. 14: 1310–1316.

Choi, E.J., J. Shin, Z.H. Khaleel, I. Cha, S.-H. Yun, S.-W. Cho et al. 2015. Synthesis of electroconductive hydrogel films by an electro-controlled click reaction and their application to drug delivery systems. Polym. Chem. 6: 4473–4478.

Cutiongco, M.F.A., B.K.K. Teo and E.K.F. Yim. 2015. Composite scaffolds of interfacial polyelectrolyte fibers for temporally controlled release of biomolecules. J. Vis. Exp. 102: e53079.

Daniel, M.-C. and D. Astruc. 2004. Gold nanoparticles: assembly, supramolecular chemistry, quantum-size-related properties, and applications toward biology, catalysis, and nanotechnology. Chem. Rev. 104: 293–346.

Daniel-da-Silva, A.L., A.M. Salgueiro and T. Trindade. 2013. Effects of au nanoparticles on thermoresponsive genipin-crosslinked gelatin hydrogels. Gold Bull. 46: 25–33.

Das, R., D. Das, P. Ghosh, S. Dhara, A.B. Panda and S. Pal. 2015. Development and application of a nanocomposite derived from crosslinked hpmc and au nanoparticles for colon targeted drug delivery. RSC Adv. 5: 27481–27490.

De Kruif, J.K., G. Ledergerber, C. Garofalo, E. Fasler-Kan and M. Kuentz. 2016. On prilled nanotubes-in-microgel oral systems for protein delivery. Eur. J. Pharm. Biopharm. 101: 90–102.

de Lima, G.G., L. Campos, A. Junqueira, D.M. Devine and M.J.D. Nugent. 2015. A novel ph-sensitive ceramic-hydrogel for biomedical applications. Polym. Adv. Technol. 26: 1439–1446.

Depan, D., A.P. Kumar and R.P. Singh. 2009. Cell proliferation and controlled drug release studies of nanohybrids based on chitosan-g-lactic acid and montmorillonite. Acta Biomater. 5: 93–100.

Donaldson, K., D. Brown, A. Clouter, R. Duffin, W. MacNee, L. Renwick et al. 2002. The pulmonary toxicology of ultrafine particles. J. Aerosol. Med. 15: 213–20.

Duncan, R. and L. Izzo. 2005. Dendrimer biocompatibility and toxicity. Adv. Drug Deliv. Rev. 57: 2215–2237.

Ge, J., E. Neofytou, T.J. Cahill, R.E. Beygui and R.N. Zare. 2012. Drug release from electric-field-responsive nanoparticles. ACS Nano. 6: 227–233.

Gheorghiu, C.C., C. Salinas-Martínez and M.C. Román-Martínez. 2014. Non-covalent immobilization of rhduphos on carbon nanotubes and carbon xerogels. Appl. Catal. A Gen. 478: 194–203.

Giammanco, G.E., C.T. Sosnofsky and A.D. Ostrowski. 2015. Light-responsive iron(III)-polysaccharide coordination hydrogels for controlled delivery. ACS Appl. Mater. Interfaces. 7: 3068–3076.

Giri, A., M. Bhowmick, S. Pal and A. Bandyopadhyay. 2011. Polymer hydrogel from carboxymethyl guar gum and carbon nanotube for sustained trans-dermal release of diclofenac sodium. Int. J. Biol. Macromol. 49: 885–893.

Giri, A., T. Bhunia, A. Pal, L. Goswami and A. Bandyopadhyay. 2016. *In situ* synthesis of polyacrylate grafted carboxymethyl guargum–carbon nanotube membranes for potential application in controlled drug delivery. Eur. Polym. J. 74: 13–25.

Goenka, S., V. Sant and S. Sant. 2014. Graphene-based nanomaterials for drug delivery and tissue engineering. J. Control. Release. 173: 75–88.

Gong, C.Y., Q. Wu, Y.J. Wang, D.D. Zhang, F. Luo, X. Zhao et al. 2013. A biodegradable hydrogel system containing curcumin encapsulated in micelles for cutaneous wound healing. Biomaterials. 34: 6377–6387.

Grubjesic, S., B.S. Ringstrand, K.L. Jungjohann, S.M. Brombosz, S. Seifert and M.A. Firestone. 2016. Cascade synthesis of a gold nanoparticle-network polymer composite. Nanoscale. 8: 2601–2612.

Hamidi, M., A. Azadi and P. Rafiei. 2008. Hydrogel nanoparticles in drug delivery. Adv. Drug Deliv. Rev. 60: 1638–1649.

Han, N., J. Johnson, J.J. Lannutti and J.O. Winter. 2012. Hydrogel-electrospun fiber composite materials for hydrophilic protein release. J. Control. Release. 158: 165–170.

Hoare, T.R. and D.S. Kohane. 2008. Hydrogels in drug delivery: progress and challenges. Polymer. 49: 1993–2007.

Hong, G., S. Diao, A.L. Antaris and H. Dai. 2015. Carbon nanomaterials for biological imaging and nanomedicinal therapy. Chem. Rev. 115: 10816 10906.

Hu, J.-S., H.-P. Liang, L.-J. Wan and C.-L. Bai. 2003. Highly dispersed metal nanoparticles in porous anodic alumina films prepared by a breathing process of polyacrylamide hydrogel. Chem. Mater. 15: 4332–4336.

Huang, Z.-M., Y.-Z. Zhang, M. Kotaki and S. Ramakrishna. 2003. A review on polymer nanofibers by electrospinning and their applications in nanocomposites. Compos. Sci. Technol. 63: 2223–2253.

Im, J.S., B.C. Bai and Y.-S. Lee. 2010. The effect of carbon nanotubes on drug delivery in an electro-sensitive transdermal drug delivery system. Biomaterials. 31: 1414–1419.

Iqbal, P.F., H. Parveen, A.R. Bhat, F. Hayat and A. Azam. 2009. Synthesis, characterization, antiamoebic activity and toxicity of novel bisdioxazole derivatives. Eur. J. Med. Chem. 44: 4747–4751.

Işıklan, N. 2007. Controlled release study of carbaryl insecticide from calcium alginate and nickel alginate hydrogel beads. J. Appl. Polym. Sci. 105: 718–725.

Ito, K., A. Saito, T. Fujie, H. Miyazaki, M. Kinoshita, D. Saitoh et al. 2016. Development of a ubiquitously transferrable silver-nanoparticle-loaded polymer nanosheet as an antimicrobial coating. J. Biomed. Mater. Res. B. Appl. Biomater. 104: 585–593.

Janiszewska, J., M. Sowińska, A. Rajnisz, J. Solecka, I. Łącka, S. Milewski et al. 2012. Novel dendrimeric lipopeptides with antifungal activity. Bioorg. Med. Chem. Lett. 22: 1388–1393.

Jansen, J.F., E.M. de Brabander-van den Berg and E.W. Meijer. 1994. Encapsulation of guest molecules into a dendritic box. Science. 266: 1226–1229.

Jayaramudu, T., G.M. Raghavendra, K. Varaprasad, R. Sadiku and K.M. Raju. 2013. Development of novel biodegradable au nanocomposite hydrogels based on wheat: for inactivation of bacteria. Carbohydr. Polym. 92: 2193–2200.

Karimi, M., P.S. Zangabad, A. Ghasemi, M. Amiri, M. Bahrami, H. Malekzad et al. 2016. Temperature-responsive smart nanocarriers for delivery of therapeutic agents: applications and recent advances. ACS Appl. Mater. Interfaces. 8: 21107–21133.

Kastellorizios, M., F. Papadimitrakopoulos and D.J. Burgess. 2015. Multiple tissue response modifiers to promote angiogenesis and prevent the foreign body reaction around subcutaneous implants. J. Control. Release. 214: 103–111.

Kim, J.I., B.S. Lee, C. Chun, J.-K. Cho, S.-Y. Kim and S.-C. Song. 2012. Long-term theranostic hydrogel system for solid tumors. Biomaterials. 33: 2251–2259.

Kim, M.-G., Y. Shon, W. Miao, J. Lee and Y.-K. Oh. 2016. Biodegradable graphene oxide and polyaptamer dna hybrid hydrogels for implantable drug delivery. Carbon. 105: 14–22.

Kryscio, D.R. and N.A. Peppas. 2012. Critical review and perspective of macromolecularly imprinted polymers. Acta Biomater. 8: 461–473.

Kwon, G.S. and T. Okano. 1996. Polymeric micelles as new drug carriers. Adv. Drug Deliv. Rev. 21: 107–116.

Kwon, G.S. 2003. Polymeric micelles for delivery of poorly water-soluble compounds. Crit. Rev. Ther. Drug Carrier Syst. 20: 357–403.

Lee, H.J., Y.H. Park and W.-G. Koh. 2013. Fabrication of nanofiber microarchitectures localized within hydrogel microparticles and their application to protein delivery and cell encapsulation. Adv. Funct. Mater. 23: 591–97.

Li, T., M. Zhang, J. Wang, T. Wang, Y. Yao, X. Zhang et al. 2016. Thermosensitive hydrogel co-loaded with gold nanoparticles and doxorubicin for effective chemoradiotherapy. AAPS J. 18: 146–155.

Li, Z., F.-L. Zhang, L.-L. Pan, X.-L. Zhu and Z.-Z. Zhang. 2015. Preparation and characterization of injectable mitoxantrone poly(lactic acid)/fullerene implants for *in vivo* chemo-photodynamic therapy. J. Photochem. Photobiol. B. 149: 51–57.

Liu, T.-Y., S.-H. Hu, T.-Y. Liu, D.-M. Liu and S.-Y. Chen. 2006. Magnetic-sensitive behavior of intelligent ferrogels for controlled release of drug. Langmuir. 22: 5974–5978.

Lu, S., K.G. Neoh, C. Huang, Z. Shi and E.-T. Kang. 2013. Polyacrylamide hybrid nanogels for targeted cancer chemotherapy *via* co-delivery of gold nanoparticles and MTX. J. Colloid Interface Sci. 412: 46–55.

Luque-Michel, E., E. Imbuluzqueta, V. Sebastián and M.J. Blanco-Prieto. 2016. Clinical advances of nanocarrier-based cancer therapy and diagnostics. Expert Opin. Drug Deliv. 1–18.

Lvov, Y., W. Wang, L. Zhang and R. Fakhrullin. 2016. Halloysite clay nanotubes for loading and sustained release of functional compounds. Adv. Mater. 28: 1227–1250.

Mandal, S.K., S. Brahmachari and P.K. Das. 2014. *In situ* synthesised silver nanoparticle-infused l-lysine-based injectable hydrogel: development of a biocompatible, antibacterial, soft nanocomposite. Chem. Plus. Chem. 79: 1733–1746.

Manzoor, A.A., L.H. Lindner, C.D. Landon, J.-Y. Park, A.J. Simnick, M.R. Dreher et al. 2012. Overcoming limitations in nanoparticle drug delivery: triggered, intravascular release to improve drug penetration into tumors. Cancer Res. 72: 5566–5575.

Memic, A., H.A. Alhadrami, M.A. Hussain, M. Aldhahri, F.A. Nowaiser, F. Al-Hazmi et al. 2015. Hydrogels 2.0: improved properties with nanomaterial composites for biomedical applications. Biomed. Mater. 11: 014104.

Milhem, O.M., C. Myles, N.B. McKeown, D. Attwood and A.D. Emanuele. 2000. Polyamidoamine starburst® dendrimers as solubility enhancers. Int. J. Pharm. 197: 239–241.

Mu, S., Y. Liang, S. Chen, L. Zhang and T. Liu. 2015. MWNT-Hybrided supramolecular hydrogel for hydrophobic camptothecin delivery. Mater. Sci. Eng. C. 50: 294–299.

O'Donnell, P.B. and J.W. McGinity. 1997. Preparation of microspheres by the solvent evaporation technique. Adv. Drug Deliv. Rev. 28: 25–42.

Otsuka, H., Y. Nagasaki and K. Kataoka. 2003. PEGylated nanoparticles for biological and pharmaceutical applications. Adv. Drug Deliv. Rev. 55: 403–419.

Pastorino, D., C. Canal and M.-P. Ginebra. 2015. Multiple characterization study on porosity and pore structure of calcium phosphate cements. Acta Biomater. 28: 205–214.

Patel, M., H.J. Moon, D.Y. Ko and B. Jeong. 2016. Composite system of graphene oxide and polypeptide thermogel as an injectable 3d scaffold for adipogenic differentiation of tonsil-derived mesenchymal stem cells. ACS Appl. Mater. Interfaces. 8: 5160–5169.

Paul, A., A. Hasan, H.A. Kindi, A.K. Gaharwar, V.T.S. Rao, M. Nikkhah et al. 2014. Injectable graphene oxide/hydrogel-based angiogenic gene delivery system for vasculogenesis and cardiac repair. ACS Nano. 8: 8050–8062.

Peng, X., C. He, J. Liu and H. Wang. 2016. Biomimetic jellyfish-like PVA/graphene oxide nanocomposite hydrogels with anisotropic and pH-responsive mechanical properties. J. Mater. Sci. 51: 5901–5911.

Peng, Z., E. Fang, C. Wang, X. Lu, G. Wang and Q. Tong. 2015. Construction of novel thermosensitive magnetic cationic liposomes as a drug and gene co-delivery system. J. Nanosci. Nanotechnol. 15: 3823–3833.

Peppas, N.A. and D.S. Van Blarcom. 2015. Hydrogel-based biosensors and sensing devices for drug delivery. J. Control. Release. 240: 142–150.

Perez, R.A., J.-H. Kim, J.O. Buitrago, I.B. Wall and H.-W. Kim. 2015. Novel therapeutic core-shell hydrogel scaffolds with sequential delivery of cobalt and bone morphogenetic protein-2 for synergistic bone regeneration. Acta Biomater. 23: 295–308.

Pérez-Martínez, C.J., S.D. Morales, T. del Castillo-Castro, T.E. Lara, M.M. Castillo-Ortega et al. 2016. Electroconductive nanocomposite hydrogel for pulsatile drug release. React. Funct. Polym. 100: 12–17.

Piao, Y. and B. Chen. 2015. Self-assembled graphene oxide-gelatin nanocomposite hydrogels: characterization, formation mechanisms, and pH-sensitive drug release behavior. J. Polym. Sci. Part B. 53: 356–367.

Popescu, M.-T., S. Mourtas, G. Pampalakis, S.G. Antimisiaris and C. Tsitsilianis. 2011. pH-responsive hydrogel/liposome soft nanocomposites for tuning drug release. Biomacromolecules. 12: 3023–3030.

Rahmani-Neishaboor, E., R. Hartwell, R. Jalili, J. Jackson, E. Brown and A. Ghahary. 2012. Localized controlled release of stratifin reduces implantation-induced dermal fibrosis. Acta Biomater. 8: 3660–3668.

Ramiro-Gutiérrez, M.L., J. Will, A.R. Boccaccini and A. Díaz-Cuenca. 2014. Reticulated bioactive scaffolds with improved textural properties for bone tissue engineering: nanostructured surfaces and porosity. J. Biomed. Mater. Res. Part A. 102: 2982–2992.

Ravi, N., H.A. Aliyar and P.D. Hamilton. 2005. Hydrogel nanocomposite as a synthetic intra-ocular lens capable of accommodation. Macromol. Symp. 227: 191–202.

Ravindra, S., A.F. Mulaba-Bafubiandi, V. Rajinikanth, K. Varaprasad, N.N. Reddy and K.M. Raju. 2012. Development and characterization of curcumin loaded silver nanoparticle hydrogels for antibacterial and drug delivery applications. J. Inorg. Organomet. Polym. Mater. 22: 1254–1262.

Richter, A.P., J.S. Brown, B. Bharti, A. Wang, S. Gangwal, K. Houck et al. 2015. An environmentally benign antimicrobial nanoparticle based on a silver-infused lignin core. Nat. Nanotech. 10: 817–823.

Ruel-Gariépy, E., G. Leclair, P. Hildgen, A. Gupta and J.-C. Leroux. 2002. Thermosensitive chitosan-based hydrogel containing liposomes for the delivery of hydrophilic molecules. J. Control. Release. 82: 373–383.

Ryu, J., J. Ko, H. Lee, T.G. Shin and D. Sohn. 2016. Structural response of imogolite-poly(acrylic acid) hydrogel under deformation. Macromolecules. 49: 1873–1881.

Saif, M.J. and H.M. Asif. 2015. Escalating applications of halloysite nanotubes. J. Chil. Chem. Soc. 60: 2949–53.

Salatin, S., J. Barar, M. Barzegar-Jalali, K. Adibkia, M.A. Milani and M. Jelvehgari. 2016. Hydrogel nanoparticles and nanocomposites for nasal drug/vaccine delivery. Arch. Pharm. Res. 39: 1181–1192.

Salgueiro, A.M., A.L. Daniel-da-Silva, S. Fateixa and T. Trindade. 2013. κ-Carrageenan hydrogel nanocomposites with release behavior mediated by morphological distinct Au nanofillers. Carbohydr. Polym. 91: 100–109.

Saravanan, P., M.P. Raju and S. Alam. 2007. A study on synthesis and properties of ag nanoparticles immobilized polyacrylamide hydrogel composites. Mater. Chem. Phys. 103: 278–282.

Satarkar, N.S. and J.Z. Hilt. 2008. Magnetic hydrogel nanocomposites for remote controlled pulsatile drug release. J. Control. Release. 130: 246–251.

Sershen, S.R., S.L. Westcott, N.J. Halas and J.L. West. 2002. Independent optically addressable nanoparticle-polymer optomechanical composites. Appl. Phys. Lett. 80: 4609.

Servant, A., C. Bussy, K. Al-Jamal and K. Kostarelos. 2013. Design, engineering and structural integrity of electro-responsive carbon nanotube-based hydrogels for pulsatile drug release. J. Mater. Chem. B. 1: 4593–4600.

Singh, R. and J.W. Lillard. 2009. Nanoparticle-based targeted drug delivery. Exp. Mol. Pathol. 86: 215–223.

Singh, S., N.K. Mehra and N.K. Jain. 2016. Development and characterization of the paclitaxel loaded riboflavin and thiamine conjugated carbon nanotubes for cancer treatment. Pharm. Res. 33: 1769–1781.

Skardal, A., J. Zhang, L. McCoard, S. Oottamasathien and G.D. Prestwich. 2010. Dynamically crosslinked gold nanoparticle-hyaluronan hydrogels. Adv. Mater. 22: 4736–4740.

Steinmetz, N.F., V. Hong, E.D. Spoerke, P. Lu, K. Breitenkamp, M.G. Finn et al. 2009. Buckyballs meet viral nanoparticles: candidates for biomedicine. J. Am. Chem. Soc. 131: 17093–17095.

Stojkovska, J., D. Kostić, Ž. Jovanović, M. Vukašinović-Sekulić, V. Mišković-Stanković and B. Obradović. 2014. A comprehensive approach to *in vitro* functional evaluation of Ag/alginate nanocomposite hydrogels. Carbohydr. Polym. 111: 305–314.

Thoniyot, P., M.J. Tan, A.A. Karim, D.J. Young and X.J. Loh. 2015. Nanoparticle-hydrogel composites: concept, design, and applications of these promising, multi-functional materials. Adv. Sci. 2: 1400010.

Tian, J., Y. Luo, L. Huang, Y. Feng, H. Ju and B.-Y. Yu. 2016. Pegylated folate and peptide-decorated graphene oxide nanovehicle for *in vivo* targeted delivery of anticancer drugs and therapeutic self-monitoring. Biosens. Bioelect. 80: 519–524.

Tomalia, D.A., A. del, M. Naylor and W.A. Goddard. 1990. Starburst dendrimers: molecular-level control of size, shape, surface chemistry, topology, and flexibility from atoms to macroscopic matter. Angew. Chemie Int. Ed. English. 29: 138–175.

Torchilin, V.P. 2001. Structure and design of polymeric surfactant-based drug delivery systems. J. Control. Release. 73: 137–172.

Wang, C., N.T. Flynn and R. Langer. 2004. Controlled structure and properties of thermoresponsive nanoparticle–hydrogel composites. Adv. Mater. 16: 1074–1079.

Wang, C., J. Mallela, U.S. Garapati, S. Ravi, V. Chinnasamy, Y. Girard et al. 2013. A chitosan-modified graphene nanogel for noninvasive controlled drug release. Nanomedicine. 9: 903–911.

Wang, J., C. Liu, Y. Shuai, X. Cui and L. Nie. 2014. Controlled release of anticancer drug using graphene oxide as a drug-binding effector in konjac glucomannan/sodium alginate hydrogels. Colloids Surf. B. Biointerfaces. 113: 223–229.

Wang, Q., J. Zhang and A. Wang. 2009. Preparation and characterization of a novel pH-sensitive chitosan-g-poly(acrylic acid)/attapulgite/sodium alginate composite hydrogel bead for controlled release of diclofenac sodium. Carbohydr. Polym. 78: 731–737.

Wang, X., Y. Du, J. Luo, B. Lin and J.F. Kennedy. 2007. Chitosan/organic rectorite nanocomposite films: structure, characteristic and drug delivery behaviour. Carbohydr. Polym. 69: 41–49.

Warheit, D.B., B.R. Laurence, K.L. Reed, D.H. Roach, G.A.M. Reynolds and T.R. Webb. 2004. Comparative pulmonary toxicity assessment of single-wall carbon nanotubes in rats. Toxicol. Sci. 77: 117–125.

Wei, L., C. Cai, J. Lin and T. Chen. 2009. Dual-drug delivery system based on hydrogel/micelle composites. Biomaterials. 30: 2606–2613.

Winnicka, K., M. Wroblewska, P. Wieczorek, P. Tomasz and E. Tryniszewska. 2012. Hydrogel of ketoconazole and PAMAM dendrimers: formulation and antifungal activity. Molecules. 17: 4612–4624.

Wu, J., S. Ding, J. Chen, S. Zhou and H. Ding. 2014. Preparation and drug release properties of chitosan/organomodified palygorskite microspheres. Int. J. Biol. Macromol. 68: 107–112.

Wu, W., J. Shen, P. Banerjee and S. Zhou. 2010. Core-shell hybrid nanogels for integration of optical temperature-sensing, targeted tumor cell imaging, and combined chemo-photothermal treatment. Biomaterials. 31: 7555–7566.

Xu, S., L. Deng, J. Zhang, L. Yin and A. Dong. 2016. Composites of electrospun-fibers and hydrogels: a potential solution to current challenges in biological and biomedical field. J. Biomed. Mater. Res. Part B. 104: 640–656.

Yadollahi, M., S. Farhoudian and H. Namazi. 2015. One-pot synthesis of antibacterial chitosan/silver bio-nanocomposite hydrogel beads as drug delivery systems. Int. J. Biol. Macromol. 79: 37–43.

Yan, H. and K. Tsujii. 2005. Potential application of poly(N-isopropylacrylamide) gel containing polymeric micelles to drug delivery systems. Colloids Surf. B Biointerfaces. 46: 142–146.

Yu, J., W. Ha, J. Sun and Y. Shi. 2014. Supramolecular hybrid hydrogel based on host–guest interaction and its application in drug delivery. ACS Appl. Mater. Interfaces. 6: 19544–19551.

Yun, J., J.S. Im, Y. Lee and H. Kim. 2011. Electro-responsive transdermal drug delivery behavior of PVA/PAA/MWCNT nanofibers. Eur. Polym. J. 47: 1893–1902.

Yun, J., D.H. Lee, J.S. Im and H. Kim. 2012. Improvement in transdermal drug delivery performance by graphite oxide/temperature-responsive hydrogel composites with micro heater. Mater. Sci. Eng. C. 32: 1564–1570.

Zhang, L., Q. Zhang, X. Wang, W. Zhang, C. Lin, F. Chen et al. 2015. Drug-in-cyclodextrin-in-liposomes: a novel drug delivery system for flurbiprofen. Int. J. Pharm. 492: 40–45.

Zhang, N., X. Xu, X. Zhang, D. Qu, L. Xue, R. Mo et al. 2016. Nanocomposite hydrogel incorporating gold nanorods and paclitaxel-loaded chitosan micelles for combination photothermal-chemotherapy. Int. J. Pharm. 497: 210–221.

Zhang, Y., J. Zhang, M. Chen, H. Gong, S. Thamphiwatana, L. Eckmann et al. 2016. A bioadhesive nanoparticle-hydrogel hybrid system for localized antimicrobial drug delivery. ACS Appl. Mater. Interfaces. 8: 18367–18374.

Zhao, F., D. Yao, R. Guo, L. Deng, A. Dong and J. Zhang. 2015. Composites of polymer hydrogels and nanoparticulate systems for biomedical and pharmaceutical applications. Nanomaterials. 5: 2054–2130.

Zhao, S., F. Zhou and R. Liu. 2013. Hybrid supramolecular hydrogels induced by au nanoparticles protected with MPEG-B -PCL copolymers with α-cyclodextrin. Supramol. Chem. 25: 767–776.

Zhou, M., S. Liu, Y. Jiang, H. Ma, M. Shi, Q. Wang et al. 2015. Doxorubicin-loaded single wall nanotube thermo-sensitive hydrogel for gastric cancer chemo-photothermal therapy. Adv. Funct. Mater. 25: 4730–4739.

Zu, S.-Z. and B.-H. Han. 2009. Aqueous dispersion of graphene sheets stabilized by pluronic copolymers: formation of supramolecular hydrogel. J. Phys. Chem. C. 113: 13651–13657.

$$3$$

Vesicles, Micelles and Cyclodextrins Immobilized into Hydrogel

Multi-component Devices for Controlled Drug Delivery

*Lorena Tavano** and *Rita Muzzalupo*

ABSTRACT

An emerging methodology to strengthen polymeric hydrogels focuses on incorporating nanomaterials within the network to obtain nanocomposites hydrogels with superior properties and tailored functionality when compared to their conventional counterparts.

Among the wide range of nanoparticles, oligosaccharides, lipid or surfactant-based systems such as cyclodextrins, liposomes, niosomes and micelles were found to be attractive in drug delivery. Their integration within the hydrogel networks results in the enhancement of the interactions between the drug and the hydrogel matrix and in the influence of drugs transport into the body and their release behaviour.

This chapter attempts to provide a brief overview of hydrogel-immobilized nanomaterials obtained by incorporation of vesicles, micelles and cyclodextrins into the gel network, analysing the potential of each combination and giving an exhaustive collection of the most relevant and recent investigations.

Keywords: multi-component hydrogels, vesicles, micelles, cyclodextrins

Department of Pharmacy, Health and Nutritional Sciences, University of Calabria, Via Pietro Bucci, Ed. Polifunzionale, 87036 Arcavacata di Rende, Italy.
* Corresponding author: uclorena@tiscali.it

1. Nanocomposite Hydrogel: Introduction

Hydrogels are three-dimensional, chemically stable, cross-linked networks that retain vast amounts of water without dissolving. Due to excellent swellability in water, softness, elasticity, and biological compatibility, hydrogels are widely used in clinical practice and experimental medicine for various applications, including drug delivery (Hoare and Kohane 2008). Indeed, hydrogels mimic native extracellular matrix, both compositionally and mechanically: their porous and hydrated molecular structure also permits drug loading into the gel matrix and its release at a rate dependent on the drug diffusion coefficient through the gel network (Akala et al. 1998).

Nevertheless, hydrogels also have several limitations. The amount and distribution of drug loading into hydrogels may be limited, mostly in the case of hydrophobic drugs. Often, the hydrogel high water content and large pore sizes result in relatively rapid drug release, although some hydrogels are sufficiently deformable to be injectable and need surgical implantation (Vashist et al. 2014). These disadvantages strongly restrict the practical use of hydrogel-based drug delivery therapies in the clinic, but over the last decades, a range of strategies have been explored to overcome them. All these approaches rely on the enhancement of the interactions between the drug and the hydrogel matrix and/or the increase of the diffusive barrier to drug release from the hydrogel (Memic et al. 2016).

An emerging methodology to strengthen polymeric hydrogels focuses on incorporating nanomaterials within the network to obtain nanocomposites hydrogels with superior properties (Haraguchi 2007). A wide range of nanoparticles such as inorganic/ceramic nanoparticles (i.e., silver, gold, or iron oxide/hydroxyapatite or silicates), polymeric materials (hyper-branched polyesters, cyclodextrins), lipid/surfactant-based systems (liposomes, niosomes and micelles) and carbon-based nanomaterials (nanodiamonds, graphene, carbon nanotubes) can be integrated within the hydrogel networks (Gaharwar et al. 2014), as illustrated in Fig. 1.

Nanocomposites hydrogels may open perspectives in various areas of advanced research and technology, because the incorporation of nanoparticles helps to better mimic the natural tissue microenvironment, to provide more precise drug release profiles also conferring stimuli-response properties (Gaharwar et al. 2014). The nature of interaction between molecular network and nanostructures can have physical or chemical character and can be stabilized by hydrogen bonds and hydrophobic interactions, influencing mechanical, chemical and biological properties all at once. The major biomedical application of nanocomposite hydrogels is in drug delivery: these multi-functional systems have been extensively used as carriers to load and transport drugs into the body and to impact its release behaviour (Merino et al. 2015).

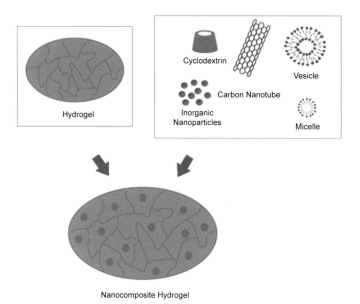

Fig. 1. Schematic representation of a nanocomposite hydrogel.

This chapter attempts to provide a brief overview of hydrogel-immobilized nanomaterials obtained by incorporation of vesicles, micelles and cyclodextrins into the gel network, analysing the potential of each combination and giving an exhaustive collection of the most relevant and recent investigations.

2. Hydrogel-Immobilized Liposomes and Niosomes

Liposomes and niosomes have lamellar (bilayer) structures composed of amphiphilic molecules, phospholipids and non-ionic surfactants respectively, surrounded by an aqueous compartment. Both vesicles are capable of encapsulating both hydrophilic (encapsulated in the inner aqueous core) and lipophilic (partitioning into the lipophilic domain of the bilayers) substances (Uchegbu and Florence 1995).

Lipid/surfactant-based vesicles can similarly be entrapped in hydrogel networks to provide prolonged drug release. The combination of vesicular systems and gel results in the so-called liposomal or niosomal gel, possessing the advantages of the individual formulations (simple vesicular suspensions and gel systems) and some other important properties (Tavano 2015). Improvement of vesicles membrane integrity and mechanical stability, enhancement of rheological characteristics and compliance for patients has been reported when liposomes and niosomes were incorporated into a gel matrix. The first study on the incorporation of liposomes in a gel was reported in 1982 by Mezei et al. (Mezei and Gulasekharam 1982), and since then many studies have been published, especially for topical applications. Several studies demonstrated that vesicular gels can be more stable to environmental stimuli compared with traditional dispersions. When the drug is placed inside the internal aqueous core and the vesicles are included in a network, the drug efflux will be through vesicular bilayer and the polymeric matrix itself (Tavano 2015). The most used polymers to obtain vesicular gels are carbomers (polymers of acrylic acid cross-linked with polyalkenyl ethers or divinyl glycol), cellulose derivatives (hydroxyethylcellulose, hydroxypropylcellulose, sodium carboxymethylcellulose) and poloxamers (PEO–PPO–PEO block copolymers).

A combination of polymers and liposomes was developed by Meyenburg et al. in order to exploit the advantageous properties of both devices for the sustained delivery of the horseradish peroxidase (HRP) (Meyenburg et al. 2000). Liposomes containing HRP were prepared from Epikuron 200 (soybean–phosphatidylcholine and *n*-Octylglucoside) and were themselves embedded inside the natural polymer fibrin. The vesicles enable horseradish peroxidase to remain in the aqueous environment and protect it during the polymerization process, while the liposomes into the network results in a depot system with sustained enzyme release.

In 2014, Alinaghi et al. proposed a combination of radiolabelled liposomes and chitosan hydrogel as a novel approach for prolonged release and delivery of glutathione, evaluating the vesicles circulation and tissue distribution in mice after intraperitoneal injection (Alinaghi et al. 2013). The results showed that liposomal gel had an appropriate gelation time both *in vitro* and *in vivo*, conferring increased durability and retention time in the peritoneal cavity respect to conventional vesicles. Moreover, RES uptake occurred less quickly than plain liposomes, suggesting that this new strategy may be useful to improve pharmacokinetics and circulation half-life of conventional vesicles.

The study of Billard and collaborators (Billard et al. 2015), deals with the design of innovative multi-component system composed of phosphatidylcholine liposomes entrapped within a chitosan physical gel. Authors demonstrated that the release profile of carboxyfluorescein (CF, used as model compound) was effectively delayed when these molecules was encapsulated into liposomal gel, in comparison with the simple CF-gel.

Calcein modulated release from small unilamellar vesicles (SUVs) and multilamellar vesicles (MLVs) entrapped in chitosan/gelatin hydrogels was demonstrated by Ciobanu and collaborators (Ciobanu et al. 2014).

Moreover, strong increase of liposomes stability was reported by inclusion in polymeric matrices. Interesting, MLV showed a better release behaviour, due to their multi-layer structure, whereby MLV-gel systems were proposed as tissue replacement or injectable depot systems in many high risk diseases including cancer.

Similar results were obtained by Peptu and collaborators entrapping calcein-loaded liposomes into gelatin-carboxymethylcellulose films: release can be controlled by modifying the vesicles bilayer composition, the network density and the film geometry (Peptu et al. 2008).

In 2007, Mourtas and collaborators performed an interesting study comparing the release of calcein and griseofulvin from conventional gels and liposomal gels (Mourtas et al. 2007). Liposomes were made of phosphatidylcholine or distearoyl-glycero-phosphatidylcholine and cholesterol and after, they were dispersed in carbopol 974, hydroxyethyl-cellulose or a mixture of the two. Results show that calcein release from liposomal gels is slower compared to control sample. Interestingly, griseofulvin release was dependent on drug loading. At high loading levels, drug was released constantly from liposomal gels irrespective of liposome type. Calcein and griseofulvin release from control carbopol gels is faster compared to hydroxyethyl-cellulose and combined gels. The same research group (Mourtas et al. 2008) studied the integrity of liposomes when dispersed in presence of various conventional formulation excipients (propyleneglycol, transcutol CG, cremophor EL and labrafac hydro WL 1219), also evaluating their effect on the release of calcein. Experimental results revealed that vesicle integrity and drug release were strongly affected by the kind of excipients: in particular, liposomes are protected from excipients when dispersed in gels compared to aqueous media.

Karimunnisa and collaborators investigated the potential of a novel mucoadhesive Ciclopirox olamine liposomal gel for vaginal use (Karimunnisa and Atmaram 2013). The liposomal formulation released about 60% of drug up to 24 h, suggesting sustained release; in addition, mucoadhesive properties prolonged the contact with vaginal wall, avoiding frequent and large dosing.

Liposomal Amphotericin B was included into thermo-sensitive gel composed of poloxamer 407 and poloxamer 188, resulting in more stable and less toxic formulation compared to free drug (Kang et al. 2010).

In 2011, Antunes and collaborators evaluated the role of nonionic vesicles (niosomes) on the rheological behaviour of Pluronic F127, demonstrating that the presence of surfactant aggregates in the network enhances the compartmentalization of Diclofenac Sodium and also gives rise to thickening effects (Antunes et al. 2011). The binary mixtures of vesicles and polymer always show a higher viscosity, indicating a stronger network due to polymer entanglements and polymer-vesicle association.

In addition, this niosomal gel can be used as successful topical formulation because of the possibility to modulate drug percutaneous permeation by changing Pluronic concentration.

Novel niosomal gel formulations as multi-functional systems for transdermal drug delivery were proposed by Tavano and collaborators in 2013 (Tavano et al. 2013). Authors made a comprehensive study, comparing the percutaneous permeation profiles of several drugs from lyotropic mesophases, niosomes and multi-component systems (niosomes incorporated into mesophases) obtained from mixture of water/AOT or Pluronic L64 as surfactants. Moreover, Deuterium resonance spectroscopy was used to evaluate if the eventual structural modifications caused by the incorporation of a third component in the formulations (drugs or drugs-loaded niosomal suspension), could influence their microstructure and then the drugs delivery across the skin. Results suggested that vehicle composition, drug solubility in the matrix and its viscosity, play an important role in the release across the stratum corneum; drugs diffusion mechanisms depend on the kind of macromolecular aggregates and its interaction with the lipid structure of the skin.

Liposomal and niosomal gels were also reported as optimal strategy to simultaneously promote drug photostabilization and the skin permeation (Ioele et al. 2016). As recently reported (Ioele et al. 2015), addition of antioxidant agents and simultaneous incorporation in Spa60-based niosomal gel were optimal approach adopted to reduce Diclofenac Sodium photo-degradation and increase its transdermal release, compared to semisolid commercial specialty or drug solution.

3. Hydrogel-Immobilized Micelles

Micelles represent one of the most versatile drug delivery systems ever since their discovery. They have a core shell structure, composed of hydrophobic internal core (providing a compartment for loading hydrophobic drug) and hydrophilic shell allows stability retention in aqueous medium (Wei et al. 2009). The development of multi-component hydrogel/micelle systems useful for drug delivery has been proved to be more efficient and possess potential application in pharmaceutical field, as illustrated in Fig. 2 (Wei et al. 2009).

Recently, Anirudhan et al. proposed a graft copolymeric micelle/hydrogel system for the dual release of drugs (Anirudhan et al. 2016). The hydrogel was prepared with poly(ethyleneglycol) and poly(vinyl alcohol), while chitosan was grafted onto oleic acid to get amphiphilic derivatives, in order to form micelles as drug carriers. The cephalosporin Cefixime trihydrate (CFX) and the analgesic Tramadol hydrochloride (TMD) were loaded into the hydrophobic micellar core and dispersed onto the polymeric

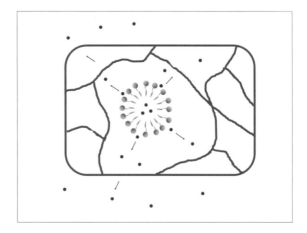

Fig. 2. Drug transport across micelles layer and polymeric matrix.

networks, respectively, resulting in the simultaneous loading of both drugs which could be delivered as a function of environmental pH and time. Results suggested that the release of TMD was controlled by the PVA/PEG hydrogel, while CFX release was dependent on the micelles; their release kinetics was independent. Additionally, the release of drugs was much more pronounced in the basic medium than in the acidic medium.

A dual-drug delivery system based on a hydrogel/micelles multi-component system was presented by Wei and collaborators for both aspirin and doxorubicin (Wei et al. 2009). Aspirin (Asp) was dispersed in PVA or Chitosan/PVA hydrogel and doxorubicin (Dox) was loaded into poly(L-glutamic acid)-b-poly(propylene oxide)-b-poly(L-glutamic acid) triblock copolymer micelles. Distinct drugs kinetics was observed: a short-term release was obtained for Asp, while Dox has a long-term and sustained release behaviour controlled by the pH and temperature sensitivity of the micelles.

Also Pluronic surfactants were used to produce polymeric micelles. Liu and collaborators encapsulated erythromycin (EM) in micelles obtained from Pluronic F127 diacrylate macromer, and then converted into hydrogel after mixing with a photoinitiator under a low-intensity UV light, with the aim to extend EM release and limited drug cytotoxicity (Liu et al. 2014).

Indeed, Poloxamer 407 was used to obtain thermo-sensitive micelles-hydrogel system for localized delivery of paclitaxel (Ju et al. 2013). Glutaraldehyde was used to generate cross-linked networks together with carboxymethyl chitosan interpenetrated in P407 gels, in which paclitaxel-loaded micelles were dispersed uniformly. After administration in tumour-bearing mice, the multi-functional system revealed a prolonged retention at tumour sites, improved efficacy and slight side effects compared with Taxol (®), drug loaded micelles and drug-loaded micelles onto unmodified P407 gels.

Chen and collaborators developed an injectable multi-component system that can undergo sol-gel phase transition by the stimulation of body temperature (Chen et al. 2013). Hexamethylene diisocyanate modified Pluronic F127 copolymer was incorporated with hyaluronic acid to develop a thermoresponsive nanocomposite material. Results showed that the multi-component device can spontaneously self-assemble into micellar structure; the release of loaded-doxorubicin was a zero-order profile and sustained for 4 weeks. *In vivo* studies revealed the viability of tumour cells decreased with incubation time (28 days), indicating a potential successful therapeutic effect in cancer treatment.

4. Hydrogel-Immobilized Cyclodextrins

One of the drawbacks in making hydrogel more hydrophobic is its significant deswelling and increasing bulk hydrophobicity, which potentially reduce its biocompatibility. The introduction of Cyclodextrins (CX) into a gel form helps to easily overcome these problems (Simões et al. 2014). CX, in fact, due to their hydrophilic exterior, could maintain the bulk hydrophilicity and swelling state of the hydrogel, and, because their hydrophobic interior, they may entrap and control the release of hydrophobic compounds (Moya-Ortega et al. 2012). Generally, CX-drug complexes can be loaded into the hydrogel during gel cross-linking, but often this strategy may result in the diffusion of the complex out of the hydrogels, resulting in a non-optimal release control. Cyclodextrins can be cross-linked directly to form a hydrogel: this approach ensures both improvement of drug loading and controlled release, compared to that achieved by simple aqueous partitioning into hydrogels.

Recently, Kuang designed an injectable and biodegradable supramolecular hydrogel, using a nucleobase (adenine/thymine)-terminated poly(ethylene oxide)s (A-PEG-A/T-PEG-T) and α-cyclodextrin (α-CD) (Kuang et al. 2014). *In vitro* studies indicated that nanocomposite hydrogels have adequate biocompatibility, and are appropriate for developing sustained and controlled-chemotherapics release. Furthermore, *in vivo* experiments employing U14 cancer cell xenograft-bearing mice, showed that the intratumoural injection of a DOX-loaded nanocomposite hydrogels inhibited tumour growth more effectively than that of free drug, DOX-loaded PEG/α-CD gel or gel alone.

Inclusion complex between the mPEG grafted polyphosphazenes and α-cyclodextrin was successful, proposed by Tian and collaborators in 2013 for the delivery of albumin as model protein (Tian et al. 2013).

Klaewklod and collaborators designed novel multi-component gels by mixing β-cyclodextrin and polyethyleneglycol (PEG) and investigated their physical-chemistry properties and their potential use for topical diclofenac delivery (Klaewklod et al. 2015). FT-IR studies showed that interactions among drug and β-cyclodextrin may include ionic attraction and hydrogen bonds. Moreover, *in vitro* drug release and skin permeation demonstrated that the multi-component gel facilitated diclofenac delivery when compared to the commercial formulation, due penetration enhancing activity of PEG and occlusion effect that enhances the penetration.

Meloxicam-gels based on complexation of four gel bases, different permeation enhancers and β-cyclodextrin were designed (Rasool et al. 2011). Best performances in terms of permeation across the skin were obtained by using hydroxypropyl methyl cellulose 15% w/w gel base containing oleic acid (1% w/w) or (5% w/w) cineol as permeation enhancers.

In 2012, cyclodextrins embebbed into liquid crystalline phases were proposed by Ammar as strategy to improve the therapeutic efficacy of lornoxicam (Ammar et al. 2012). The formulation based of Brij 97 and glycerol in 3:1 weight ratio, 10% Miglyol® 812 and 40% water, showed higher drug release and low *ex vivo* permeation, offering high topical effect with low systematic side effects. Additionally, the same sample showed superior anti-inflammatory activity when applied topically, compared to that of Feldene® gel.

An interesting application of drug loaded cyclodextrins-gel was proposed by Fernández-Ferreiro et al. for the ocular delivery of fluconazole (Fernández-Ferreiro et al. 2014). Drug loaded hydroxypropyl-β-cyclodextrins were incorporated into an ion-sensitive ophthalmic gel composed of gellan gum and κ-carrageenan (natural polysaccharides), showing good bioadhesive properties and effective control of antifungal release.

In 2014, Choi aimed to improve the solubility of paclitaxel using cyclodextrins and incorporating them into a mucoadhesive and thermoreversible hydrogel (obtained from mixture of multiblock copolymer F127 and PEO) for oral topical delivery (Choi et al. 2014). Results demonstrated that inclusion complex improved drug solubility, while the multi-component formulation underwent gelation at physiological temperature. *In vitro* release was sustained due to the presence of PEO and cell cytotoxicity (evaluated by a MTT assay, using KB cells) was not significant.

Similar strategy was proposed by Bilensoy in 2006 (Bilensoy et al. 2006). A vaginal gel obtained from the thermo-sensitive Pluronic F127, the mucoadhesive polymers Carbopol 934 and hydroxypropylmethylcellulose was designed and Clotrimazole was incorporated into β-cyclodextrins to increase its aqueous solubility. The complexation with cyclodextrins strongly decreased drug release, while the gel dosage form containing Pluronic F127 gel (20% w/w), was found to provide continuous and prolonged release of drug above Minimal Inhibitory Concentration (MIC) values.

In 2007, the same authors successfully formulated 5FU-β-cyclodextrins in a vaginal gel, obtained from mixture of F127 together with alternative mucoadhesive polymers, e.g., hyaluronic acid, Carbopol 934 and hydroxyl propylmethylcellulose (Bilensoy et al. 2007).

Considering that cyclodextrins-based hydrogels have been described as suitable formulation to be used as wound dressing, Pinho and collaborators (Pinho et al. 2014) developed a novel system capable of forming inclusion complexes with gallic acid (as antibacterial agent), for the treatment of infected wounds and enhancement of healing process. Designed materials were suitable for the contact with injured skin because they were easy to handle and soft; the antibacterial activity of gallic acid was maintained after its incorporation within the network gel and its release was sustained for 48 h.

5. Conclusions

Incorporation of nanomaterials was recently proposed as an emerging strategy to strengthen polymeric networks, resulting in nanocomposite hydrogels with superior properties and tailored functionality when compared to their conventional counterparts. In particular, nanocomposite hydrogels were found to be attractive in a wide range of applications, including drug delivery, tissue engineering, bio-sensing, regenerative medicine, and other biomedical applications. Although extensive research has been carried out, many obstacles remain to be overcome and many other aspects including long-term biocompatibility and biodegradability need to be investigated before they can be used in clinical applications and tissue replacement.

Acknowledgment

MIUR, the Italian Ministry for University, is acknowledged for financial support.

References

Akala, E.O., P. Kopecková and J. Kopecek. 1998. Novel pH-sensitive hydrogels with adjustable swelling kinetics. Biomaterials. 19: 1037–1047.
Alinaghi, A., M.R. Rouini, F. Johari Daha and H.R. Moghimi. 2013. Hydrogel-embeded vesicles, as a novel approach for prolonged release and delivery of liposome, *in vitro* and *in vivo*. J. Liposome Res. 23: 235–243.

Ammar, H.O., M. Ghorab, A.A. Mahmoud, T.S. Makram and S.H. Noshi. 2012. Topical liquid crystalline gel containing lornoxicam/cyclodextrin complex. J. Incl. Phenom. Macro. 73: 161–175.

Anirudhan, T.S., J. Parvathy and A.S. Nair. 2016. A novel composite matrix based on polymeric micelle and hydrogel as a drug carrier for the controlled release of dual drugs. Carbohydr. Polym. 136: 1118–1127.

Antunes, F.E., L. Gentile, C.O. Rossi, L. Tavano and G.A. Ranieri. 2011. Gels of Pluronic F127 and nonionic surfactants from rheological characterization to controlled drug permeation. Colloids Surf. B. Biointerfaces. 87: 42–48.

Bilensoy, E., M.A. Rouf, I. Vural, M. Şen and A.A. Hıncal. 2006. Mucoadhesive, thermosensitive, prolonged-release vaginal gel for clotrimazole: β-cyclodextrin complex. AAPS Pharm. Sci. Tech. 14: 38.

Bilensoy, E., Y. Çirpanli, M. Şen, A.L. Doğan and S. Çaliş. 2007. Thermosensitive mucoadhesive gel formulation loaded with 5-Fu: cyclodextrin complex for HPV-induced cervical cancer. Phenom. Macrocycl. Chem. 57: 363–370.

Billard, A., L. Pourchet, S. Malaise, P. Alcouffe, A. Montembault and C. Ladavière. 2015. Liposome-loaded chitosan physical hydrogel: toward a promising delayed-release biosystem. Carbohydr. Polym. 115: 651–657.

Chen, Y.Y., H.C. Wu, J.S. Sun, G.C. Dong and T.W. Wang. 2013. Injectable and thermoresponsive self-assembled nanocomposite hydrogel for long-term anticancer drug delivery. Langmuir. 29: 3721–3729.

Choi, S.G., S.E. Lee, B.S. Kang, C.L. Ng, E. Davaa and J.S. Park. 2014. Thermosensitive and mucoadhesive sol-gel composites of paclitaxel/dimethyl-β-cyclodextrin for buccal delivery. PLoS ONE. 9: 109090.

Ciobanu, B.C., A.N. Cadinoiu, M. Popa, J. Desbrières and C.A. Petu. 2014. Modulated release from liposomes entrapped in chitosan/gelatin hydrogels. Mater. Sci. Eng. C. Mater. Biol. Appl. 43: 383–391.

Fernández-Ferreiro, A., N. Fernández Bargiela, M.S. Varela, M.G. Martínez, M. Pardo, A. Piñeiro Ces et al. 2014. Cyclodextrin-polysaccharide-based, *in situ*-gelled system for ocular antifungal delivery. Beilstein J. Org. Chem. 10: 2903–2911.

Gaharwar, A.K., N.A. Peppas and A. Khademhosseini. 2014. Nanocomposite hydrogels for biomedical applications. Biotechnol. Bioeng. 111: 441–452.

Haraguchi, K. 2007. Nanocomposite hydrogels. Current Opinion in Solid State and Materials Science. 11: 47–54.

Hoare, T.R. and D.S. Kohane. 2008. Hydrogels in drug delivery: Progress and challenges. Polymer. 49: 1993–2007.

Ioele, G., L. Tavano, M. De Luca, G. Ragno, N. Picci and R. Muzzalupo. 2015. Photostability and *ex vivo* permeation studies on diclofenac in topical niosomal formulations. Int. J. Pharm. 494: 490–497.

Ioele, G., L. Tavano, R. Muzzalupo, M. De Luca and G. Ragno. 2016. Stability-indicating methods for NSAIDs in topical formulations and photoprotection in host-guest matrices. Mini. Rev. Med. Chem. 16: 676–682.

Ju, C., J. Sun, P. Zi, X. Jin and C. Zhang. 2013. Thermosensitive micelles_hydrogel hybrid system based on poloxamer 407 for localized delivery of paclitaxel. J. Pharm. Sci. 2013. 102: 2707–2717.

Kang, J.W., E. Davaa, Y.T. Kim and J.S. Park. 2010. A New Vaginal Delivery System of Amphotericin B: A Dispersion of Cationic Liposomes in a Thermosensitive Gel. 18: 637–644.

Karimunnisa, S. and P. Atmaram. 2013. Mucoadhesive nanoliposomal formulation for vaginal delivery of an antifungal. Drug Dev. Ind. Pharm. 39: 1328–1337.

Klaewklod, A., V. Tantishaiyakul, N. Hirun, T. Sangfai and L. Li. 2015. Characterization of supramolecular gels based on β-cyclodextrin and polyethyleneglycol and their potential use for topical drug delivery. Mater Sci. Eng. C. Mater Biol. Appl. 50: 242–250.

Kuang, H., H. He, Z. Zhang, Y. Qi, Z. Xie, X. Jing et al. 2014. Injectable and biodegradable supramolecular hydrogels formed by nucleobase-terminated poly(ethylene oxide)s and R-cyclodextrin. J. Mater. Chem. B. 2: 659–667.

Liu, T., T. Wu, H. Liu, B. Ke, H. Huang, Z. Jiang et al. 2014. Ultraviolet-crosslinked hydrogel sustained-release hydrophobic antibiotics with long-term antibacterial activity and limited cytotoxicity. J. Appl. Polym. Sci. 131: 40438–40444.

Memic, A., H.A. Alhadrami, M.A. Hussain, M.F. Aldhahri, F. Al Nowaiser, F. Al-Hazmi et al. 2016. Hydrogels 2.0: improved properties with nanomaterial composites for biomedical applications. Biomed. Mater. 11: 014104.

Merino, S., C. Martin, K. Kostarelos, M. Prato and E. Vazquez. 2015. Nanocomposite hydrogels: 3D polymer_nanoparticle synergies for on-demand drug delivery. ACS Nano. 9: 4686–4697.

Meyenburg, S., H. Lilie, S. Panzner and R. Rudolph. 2000. Fibrin encapsulated liposomes as protein delivery system studies on the *in vitro* release behavior. J. Control. Rel. 69: 159–168.

Mezei, M. and V. Gulasekharam. 1982. Liposomes-a selective drug delivery system for the topical route of administration. J. Pharm. Pharmacol. 34: 473–474.

Mourtas, S., S. Fotopoulou, S. Duraj, V. Sfika, C. Tsakiroglou and S.G. Antimisiaris. 2007. Liposomal drugs dispersed in hydrogels. Effect of liposome, drug and gel properties on drug release kinetics. Colloids Surf. B. Biointerfaces. 55: 212–21.

Mourtas, S., S. Duraj, S. Fotopoulou and S.G. Antimisiaris. 2008. Integrity of liposomes in presence of various formulation excipients, when dispersed in aqueous media and in hydrogels. Colloids Surf. B. Biointerfaces. 61: 270–276.

Moya-Ortega, M.D., C. Alvarez-Lorenzo, A. Concheiro and T. Loftsson. 2012. Cyclodextrin-based nanogels for pharmaceutical and biomedical applications. Int. J. Pharm. 428: 152–163.

Peptu, C., M. Popa and S.G. Antimisiaris. 2008. Release of liposome-encapsulated calcein from liposome entrapping gelatin-carboxymethylcellulose films: a presentation of different possibilities. J. Nanosci. Nanotechnol. 8: 2249–58.

Pinho, E., M. Henriques and G. Soares. 2014. Cyclodextrin/cellulose hydrogel with gallic acid to prevent wound infection. Cellulose. 21: 4519–4530.

Rasool, B.K., R.H. Gareeb, S.A. Fahmy and A.A. Rasool. 2011. Meloxicam β-cyclodextrin transdermal gel: physicochemical characterization and *in vitro* dissolution and diffusion studies. Curr. Drug Deliv. 8: 381–391.

Simões, S.M., F. Veiga, J.J. Torres-Labandeira, A.C. Ribeiro, A. Concheiro and C. Alvarez-Lorenzo. 2014. Syringeable self-assembled cyclodextrin gels for drug delivery. Curr. Top. Med. Chem. 14: 494–509.

Tavano, L., L. Gentile, C. Oliviero Rossi and R. Muzzalupo. 2013. Novel gel-niosomes formulations as multi-component systems for transdermal drug delivery. Colloids Surf. B. Biointerfaces. 110: 281–288.

Tavano, L. 2015. Liposomal gels in enhancing skin delivery of drugs. pp. 329–341. *In*: Dragicevic-Curic, N. and H. Maibach [eds.]. Chemical Methods in Penetration Enhancement: Drug Manipulation Strategies and Vehicle Effects. Percutaneous Permeation Enhancer. Springer Berlin Heidelberg.

Tian, Z., C. Chen and H.R. Allcock. 2013. Injectable and biodegradable supramolecular hydrogels by inclusion complexation between poly(organophosphazenes) and α-cyclodextrin. Macromolecules. 46: 2715–2724.

Uchegbu, I.F. and A.T. Florence. 1995. Nonionic surfactant vesicles (niosomes): physical and pharmaceutical chemistry. Adv. Colloid Interface Sci. 58: 1–55.

Vashist, A., A. Vashist, Y.K. Gupta and S. Ahmad. 2014. Recent advances in hydrogel based drug delivery systems for the human body. J. Mater. Chem. B. 2: 147–166.

Wei, L., C. Cai, J. Lin and T. Chen. 2009. Dual-drug delivery system based on hydrogel/micelle composites. Biomaterials. 30: 2606–2613.

Molecularly Imprinted Hydrogels for the Selective Release of Therapeutics

*Piotr Luliński** and *Marcin Woźnica*

ABSTRACT

Imprinting technology involves the creation of specific binding sites in the polymeric network during polymerization in the presence of the template molecule. The major advantage of molecularly imprinted polymers formed after final template removal is high selectivity of material. The incorporation of imprinting technology into the synthesis of hydrophilic and biocompatible hydrogels can provide highly sophisticated carriers for drugs with prolonged release profiles. Moreover, molecularly imprinted hydrogels have attracted attention as the versatile biomaterials for the stereoselective release of chiral therapeutics. This extremely important property can maximize the delivery of eutomer, the pharmacologically active isomer of interest and reduce or even eliminate the delivery of the distomer, the undesirable isomer. Nowadays, the application of molecularly imprinted hydrogels in this field is still at the development stage. In this chapter, the principles of imprinting technology, the synthetic aspects and the drug-release behaviour of molecularly imprinted hydrogels are discussed. A brief survey of recent published studies

Department of Organic Chemistry, Faculty of Pharmacy, Medical University of Warsaw, Banacha 1, 02-097 Warsaw, Poland.
* Corresponding author: piotr.lulinski@wum.edu.pl

emphasizes the possible utility of molecularly imprinted hydrogels as the drug delivery devices in various administering routes. Finally, some current limitations and future prospects for the molecularly imprinted hydrogels are outlined.

Keywords: drug delivery, hydrogel, molecular imprinting, ocular administration, sustained release

1. Introduction

Just a few days before the beginning of 1960 a famous physicist Richard Phillip Feynman presented a lecture at the American Physical Society devoted to a new field of science that is nowadays known as nanoscience. During his talk, one bright idea was suggested: "It would be very interesting in surgery if you could swallow the surgeon. You put the mechanical surgeon inside the blood vessel and it goes into the heart and looks around. It finds out which valve is the faulty one and takes a little knife and slices it out" (Feynman 1960). This idea has become a keystone of nanomedicine as well as the medicinal model currently known as a personalized medicine, precision therapy or stratified medicine. The concept of personalized medicine is inextricably related to the personalized pharmacotherapy based on targeted drug delivery devices and thus an advanced, so-called "intelligent" drug delivery carrier, corresponds to "mechanical surgeon" cited above.

A vast number of diseases are still diagnosed in late symptomatic stage when various biochemical cascades are at different levels depending on the individual variability. The current model of therapy known as one-size-fits-all has resulted in moderate success for the predominant group of patients. Personalized pharmacotherapy allows for applying, to a single patient, the best suited drug which needs to be delivered at the right time and specific place in order to increase drug efficacy, to minimize the side effects of the dose and to facilitate fast patient recovery. However, the traditional pharmaceutical formulations do not fulfill the current demands of personalized pharmacotherapy. Polymers are a group of chemicals that presents great potential for drug delivery devices for personalized pharmacotherapy. Synthetic polymeric matrices have been intensively examined for many years but their successful implementation is hampered by the use of organic solvents for synthesis and the toxicity of degradation products (Koutsopoulos 2012, Wani 2015). The advanced technological progress allows developing the new platform of polymer-based biomaterials for drug carriers *viz.* hydrogels. The polymeric hydrogels have attracted attention as versatile carriers in drug delivery because they meet the rigorous criteria such as non-toxicity, non-immunogenicity, biocompatibility as well as comply with additional demands such as delivering of therapeutics in a sustained mode, achieving of maximum therapeutic efficiency with minimal toxic side effects.

The term "hydrogel" was originally used by Jacob Maarten van Bemmelen to define an inorganic hydrate of copper oxide (van Bemmelen 1894). However, it was the idea of Otto Wichterle and Drahoslav Lim that allows designing the synthetic material for living tissues which presents mechanical properties compatible to the natural environment, sufficient permeability for water-soluble compounds, resistance to enzymatic degradation and the absence of harmful impurities. This polymeric hydrogel consisted of 2-hydroxyethyl methacrylate and ethylene glycol dimethacrylate (Wichterle and Lim 1960). Over the next decades, significant progress has been made in the chemistry of hydrogels. Hydrogels were identified as very important functionalized biomaterials. Both natural and synthetic hydrogels have gained attention due to their properties such as reversible swelling behaviour, high water capacity, stability, long shelf life as well as well-defined structure. The enormous interest in the synthesis and application of hydrogels is reflected in the large number of articles that have been published since 1960. Despite the fact that more than fifty thousand articles have been published in the last half century, only an infinitesimal number of hydrogel formulations has been approved by various government agencies for the evaluation and control of medicinal products (Calo and Khutoryanskiy 2015). Thus, the practical utility of novel hydrogel based materials in the personalized pharmacotherapy still remains an important challenge. The control of drug release kinetics is the property of hydrogels that still needs to be improved. The optimal drug delivery carrier should be synchronized with the physiological status of the patient and should provide drug as the response to changes in the intracorporeal environment (Lee et al. 2013, Buwalda et al. 2014, Ullah et al. 2015). Environmental sensitivity has been identified as a significant property of the novel generation of hydrogels responsive to the variety of physical, chemical or biological stimuli such as temperature, electric or magnetic field, light, pressure, sound, ionic strength or pH of solvent, endogenous biomolecule or enzyme. Here, molecularly imprinted hydrogels have found a prominent role.

In this chapter, the principles of imprinting technology, the synthetic aspects and the drug-release behaviour of molecularly imprinted hydrogels will be discussed, followed by the short description of safety measures that have to be considered during the application of imprinted hydrogels as drug delivery devices. A brief survey of the recent literature will emphasize the possible utility of molecularly imprinted hydrogel drug carriers in various administering routes. Finally, some current limits and future prospects for the molecularly imprinted hydrogels will be outlined.

2. Principles of Imprinting Process

The molecularly imprinted polymers are characterized by the high level of selectivity due to the presence of specific recognition sites formed in the polymer network by the template-tailored synthesis. The synthesis of imprinted materials consists of three steps: the formation of prepolymerization structure, the polymerization reaction and the template removal (Fig. 1). The formation of the prepolymerization structure can be obtained by the covalent or non-covalent strategies. The covalent approach assumes the chemical reaction between template molecule and functional monomer in order to form functionalized compound prior to the polymerization. This approach was first introduced by Gunter Wulff and co-workers (Wulff et al. 1972). The non-covalent approach utilizes the range of weak intermolecular interactions such as ionic forces, hydrogen bonds, van der Waals forces or π-π interactions that can exist between the template molecule and functional monomer in order to form the prepolymerization complex prior to the polymerization. The non-covalent strategy was proposed by Klaus Mosbach and co-workers (Arshady and Mosbach 1981).

There are four critical factors during the imprinting process that can strongly affect the property of imprinted materials and the effectiveness of imprinting. They are: the choice of template, the preselection of functional monomer, the conditions of polymerization reaction and the effective template removal.

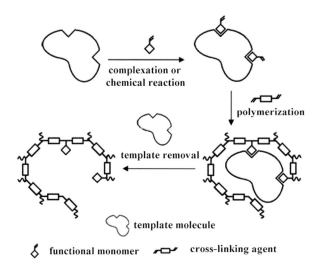

Fig. 1. The schematic idea of the imprinting process.

The choice of template is one of the crucial factors in the synthesis of imprinted materials. Certain structural elements of the template molecule are required to facilitate the imprinting process. The presence of functional groups or/and heteroatoms that could form covalent bonds or that could non-covalently interact with functional monomers is the main factor responsible for the stabilization of the prepolymerization structure. The aromatic, heteroaromatic or polyaromatic rings enhance the stabilization and together with cyclic systems as well as aliphatic chains are responsible for the formation of steric effects inside the polymeric network.

It is well known that the template and the target molecule should be the same (the target molecule is defined as the bioanalyte or pharmacologically active compound to which the imprinted polymer is dedicated). However, a majority of biocompounds or drugs possess the physico-chemical properties that limit their application in the synthesis of molecularly imprinted polymers, mainly due to insufficient solubility in organic solvents. The economic reasons have to be taken into account too because a lot of biocompounds or drugs are rarely available or expensive. Thus, the structural analogues of target molecule are widely applied as the template during the imprinting process (Sreenivasan 1999).

The critical moment in the design of imprinted materials is the selection of functional monomer that should interact with the template molecule *via* complementary functionalities. The selection of appropriate functional monomer could be a laborious process. The validation of the choice of proper monomer can proceed after the synthesis and analysis of binding properties of the imprinted polymer. Here, the theoretical studies have been employed as a powerful tool in the preselection of functional monomers (Nicholls et al. 2015).

Next, the polymerization reaction conditions such as the presence of cross-linkers, solvents or initiators (elevated temperature or ultra-violet irritation) have to be optimized. Here again the choice of covalent or non-covalent strategy ought to be considered. The covalent approach allows the unrestricted choice of polymerization conditions. When the non-covalent approach is employed, the harsh conditions of polymerization reaction can destabilize the prepolymerization systems, resulting in the failure of imprinting process. On the other hand, the ease of formation of the prepolymerization complex *via* non-covalent approach makes this strategy the most commonly used to provide the imprinted material.

Finally, the template molecule has to be removed from the polymer matrix to leave three-dimensional cavities empty (Lorenzo et al. 2011). This stage is the final critical factor of the synthesis because only total removal of the template molecule allows obtaining specific binding sites in the imprinted polymer network. Thus, the imprinting process is considered as the process that allows for modifying the surface of polymer by the template molecule.

The main parameter describing the efficacy of imprinting process is the imprinting factor. In the simplest way, the imprinting factor is defined as ratio of the binding capacity of the template on the imprinted polymer to the binding capacity of the template on the reference non-imprinted polymer. Hence, the synthesis of non-imprinted polymer has to be carried out in the same conditions omitting the addition of template molecule.

The brief overview of the synthesis of imprinted polymers above outlined the most important moments of the imprinting process. The imprinting technique has gained widespread attention mainly due to its application in the fabrication of molecularly imprinted sorbents for the purpose of the selective separation of compounds. There are some excellent books and reviews that provide more detailed information regarding the synthesis and application of imprinted polymers (Wulff 1995, 2002, Alexander et al. 2006, Alvarez-Lorenzo and Concheiro 2013a, Whitcombe et al. 2014). Apart from the use of imprinted polymers in the separation science, the new promising area of application has been explored. Molecularly imprinted polymers could serve as the drug delivery devices because they can provide high selectivity towards the particular drug. Moreover, they also show high stereoselectivity that is extremely important property in drug delivery forms. The majority of drugs possess chiral atoms in their molecule and their pharmacological activity is demonstrated only by one isomer or only one isomer shows the significantly higher activity. The ability to maximize the delivery of given eutomer (the isomer of interest) and reduce or even eliminate the delivery of the distomer (the undesirable isomer) is an enormous advantage of imprinted polymers. Molecularly imprinted polymers as the drug delivery devices have yet not found any commercial applications. There are still a lot of limitations that ought to be overcome. Some of the problems are pointed out in numerous books and reviews (Alvarez-Lorenzo 2004, 2013b, Luliński 2013). However, interesting investigations are in progress showing the possibility for application of molecularly imprinted hydrogels as the drug dosage forms. The most advanced experiments and the recent results are discussed below.

3. Macromolecular Memory of Hydrogels

Hydrogels are defined as water-swollen and cross-linked polymeric networks that are produced from one or more monomers or are the polymeric materials that exhibit the ability to swell and retain a significant fraction of water within their structure without dissolving. Recently, hydrogels have been defined as two- or multicomponent systems containing three-dimensional network of polymer chains and water that fills the regions between macromolecules (Ahmed 2015).

Different classifications of hydrogels have been proposed. In terms of composition, hydrogels can be divided into homopolymeric hydrogels which are derived from uniform monomer, copolymeric hydrogels which refer to at least two various monomers randomly located in the polymeric network (one should possess hydrophilic character) and multipolymer (interpenetrating) hydrogels that comprise of two different cross-linkers. A more important categorization is based on the type of interactions during the cross linking step. The physical cross linking of hydrogels provides transient junctions in the polymer network that exists due to the weak intermolecular interaction such as ionic forces, hydrogen bonds or hydrophobic interactions. The chemical cross linking resulted in permanent junctions in the polymer network that involves covalent bonds in the cross-linked hydrogel (Hennink and van Nostrum 2012, Ahmed 2015, Ullah et al. 2015). The molecularly imprinted hydrogels are mainly synthesized as chemically cross-linked polymers.

The idea of molecular imprinting involves the creation of three-dimensional cavities in the most rigid highly cross-linked polymeric network. In the case of low cross-linked hydrogels that possess relatively high degree of flexibility of polymer chains, the process of imprinting can be more properly define as the process of creation of the macromolecular memory in the hydrogel network (Byrne and Salian 2008). Once the imprinting process proceeds, the complementary interactions of various functionalities between the target molecule and the polymer network as well as the spatial or configurational specificity governed the recognition mechanism. It could be questionable that the flexibility of polymeric chains in hydrogels can provide the macromolecular memory of the conformations of chains since the relaxation of network can diminish the spatial effects of imprinting. However, the multiple interactions during the imprinting stage between the template and monomers evoke the incorporation of mer units into the polymeric chain in the conformation form which is characterized by low energy. When the polymerization is finished, the global energy minimum of growing polymer chains with template complexes is achieved promoting the memorization of the chain conformation. Then, the molecular recognition of target molecule by the flexible structure of hydrogel occurs as the dynamic process that comprises the successive steps of mutual conformational adaptations. Such process allows to modify the specificity and affinity of interactions with target molecule by many trial-and-error steps until the high energy interactions are favored and compound is bound (Demchenko 2001).

The recognition of target molecule by the imprinted hydrogel takes place in the swollen state including water as the medium. The swollen volume at equilibrium has to be very similar to the relaxed polymer volume fraction during the imprinting stage. The hydrophilic groups in the polymer backbone and the hydrophobic regions of cross-linked junctions are responsible for the preservation of macromolecular memory and imprinting effect. Thus, the optimization of synthetic parameters is necessary to provide the imprinted hydrogel with controlled swelling.

The main factors that have to be considered during the synthesis of imprinted hydrogels are as follows: the ratio between the template and monomer, the diversity of monomers, the density of cross-linker, and the polymerization reaction conditions.

A very important factor is the optimal ratio between the template molecule and the functional monomers which is responsible for the enhancement of the interactions between the respective chemicals. This is the major variable responsible for the effective imprinting of hydrogels. The large excess of monomers provides randomly incorporated monomer functionalities similarly to the non-imprinted hydrogel affecting the macromolecular memory of polymer chains and diminishing the imprinting effect. On the contrary, the low ratio of monomer to the template results in the insufficient effectiveness of simultaneous interactions that has to occur to enhance the macromolecular memory in the polymer chain resulting in the disappearance of imprinting effect, too. This phenomenon was observed during the optimization of prepolymerization conditions with timolol as the template. In the experiments, the various ratios of timolol to the functional monomer were employed. The optimized stoichiometry of the complexation was equal to one molecule of timolol to eight molecules of monomer and it was confirmed by isothermal titration calorimetry. After the polymerization was finished, the binding capacities of the resulted imprinted hydrogels towards timolol were determined. It was proved that the increase in the amount of monomer functionalities (the stoichiometry of prepolymerization complex was more than one timolol to eight monomers) as well as decrease in the amount of monomer functionalities (the stoichiometry of prepolymerization complex was less than one timolol to six monomers) resulted in a significant increase of the non-specific adsorption. As a consequence, the disappearance of imprinting effect was observed due to similar binding ability of the imprinted and non-imprinted hydrogels (Yanez et al. 2011a).

The next important factor is the diversity of monomers that form heteropolymeric system. The employment of different monomers in the formation of the prepolymerization complexes enhances the strength of interactions with the template molecule. After the hydrogel is created, the diverse monomer functionalities play a crucial role in the recognition of the target molecule which based on the complementarity. This factor was analyzed during the determination of the diffusion coefficients of four ketotifen imprinted hydrogels possessing different composition: poly(N-vinylpirrolidone-*co*-2-hydroxyethyl methacrylate-*co*-polyethylene glycol dimethacrylate), poly(acrylamide-*co*-2-hydroxyethyl methacrylate-*co*-polyethylene glycol dimethacrylate), poly(acrylic acid-*co*-2-hydroxyethyl methacrylate-*co*-polyethylene glycol dimethacrylate), and poly(N-vinylpirrolidone-*co*-acrylamide-*co*-acrylic acid-*co*-2-hydroxyethyl methacrylate-*co*-polyethylene glycol dimethacrylate). The following diffusion coefficients were determined: 80, 34, 54, and 0.7 x 10^{-9} cm^2/s, respectively. The slowest diffusion was noted for the ketotifen imprinted hydrogel with the most complex composition. It should be added that the simultaneous determination of structural parameters of the imprinted and non-imprinted hydrogels revealed no significant difference between them. It was concluded that the imprinting technique resulted in the structural plasticity of polymeric chains and the imprinting process is responsible for the formation of macromolecular memory due to the organization of the diverse functionalities in the polymer architecture. The multiplicity and diversity of functionalities are responsible for binding events that affect the transport throughout the imprinted hydrogel and delay the diffusion of drugs (Venkatesh et al. 2008).

Then, the density of cross-linker or the molar percentage of cross linking agents in the total mass of polymer is very important. In the highly cross-linked rigid polymers, the movement of the functional residues is strongly restricted. In contrast, the low cross-linked swellable systems such as hydrogels, ensure facile diffusion of the compound to the inner regions of the net. A higher ratio of cross-linker affects the swelling property of imprinted hydrogel because it hampers the mobility of the polymer chains. As a consequence, it prevents vast imbibe of water and counteracts against the destruction of imprinted sites. This problem was considered in the analysis of timolol imprinted hydrogel. The different molar concentrations of ethylene glycol dimethacrylate cross-linker were used in the synthesis of imprinted hydrogels. Then, Langmuir isotherms were determined and maximum binding capacities of hydrogels as well as the dissociation constant were calculated. It was found that the dissociation constants were similar for all imprinted hydrogels in all tested molar concentrations of cross-linker. The maximum binding capacities of all imprinted hydrogels were very similar and independent of the cross-linker molar concentration. On the contrary, the non-imprinted hydrogels possessed ten times lower values of the maximum binding capacity. Moreover, the non-imprinted hydrogels revealed the decrease of maximum binding capacity with the increase of concentration of the cross-linker. It was explained that in the non-imprinted systems, the functionalities from monomer are randomly distributed in the hydrogel net and they are separated by the cross-linker chains which prevent interactions with timolol (Alvarez-Lorenzo et al. 2002).

The polymerization reaction can affect the sequence of imprinted hydrogel network. The polymerization is mainly carried out as a free-radical process that is difficult to control. The resulted cross linking polymeric structure could possess multiple defects. The formation of primary and secondary loops, entanglements and dangling ends can affect the recognition process. Here, an interesting technique involving the living radical polymerization was introduced to overcome the problem. This technique provides better memorization of the hydrogel chain conformations (Salian et al. 2012).

The presence of solvent during polymerization also plays important role. The imprinted hydrogels that are prepared in the absence of solvent (or more precisely the largest volume of hydrophilic monomer plays a role of solvent) are characterized by relatively high binding capacity and high imprinting effect. On the contrary, the presence of solvent (mostly protic and polar one) provides a macro- or microstructure of hydrogel. The porous system is responsible for the transport of solutes inside the hydrogel network and is closely related to the water swellability.

Once the imprinted hydrogel is obtained, it should be characterized by the determination of imprinting efficacy, swelling properties as well as the structural and mechanical properties. The effectiveness of imprinting process is estimated based upon the imprinting effect which was described above. The specific parameter devoted to hydrogels is the swelling ratio describing the ability of dry polymer to swell and retain water. In the absence of cross linking points (junctions) the linear polymeric chains dissolve in water due to thermodynamic compatibility. The cross linking provides heterogeneous matrix with low water swelling (high cross-link density) hydrophobic regions and the solubility is counterbalanced by the retractive forces of the elasticity of junctions in the polymer network. In the equilibrium swollen state, the thermodynamic forces of mixing and retractive forces of the polymeric chains are balanced. However, the swelling of hydrogels is a complex process. Firstly, the polar hydrophilic groups of imprinted hydrogel matrix are hydrated by water (primary bound water), followed by the swelling of the hydrophobic regions of hydrogel (secondary bound water). The primary and secondary bound water comprise the total bound water. Finally, the osmotic driving forces of the hydrogel network to imbibe additional water are hampered by chemical cross linking providing equilibrium swelling state with additional bulk or free water which fills the regions between the cross-linked points (Hoffman 2012).

Finally, the structure and mechanical properties of hydrogel should be defined. The structural determination of hydrogels can be done by the analysis of the polymer volume fraction in swollen state, the average molecular weight and the average distance between two cross linking junctions. The polymer volume fraction in the swollen state is defined as the amount of liquid phase imbibed and retained in the hydrogel network. The average molecular weight is a measure of the polymer cross linking degree. The average distance (mesh size) describes the intervals between two neighboring junctions in the cross linking net and this value determines the space available between macromolecular chains that can be filled with water (Peppas et al. 2000).

The additional characterization included scanning electron microscopy analysis to reveal the surface of dry hydrogels. In general, the micrographs reveal very regular, smooth and poreless surface on both imprinted and non-imprinted polymers. The infra-red spectroscopy analysis can also be employed to confirm the completion of the polymerization reaction and the lack of unreacted double bonds from the monomers. The differential scanning calorymetry analysis can reveal the thermal behaviour of hydrogels (Alvarez-Lorenzo et al. 2002).

The mechanical properties are mainly related to the viscoelastic behaviour of hydrogels which plays significant role when hydrogels are considered for the pharmaceutical formulations. Here, the standard mechanical tests can be carried out and the parameters such as the elastic modulus, viscous modulus and loss modulus should be determined (Koetting et al. 2015). A set of rheological analyses was performed on timolol imprinted poly(methacrylic acid-*co*-2-hydroxyethyl methacrylate) and poly(methyl methacrylate-*co*-2-hydroxyethyl methacrylate) hydrogels. The dependence between the elastic and viscous moduli and the angular frequency showed similar pattern for imprinted and non-imprinted hydrogels. It was concluded that timolol did not modify the mechanical properties. The plot of dissipation factor (tan δ) against temperature for dry hydrogels at fixed angular frequency revealed peaks that indicate the glass transition temperature of imprinted hydrogel. It was also stated that the rheological analysis can indicate modification of the inter- and intrachain interactions due to the presence of the template molecule (Alvarez-Lorenzo et al. 2002).

4. Release of Drugs from Imprinted Hydrogels

The characterization of transport parameters as well as the determination of drug release kinetics from the imprinted hydrogel is very important considering their application as the drug carriers. The vast amount of hydrogel drug delivery forms represent swelling controlled systems. During the penetration of water into the polymer network, the hydrogel starts to swell and the glass transition temperature of polymer is lowered. It results in the transformation of imprinted hydrogel to rubberlike form. The drug that is embedded inside the polymeric network dissolves in water and the diffusion process is initiated (Fig. 2). In the swelling controlled systems, three variables play a crucial role: the diffusion concentration gradient, the polymer stress gradient and the osmotic forces. The selected hydrogels present the non-swelling controlled systems. Here, the relaxation of the polymer matrix governed water penetration inside the net and the transport is characterized by Fick's laws of diffusion. However, in various imprinted hydrogel systems, the anomalous transport mechanisms are observed (Serra et al. 2006).

The detailed discussion of relations between the imprinting effects and the transport of drugs with the context of structural characterization of the imprinted hydrogels is scarce in literature. However, a few important reviews and papers describe the different mathematic models as well as the details of theory related to the transport of drug within the imprinted hydrogels (Bayer and Peppas 2008, Byrne et al. 2002, 2008, Venkatesh et al. 2008, Puoci et al. 2011, Koetting et al. 2015).

The release of drug from pharmaceutical form is performed through different routes (Byrne et al. 2002, Hilt and Byrne 2004, Serra et al. 2006, Hoare and Kohane 2008) and different mathematic models are employed to the analysis of drug release profiles (Dash et al. 2010). In the imprinted hydrogels, the numerous complementary or sterically oriented functionalities interact with the drug. The interactions in the macromolecular memory sites delay the release of the drug from the imprinted hydrogel despite of the swelling degree of polymer. The strength of those interactions can be responsible for the delayed release. The sustained release can be also explained by so-called "tumbling effect" which is described as the migration of the drug from one macromolecular memory site to another. The functionally diverse hydrogel system is able to do multiple contacts with the drug to create efficient complexation due to the reduction of the entropically unfavorable translational and rotational free energies. The phenomenon was analyzed in the timolol imprinted poly(N-vinylpirrolidone-*co*-acrylamide-*co*-acrylic acid-*co*-2-hydroxyethyl methacrylate-*co*-polyethylene glycol dimethacrylate)

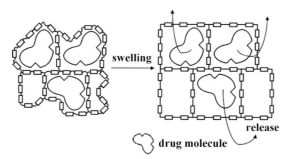

Fig. 2. The schematic idea of drug release from hydrogels due to swelling or/and relaxation of the polymer.

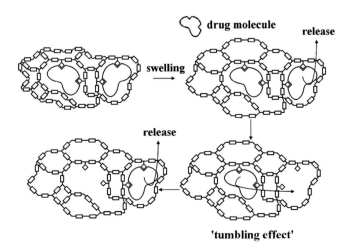

Fig. 3. The schematic idea of release of drug from imprinted hydrogel involving "tumbling effect".

hydrogel that consisted of three various functional monomers (Venkatesh et al. 2008, Yanez et al. 2011a). It was proposed that the imprinting effect is responsible for delay transport. The sustained release of drug occurs due to the random interactions through the network imprinted by it. The drug itinerates from one macromolecular memory site to another high affinity region where the complexation takes place and then escapes from it and itinerates to another one and so on. This behaviour is responsible for increasing of mean residence time of the drug in the hydrogel net (Fig. 3).

In another mechanism, the competitive binding of structurally related compound that is presented in the intracorporeal environment promotes the release of the drug. This mechanism was investigated with hydrocortisone imprinted polymer. This imprinted system showed the ability to adsorb a considerable amount of testosterone due to the structural similarity of both compounds. The release of testosterone in water was very slow and even after 24 hr only 45% of testosterone was released. However, in the presence of hydrocortisone (which was also used as the template molecule during the synthesis of polymer) the competitive binding was promoted and the rapid release of testosterone from the binding sites occurred, completing the total release of testosterone within four hours (Sreenivasan 1999). Those imprinting systems are extremely interesting as the drug carriers because they can respond for the alterations of the concentration of important bioanalyte or biomarker (Fig. 4).

There are also mechanisms that involve the hydrolytically induced releasing of drug or release in the physical stimuli responsive manner. The first approach required the use of the erodible imprinting system from which the drug cannot be released unless the whole (or a part of) the polymer

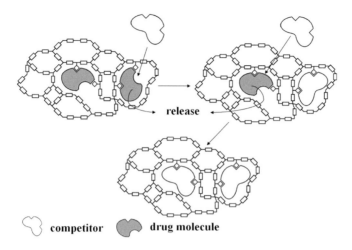

competitor   drug molecule

Fig. 4. The schematic idea of the stimuli responsive release of the drug from imprinted hydrogel after swelling in the presence of competitor.

degrades. The latter describes the release of drug after the response to shift of the physicochemical properties of external fluids (Li et al. 2010).

5. Safety Measures for Imprinted Hydrogels

It is necessary to discuss the additional precautions related to the applications of imprinted hydrogels as the drug delivery devices. These include: biocompatibility and toxicity, capacity of the formulation and stability of the imprinted material.

The synthetic monomers and cross-linkers that are used during the preparation of imprinted hydrogels for the dosage forms have to be biocompatible because they are in contact with sensitive tissues. This requirement significantly reduces the choice of effective functional monomers for the imprinting process because many of them are toxic ones. Only the application of the well-known and previously tested reagents could prevent any unexpected incompatibility. The reagents of interest are mostly methacrylic acid and ethylene glycol dimethacrylate or their analogues. They are commonly used in the preparation of imprinted materials and they are also used in the production of commercial pharmaceutical formulations such as Eudragit® (copolymer of ethyl acrylate, methyl methacrylate and a low-content of methacrylic acid ester with quaternary ammonium groups) or contact lenses such as Ocufilcon D® (copolymer of 2-hydroxyethyl methacrylate, methacrylic acid and ethylene glycol dimethacrylate). The most probable impurity of imprinted hydrogels can be caused by leaching of the template molecule or so-called "bleeding effect". This phenomenon is an undesirable corollary of the use of template in the prepolymerization mixture. Numerous approaches were introduced to overcome the "bleeding effect" such as continuous extraction, thermal annealing, microwave assisted extraction and supercritical fluid desorption (Ellwanger et al. 2001, Lorenzo et al. 2011). The residual impurities in the hydrogel matrix could be derived also from unreacted monomers, initiators or solvents. Substantial progress was observed in the improvement of purification processes of hydrogels. Additional steps, which lead to the highest possible degree of monomer conversion, can be applied such as the post-polymerization thermal treatment of products. This excellent approach includes cross linking of water-soluble polymers by the thermal treatment under high pressure *via* autoclaving or microwave radiation (Cook et al. 2012). The very promising technique to overcome the utilization of toxic solvents during synthesis of imprinted materials is to carry out the polymerization process in the presence of supercritical carbon dioxide (da Silva et al. 2011).

Biocompatibility can be proved involving cytotoxicity assays. Here, an example could be the analysis of cytotoxicity of the moderately cross-linked ibuprofen imprinted poly(2-dimethylamino)ethyl methacrylate-*co*-ethylene glycol dimethacrylate hydrogel prepared with the support of the supercritical carbon dioxide technology. The cytotoxicity tests were carried out with human colorectal carcinoma-derived Caco-2 cells confirming the biocompatibility of hydrogel. The experiment revealed the higher number of cells in the vicinity of imprinted hydrogel. The zeta potentials of imprinted hydrogel and non-imprinted ones were determined (6.7 and 17.5 mV, respectively). The observation was explained by the interaction of positively charged hydrogel with the negatively charged surface of the cell by the electrostatic forces. It means that the presence of ibuprofen during the synthesis and its subsequent removal induced the modification of the surface of imprinted hydrogel with positive charge. The microscopic photographs were presented in order to support the results (da Silva et al. 2011).

The sufficient binding capacity of imprinted hydrogel is necessary to ensure the required dose of drug that has to be released. In the most common way, after the synthesis and template removal step, the drug has to be loaded to imprinted hydrogel. This approach includes the soaking of hydrogel in the drug standard solution for the defined period of time to achieve the equilibrium. Second approach includes *in situ* loading of drug during the fabrication of imprinted material (drug is a part of the prepolymerization complex). The latter procedure increases the loading capacity of imprinted hydrogel but it is limited to drugs which can survive the polymerization process. Another problem arises from the fact that there is no guarantee that the whole amount of the drug is introduced to the polymer network during the preparation of imprinted material (Byrne et al. 2008). The precise determination of amount of the drug after the polymerization and post-polymerization preparation may be difficult to perform. The non-specific adsorption is another problem during drug loading procedure (the drug is adsorbed on the hydrogel but not in the specific macromolecular memory sites). It has to be excluded because it can provoke unexpected expulsion or so-called "burst effect" of drug during hydrogel swelling (Norell et al. 1998). The "burst effect" could leads to serious consequences after the administrating, especially when the drug is characterized by the narrow therapeutic index.

Finally, the long-term stability of imprinted hydrogels has to be determined. The immutability of the hydrogel drug carrier during the lifespan of application has to be constant. It is well-known that highly cross-linked imprinted polymers possess long-life stability and the adsorption tests that were carried out several years after the synthesis revealed very similar adsorption characteristic. However, a detailed analysis of the drug release behaviour from the imprinted hydrogel after prolonged time is rather scarce.

6. Application of Imprinted Hydrogels for Ocular Administration

The available ocular pharmaceutical formulations such as eye drops are characterized by the low effectiveness of ophthalmic drug delivery. The protective mechanisms of lacrimal apparatus and the fast removal of drugs from anterior segments of eye by the nasolacrimal drainage are responsible for low bioavailability. The application of ophthalmic ointments and gels only slightly improve the therapeutic effects. The bioavailability of ophthalmic drugs significantly increased when ophthalmic drug delivery systems based on the contact lenses were introduced into the treatment. However, the low loading capacity of such devices is a main limitation (Xinming et al. 2008, Bengani et al. 2013, Kirchhof et al. 2015).

Molecularly imprinted hydrogels were extensively investigated as the ocular drug delivery forms with a hope to overcome existing problems. Carmen Alvarez-Lorenzo and co-workers (Alvarez-Lorenzo et al. 2002) prepared the imprinted soft contact lenses able to deliver timolol in sustained mode. Timolol is a non-selective β-adrenergetic receptor antagonist that is widely applied in the treatment of glaucoma. The molecule of timolol possesses chiral carbon atom and only S enancjomer possesses high pharmacological activity. Therefore, the design of drug delivery form to deliver necessary eutomer is an important scientific challenge. The authors evaluated the influence of the composition of the matrix and the loading capacity of 2-hydroxyethyl methacrylate (backbone monomer) hydrogels weakly cross-linked with ethylene glycol dimethacrylate and with the presence or the absence of methacrylic acid and methyl methacrylate (functional monomers). The dry hydrogels were clear and smooth with poreless surface and presented appropriate properties required for the contact lenses. The diffusion of S-timolol into the physiological saline from imprinted hydrogel build up from 2-hydroxyethyl methacrylate or combined 2-hydroxyethyl methacrylate and methacrylic acid was slow. The latter hydrogel presented the highest loading capacity equal to 12 µg of S-timolol in 1 mg of dry hydrogel. In the following study, the effects of different monomers on the binding capacity as well as the impact of the stoichiometry of reagents and the polymerization conditions were investigated (Hiratani and Alvarez-Lorenzo 2002, 2004, Hiratani et al. 2005a, Yanez et al. 2011a). The prepolymerization systems including methacrylic acid (functional monomer), N,N-diethylacrylamide (backbone monomer as well as solvent), ethylene glycol dimethacrylate (cross-linker at various concentrations) and S-timolol (template) were investigated. The polymerization was proceeded in the mould that forms final contact lenses with diameter of 16 mm and thickness of 0.3 mm. The adsorption of the target drug (S-timolol) was carried out after the template removal step by the soaking procedure. The binding capacities of imprinted hydrogels were satisfied and were more than two times higher than the non-imprinted ones. The dissociation constants were between 5.0 and 8.9 µmol/L (depending on the concentration of cross-linker) for imprinted hydrogels and between 6.3 and 29.4 µmol/L for non-imprinted hydrogels. The release was carried out in 0.9% sodium chloride aqueous medium imitating the physiological conditions of the ocular surface. The profiles of S-timolol release were analyzed. The Higuchi model was employed for the analysis of drug release kinetics. The transport of the drug from imprinted hydrogel was characterized by Fick's laws of diffusion. Moreover, the presence of physiological saline strongly affected the diffusion of drug retarding the release process. However, the composition of imprinted hydrogels has to ensure appropriate permeability of oxygen and carbon dioxide recommended for safe day or month-wearing soft contact lenses. Therefore, the nature of monomers on the profiles of S-timolol release was investigated and 3-[tris(trimethylsiloxy)silyl]propyl methacrylate was selected as the functional monomer for analysis. This monomer provides hydrogel with very good permeability of oxygen and is often used as the component of month-wearing soft contact lenses. The imprinted hydrogel matrix was built up from 3-[tris(trimethylsiloxy)silyl] propyl methacrylate as well as methacrylic acid (both used as functional monomers), N,N-diethylacrylamide (backbone monomer) and ethylene glycol dimethacrylate (cross-linker). The diffusion coefficient obtained for imprinted hydrogel confirmed that S-timolol was released in sustained mode. Thus, the modulation of the composition of hydrogel was possible to adapt the drug release behaviour for imprinted soft contact lenses with better oxygen permeability. Finally, the dissolution of S-timolol in the mixture of monomers, which allowed to exclude organic solvents at the minimum of cross linking is necessary to secure macromolecular memory sites in the hydrogel network. The *in vivo* experiments of releasing S-timolol from the imprinted contact lenses instilled in cornea were carried out (Hiratani et al. 2005b). S-Timolol was detected in the tear fluid for a period of 180 min, which was two-fold longer than that from the non-imprinted hydrogel. The comparative analysis of S-timolol released from the eye drops containing 0.068% and 0.25% of S-timolol showed the presence of the drug in the tear fluid for only 60 min. It was also found that the ocular bioavailability of S-timolol from the eye drops only slightly depended on the dose, but the corresponding bioavailability from the presoaked imprinted soft contact lenses increased significantly (for 34 µg of timolol the AUC—area under curve values were 1.24 and 10.76 mmol min/L, respectively). However, the loading capacity of the imprinted soft contact lenses was insufficient to *in vivo* release due the effect of the release medium, the continuous renovation of the lacrimal fluid and the blinking. In order to improve the loading capacity, an innovative method using a supercritical fluid technology was proposed (Braga et al. 2010, Yanez et al. 2011b). This method employed hydrogel based commercial soft contact lenses (Hilafilcon B®) and selected drug. The sequential impregnation-imprinting and extraction steps were performed with the non-steroid anti-inflammatory drug R/S-flurbiprofen as the template using the supercritical carbon dioxide technology. The rearrangement of polymeric regions of soft contact lenses in the presence of the template as well as the effect of supercritical carbon dioxide on the plasticization of hydrogel was responsible for imprinting effect. It was observed that each consequent impregnation step resulted in the increase of binding capacity of the imprinted soft contact lenses. The comprehensive analysis of the structure and binding experiments with some structurally related compounds revealed the recognition ability and a higher affinity for R/S-flurbiprofen in aqueous solutions. The release profiles were investigated revealing the sustained release of R/S-flurbiprofen for six hours in aqueous medium. The study of S-ibuprofen release from soft contact lenses prepared using supercritical fluid technology was also provided (da Silva et al. 2011). The imprinted hydrogel was build up only from 2-(dimethylamino)ethyl methacrylate (functional as well as backbone monomer) and ethylene glycol dimethacrylate (cross-linker). The release behaviour showed strong dependence on pH of releasing medium. In the neutral pH the anomalous transport was observed and the release of S-ibuprofen after 24 h was equal to 181 mg/g for imprinted hydrogel and only 65 mg/g for non-imprinted one. In the acidic pH, the release was close to the kinetic of zero-order according to Korsmeyer-Peppas model which was employed for the analysis of drug release profile. The lower diffusion coefficient of S-ibuprofen from imprinted hydrogel in acidic pH (0.0357 versus 0.1337 h^{-1} in neutral pH) was explained by the lower solubility of

S-ibuprofen in acidic medium and enhancement of hydrophobic interactions between the drug and hydrogel. It was concluded that different interactions (hydrogen bond and hydrophobic forces) are involved in the stabilization of the complex between the S-ibuprofen and imprinted hydrogel. Nevertheless, the procedure is not effective for monthly-wearing soft contact lenses probably due to the different composition of hydrogel. The imprinted soft contact lenses were also investigated for various anti-inflammatory drugs as well as antibiotics carriers (Alvarez-Lorenzo et al. 2006, Maryam et al. 2007, Malaekeh-Nikouei et al. 2012, Tieppo et al. 2012, Malakooti et al. 2015).

There are also patents and patent applications presenting inventions related to ocular drug delivery systems based on the imprinted technology. An interesting invention is devoted to the extended or continuous wear imprinted hydrogels dedicated to delivery of various drugs and comfort compounds. One of the examples described in this patent is dedicated to the imprinted hydrogel drug carrier for ketotifen and other anti-histamine drugs. Here, the hydrogel build up from acrylic acid, acrylamide, and N-vinylpirrolidone as the functional monomers as well as poly(2-hydroxyethyl methacrylate) as the backbone monomer and poly(ethylene glycol dimethacrylate) as the cross-linker presented the highest binding capacity and specificity. The optimum percentage of cross-linker was set at 5%. Another example describes the imprinted hydrogel for delivery of fluconazole or other anti-fungal drugs. Here, on the contrary, the most suitable system consists of acrylamide, 2-(diethylamino)ethyl methacrylate and N-vinylpirrolidone as the functional monomers (the backbone monomer and the cross-linker were the same as above). Finally, the latter system was also effective for the preparation of drug delivery system for hyaluronic acid (Byrne and Venkatesh 2012, Byrne et al. 2013, Maryam and Byrne 2013).

7. Other Examples of Imprinted Hydrogels for Drug Delivery

The investigations of imprinted hydrogels as the drug delivery forms for other administrating route are rather scarce and limited to selected important pharmacological agents. There is also the insufficiency in the analysis of release profiles *in vivo* which indisposes further development or commercialization of imprinted hydrogels. However, there are a few interesting examples that can be found in the literature describing imprinted hydrogel systems dedicated to the delivery of selected anti-cancer drugs, antibiotics or insulin. 5-Fluorouracil is an anti-cancer drug that is used in treatment of breast, colorectal, liver or brain carcinoma. This compound undergoes fast transformation due to the high rate of metabolism in the human body. However, the high concentration of this agent in serum is necessary to achieve sufficient therapeutic effect. Such concentration has to be maintained for a prolonged time but cannot exceed a certain value to avoid severe side effects. Hence, the imprinted hydrogel was designed for sustained release of 5-fluorouracil (Singh and Chauhan 2008, Cirillo et al. 2009). The hydrogel was build up from 2-hydroxyethyl methacrylate (backbone monomer), acrylic acid (functional monomer) and N,N'-methylenebisacrylamide (cross-linker). The different concentrations of 5-fluorouracil (template) were applied to observe the effect of the number of recognition sites in the imprinted net on the entrapment of drug and the release profile. As it was expected, the higher binding capacity was noted for the imprinted hydrogel prepared in the presence of higher concentration of 5-fluorouracil. However, *in vitro* release profiles revealed non-Fickian diffusion of the drug from hydrogel with n values below 0.5 for both imprinted hydrogels. It was supposed that the release of drug is also controlled by the degradation of the covalent linkage of the hydrogel network. Recently, the uniform and spherical hydrophilic nanoparticles (diameter ca 250 nm) were obtained for delivery of 5-fluorouracil. The hydrogel was a copolymer of methacrylic acid and ethylene glycol dimethacrylate with nearly equimolar amount of each reagent. The *in vitro* release experiments revealed complete desorption of the drug from non-imprinted hydrogel within five hours but in case of imprinted hydrogel the release was continued for more than two days. In another interesting work, the metal coordinate bond strategy was employed to prepare imprinted hydrogel with pH-responsive property for controlled release of the antibiotic, doxorubicin (Zhang et al. 2014). The hydrogel was built up from 4-vinylpyridine (functional monomer), 2-hydroxyethyl methacrylate (backbone monomer) and N,N-methylenebisacrylamide (cross-linker). Additionally, the cupric ions were used to serve as the bridge between the functional monomer and the template. The strong coordinate interactions enhanced the stability of the prepolymerization complex of 4-vinylpyridine and doxorubicin. The strong pH-dependence of the release of doxorubicin from the imprinted hydrogel was observed. At pH 6 or at pH 7.2, approximately 10% of the loaded drug was released to medium but at pH 5 the release was accelerated to nearly 60%. The pH value affected the coordinate interactions between the cupric ions and doxorubicin which are steady in the basic or neutral range. In lower pH values, the protonation of 4-vinylpyridine resulted in the cleavage of coordinate bonds and the release of doxorubicin. The analysis of *in vitro* release profiles revealed that the drug was released from imprinted hydrogel for seven days and only for one day from non-imprinted counterpart. Finally, low cross-linker and also pH-responsive insulin delivery system was proposed (Li et al. 2010) based on methacrylic acid and poly(ethylene glycol dimethacrylate) as functional and backbone monomers as well as N,N-methylenebisacrylamide as the cross-linker. The imprinted hydrogel showed the sustained release of insulin only in acidic medium but more detailed studies were omitted.

8. Current Status and Future Prospects

Molecularly imprinted hydrogels are promising materials in the construction of future drug delivery devices because they can provide improved delivery profiles, prolonged releasing times and extended residency of the drug. This class of hydrogels could release the drugs in the feedback regulated way which is extremely required in modern pharmacotherapy. Most importantly, the imprinted hydrogels are highly selective materials capable of providing the appropriate enantiomeric form of the drug. The future perspectives for imprinted hydrogels as the drug delivery forms are very promising, mostly for ocular administrating route. The extensive investigations that have been published recently allowed overcoming some existing problems such as low bioavailability. However, further investigations are necessary to obtain the ideal imprinted hydrogel based soft contact lenses which will be characterized by sufficient loading capacity, controllable zero-order release profile below the toxic limits or the release during entire wear time within the therapeutic window. The synchronization of the drug release with the patient intracorporeal environment will be additional advantage. The requirements for elder people arising from lower volume of tears or higher risk of infections have to be adopted, too. A majority of original articles devoted to hydrogels describes the development of new materials and their detailed characterization but the safety measures and clinical studies of new drug delivery devices are often omitted. Thus, the *in vivo* release profiles, cytotoxicity tests, long-term compatibility and clinical performance should become a standard in the future studies to facilitate the commercialization of novel imprinted hydrogel drug delivery forms. However, the regulatory affairs as well as the high costs of the clinical studies can be a major barrier to commercialization. Nevertheless, the significant progress in the field of molecular imprinting of hydrogels and the current requirement of the drug delivery form could prompt the imprinted drug delivery devices more sophisticated and capable for personalized or for individual treatment.

Acknowledgement

Authors would like to thanks Prof. Dorota Maciejewska for her fruitful discussions during the preparation of the chapter.

References

Ahmed, E.M. 2015. Hydrogel: preparation, characterization and applications: a review. J. Adv. Res. 6: 105–121.
Alexander, C., H.S. Andersson, L.I. Andersson, R.J. Ansell, N. Kirsch, I.A. Nicholls et al. 2006. Molecular imprinting science and technology: a survey of the literature for the years up to and including 2003. J. Mol. Recognit. 19: 106–180.

Alvarez-Lorenzo, C., H. Hiratani, J.L. Gomez-Amoza, R. Martinez-Pacheco, C. Souto and A. Concheiro. 2002. Soft contact lenses capable of sustained delivery of timolol. J. Pharm. Sci. 91: 2182–2192.

Alvarez-Lorenzo, C. and A. Concheiro. 2004. Molecularly imprinted polymers for drug delivery. J. Chromatogr. B. 804: 231–245.

Alvarez-Lorenzo, C., F. Yanez, R. Barreiro-Iglesias and C. Concheiro. 2006. Imprinted soft contact lenses as norfloxacin delivery systems. J. Control. Release. 113: 236–244.

Alvarez-Lorenzo, C. and A. Concheiro. 2013a. Handbook of molecularly imprinted polymers. Smithers Rapra, Shawbury, United Kingdom.

Alvarez-Lorenzo, C., C. González-Chomón and A. Concheiro. 2013b. Molecularly imprinted hydrogels for affinity-controlled and stimuli-responsive drug delivery. pp. 228–260. *In*: Alvarez-Lorenzo, C., A. Concheiro, H.J. Schneider and M. Shahinpoor [eds.]. Smart Materials for Drug Delivery. Volume 1. RSC, Cambridge, United Kingdom.

Arshady, R. and K. Mosbach. 1981. Synthesis of substrate-selective polymers by host-guest polymerization. Macromol. Chem. Phys. – Makromol. Chem. 182: 687–692.

Bayer, C.L. and N.A. Peppas. 2008. Advances in recognitive, conductive and responsive delivery systems. J. Control. Release. 132: 216–221.

Bengani, L.C., K.-H. Hsu, S. Gause and A. Chauhan. 2013. Contact lenses as a platform for ocular drug delivery. Expert Opin. Drug Deliv. 10: 1483–1496.

Braga, M.E.M., F. Yanez, C. Alvarez-Lorenzo, D. Concheiro, C.M.M. Duarte, M.H. Gil et al. 2010. Improved drug loading/release capacities of commercial contact lenses obtained by supercritical fluid assisted molecular imprinting method. J. Control. Release. 148: e102–e104.

Buwalda, S.J., K.W.M. Boere, P.J. Dijkstra, J. Feijen, T. Vermonden and W.E. Hennink. 2014. Hydrogels in a historic perspective: from simple network to smart materials. J. Control. Release. 190: 254–273.

Byrne, M.E., K. Park and N.A. Peppas. 2002. Molecular imprinting within hydrogels. Adv. Drug Deliv. Rev. 54: 149–161.

Byrne, M.E. and V. Salian. 2008. Molecular imprinting within hydrogels II: progress and analysis of the field. Int. J. Pharm. 364: 188–212.

Byrne, M.E., J.Z. Hilt and N.A. Peppas. 2008. Recognitive biomimetic networks moiety imprinting for intelligent drug delivery. J. Biomed. Mater. Res. 84A: 137–147.

Byrne, M.E. and S. Venkatesh. 2012. Contact drug delivery systems. U.S. Patent Appl. # 2012/0087971 A1.

Byrne, M.E., S. Venkatesh, C. White and A. Maryam. 2013. Extended or continuous wear silicone hydrogel contact lenses for the extended release of comfort molecules. U.S. Patent Appl. # 2013/0195952 A1.

Calo, E. and V.V. Khutoryanskiy. 2015. Biomedical applications of hydrogels: a review of patents and commercial products. Eur. Polym. J. 65: 252–267.

Cirillo, G., F. Iemma, F. Puoci, O.I. Parisi, M. Curcio, U.G. Spizzirri et al. 2009. Imprinted hydrophilic nanospheres as drug delivery systems for 5-fluorouracil sustained release. J. Drug Target. 17: 72–77.

Cook, J.P., G.W. Goodall, V. Olga, O.V. Khutoryanskaya and V.V. Khutoryanskiy. 2012. Microwave-assisted hydrogel synthesis: a new method for crosslinking polymers in aqueous solutions. Macromol. Rapid Commun. 33: 332–336.

da Silva, M.S., R. Viveiros, P.I. Morgado, A. Aguiar-Ricardo, I.J. Correia and T. Casimiro. 2011. Development of 2-(dimethylamino)ethyl methacrylate-based molecular recognition devices for controlled drug delivery using supercritical fluid technology. Int. J. Pharm. 416: 61–68.

Dash, S., P.N. Murthy, L. Nath and P. Chowdhury. 2010. Kinetic modeling on drug release from controlled drug delivery systems. Acta Pol. Pharm. 67: 217–223.

Demchenko, A.P. 2001. Recognition between flexible protein molecules: induced and assisting folding. J. Mol. Recognit. 14: 42–61.

Ellwanger, A., C. Berggren, S. Bayoudh, C. Crecenzi, L. Karlsson, P.K. Owens et al. 2001. Evaluation of methods aimed at complete removal of template from molecularly imprinted polymers. Analyst. 126: 784–792.

Feynman, R.P. 1960. There's plenty of room at the bottom. Eng. Sci. 23: 22–36.

Hennink, W.E. and C.F. van Nostrum. 2012. Novel crosslinking methods to design hydrogels. Adv. Drug Deliv. Rev. 64: 223–236.

Hilt, J.Z. and M.E. Byrne. 2004. Configurational biomimesis in drug delivery: molecular imprinting of biologically significant molecules. Adv. Drug Deliv. Rev. 56: 1599–1620.

Hiratani, H. and C. Alvarez-Lorenzo. 2002. Timolol uptake and release by imprinted soft contact lenses made of N,N-diethylacrylamide and methacrylic acid. J. Control. Release. 83: 223–230.

Hiratani, H. and C. Alvarez-Lorenzo. 2004. The nature of backbone monomers determines the performance of imprinted soft contact lenses as timolol drug delivery system. Biomaterials. 25: 1105–1113.

Hiratani, H., Y. Mizutani and C. Alvarez-Lorenzo. 2005a. Controlling drug release from imprinted hydrogels by modifying the characteristics of the imprinted cavities. Macromol. Biosci. 5: 728–733.

Hiratani, H., A. Fujiwara, Y. Tamiya, Y. Mizutani and C. Alvarez-Lorenzo. 2005b. Ocular release of timolol from molecularly imprinted soft contact lenses. Biomaterials. 26: 1293–1298.

Hoare, T.R. and D.S. Kohane. 2008. Hydrogels in drug delivery: progress and challenges. Polymer. 49: 1993–2007.

Hoffman, A.S. 2012. Hydrogels for biomedical application. Adv. Drug Deliv. Rev. 64: 18–23.

Kirchhof, S., A.M. Goeperich and F.P. Brandl. 2015. Hydrogels in ophthalmic applications. Eur. J. Pharm. Biopharm. 95: 227–238.

Koetting, M.C., J.T. Peters, S.D. Steichen and N.A. Peppas. 2015. Stimuli-responsive hydrogels: theory, modern advances and applications. Mater. Sci. Eng. R 93: 1–49.

Koutsopoulos, S. 2012. Molecular fabrications of smart nanobiomaterials and applications in personalized medicine. Adv. Drug Deliv. Rev. 64: 1459–1476.

Lee, S.C., I.K. Kwon and K. Park. 2013. Hydrogels for delivery of bioactive agents: a historical perspective. Adv. Drug. Deliv. Rev. 65: 17–20.

Li, S., A. Tiwari, Y. Ge and D. Fei. 2010. A pH-responsive, low crosslinked, molecularly imprinted insulin delivery system. Adv. Mater. Lett. 1: 4–10.

Lorenzo, R.A., A.M. Carro, C. Alvarez-Lorenzo and A. Concheiro. 2011. To remove or not to remove? The challenge of extracting the template to make the cavities available in molecularly imprinted polymers (MIPs). Int. J. Mol. Sci. 12: 4327–4347.

Luliński, P. 2013. Molecularly imprinted polymers as the future drug delivery devices. Acta Pol. Pharm. 70: 601–609.

Malaekeh-Nikouei, B., F.A. Ghaeni, V.S. Motamedshariaty and S.A. Mohajeri. 2012. Controlled release of prednisolone acetate from molecularly imprinted hydrogel contact lenses. J. Appl. Polym. Sci. 126: 387–394.

Malakooti, N., C. Alexander and C. Alvarez-Lorenzo. 2015. Imprinted contact lenses for sustained release of polymyxin B and related antimicrobial peptides. J. Pharm. Sci. 104: 3386–3394.

Maryam, A., S. Horikawa, S. Venkatesh, J. Saha, J.W. Hong and M.E. Byrne. 2007. Zero order therapeutic release from imprinted hydrogel contact lenses within *in vitro* physiological ocular tear flow. J. Control. Release. 124: 154–162.

Maryam, A. and M.E. Byrne. 2013. Controlled and extended delivery of hyaluronic acid and comfort molecules *via* a contact lens platform. U.S. Patent # 8,388,995.

Nicholls, I.A., S. Chavan, K. Golker, B.C.G. Karlsson, G.D. Olsson, A.M. Rosengren et al. 2015. Theoretical and computational strategies for the study of the molecular imprinting process and polymer performance. pp. 25–50. *In*: Mattiasson, B. and L. Ye [eds.]. Molecularly Imprinted Polymers in Biotechnology. Springer, Berlin-Heidelberg, Germany.

Norell, M.C., H.S. Andersson and I.A. Nicholls. 1998. Theophilline molecularly imprinted polymer dissociation kinetics: a novel sustained release drug dosage mechanism. J. Mol. Recognit. 11: 98–102.

Peppas, N.A., P. Bures, W. Leobandung and H. Ichikawa. 2000. Hydrogels in pharmaceutical formulations. Eur. J. Pharm. Biopharm. 50: 27–46.

Puoci, F., G. Cirillo, M. Curcio, O.I. Parisi, F. Iemma and N. Picci. 2011. Molecularly imprinted polymers in drug delivery: state of art and future perspectives. Expert Opin. Drug Deliv. 8: 1379–1393.

Salian, V.D., A.D. Vaughan and M.E. Byrne. 2012. The role of living/controlled radical polymerization in the formation of improved imprinted polymers. J. Mol. Recognit. 25: 361–369.

Serra, L., J. Domenech and N.A. Peppas. 2006. Drug transport mechanism and release kinetics from molecularly imprinted designed poly(acrylic acid-*g*-ethylene glycol) hydrogels. Biomaterials. 27: 5440–5451.

Singh, B. and N. Chauhan. 2008. Preliminary evaluation of molecular imprinting of 5-fluorouracil within hydrogels for use as drug delivery systems. Acta Biomater. 4: 1244–1254.

Sreenivasan, K. 1999. On the application of molecularly imprinted poly(HEMA) as a template responsive release system. J. Appl. Pol. Sci. 71: 1819–1821.

Tieppo, A., K.M. Pate and M.E. Byrne. 2012. *In vitro* controlled release of an anti-inflammatory from daily disposable therapeutic contact lenses under physiological ocular tear flow. Eur. J. Pharm. Biopharm. 81: 170–177.

Ullah, F., M.B.H. Othman, F. Javed, Z. Ahmad and H.M. Akil. 2015. Classification, processing and application of hydrogels: a review. Mater. Sci. Eng. C 57: 414–433.

van Bemmelen, J.M. 1894. Das Hydrogel und das kristallinische Hydrat des Kupferoxyds. Z. Anorg. Chem. 5: 466–483.

Venkatesh, S., J. Saha, S. Pass and M.E. Byrne. 2008. Transport and structural analysis of molecularly imprinted hydrogels for controlled drug delivery. Eur. J. Pharm. Biopharm. 69: 852–860.

Wani, A.L. 2015. Personalized medicine: a near future or yet miles to go? Adv. Integr. Med. 2: 112–113.

Whitcombe, M.J., N. Kirsch and I.A. Nicholls. 2014. Molecular imprinting science and technology: a survey of the literature for the years 2004–2011. J. Mol. Recognit. 27: 297–401.

Wichterle, O. and D. Lim. 1960. Hydrophilic gels for biological use. Nature. 185: 117–118.

Wulff, G., A. Sarhan and K. Zabrocki. 1972. Über die Anwendung von enzymanalog gebauten polymeren zur racemattrennung. Angew. Chem. 84: 364–364.

Wulff, G. 1995. Molecular imprinting in cross-linked materials with the aid of molecular templates—a way towards artificial antibodies. Angew. Chem. Int. Ed. 34: 1812–1832.

Wulff, G. 2002. Enzyme-like catalysis by molecularly imprinted polymers. Chem. Rev. 102: 1–27.

Xinming, L., C. Yingde, A.W. Lloyd, S.V. Mikhalovsky, S.R. Sandeman, C.A. Howel et al. 2008. Polymeric hydrogels for novel contact lens-based ophthalmic drug delivery systems: a review. Cont. Lens Anterior Eye. 31: 57–64.

Yanez, F., A. Chauhan, A. Concheiro and C. Alvarez-Lorenzo. 2011a. Timolol-imprinted soft contact lenses: influence of the template: functional monomer ratio and the hydrogel thickness. J. Appl. Polym. Sci. 122: 1333–1340.

Yanez, F., L. Martikainen, M.E.M. Braga, C. Alvarez-Lorenzo, C. Concheiro, C.M.M. Duarte et al. 2011b. Supercritical fluid-assisted preparation of imprinted contact lenses for drug delivery. Acta Biomaterialia. 7: 1019–1030.

Zhang, Q., L. Zhang, P. Wang and S. Du. 2014. Coordinate bonding strategy for molecularly imprinted hydrogels: toward pH-responsive doxorubicin delivery. J. Pharm. Sci. 103: 643–651.

5

Prodrugs and Bioconjugate Hydrogels

A Valuable Strategy for the Prolonged-Delivery of Drugs

Ankit Jain,[2] *Anamika Sahu,*[3,a] *Aviral Jain*[3,b] and *Arvind Gulbake*[1,*]

ABSTRACT

Hydrogels have received considerable attention in recent years as one of the promising novel drug delivery systems and also for their role as scaffolds for cells, owing to their unique potentials. A number of crosslinking methods have been used for development of the hydrogel matrix structures which can be classified in two groups of chemically- and physically-induced crosslinking. Prodrug-based self-assembled hydrogels represent a novel class of active biomaterials, exploited for biomedical applications especially for stimuli responsive drug delivery devices. The prodrug-based self-assembled hydrogels show many advantages such as enhanced drug loading, controlled drug delivery, reduction of burst

[1] Centre for Interdisciplinary Research, D. Y. Patil University, Kolhapur - 416006 (M.S.) India.
[2] Pharmaceutics Research Laboratory, Department of Pharmaceutical Sciences, Dr. Hari Singh Gour Central University, Sagar (M.P.), India - 470 003.
   Email: ankitjainsagar@gmail.com
[3] Pharmaceutics Research Laboratory, Department of Pharmaceutics, Ravishankar College of Pharmacy, Bhopal (M.P.) 462010, India.
[a] Email: nmksahu@gmail.com
[b] Email: draviraljain@gmail.com
[*] Corresponding author: arvind.gulbake@gmail.com

release, and simultaneous delivery of multiple drugs. The performance of hydrogels can be enhanced by bioconjugation approach using proteins and peptides. Micro and nanofabrication techniques have been used to manipulate bioconjugated hydrogels for modulating cellular function and tissue morphogenesis. The aim of this chapter is to introduce a novel kind of biomaterial-molecular hydrogel especially prodrug and bioconjugated hydrogel for biomedical applications.

Keywords: hydrogel, prodrugs, bioconjugate

1. Introduction

The development of biodegradable polymers has evoked great interest for pharmaceutical, veterinary, agricultural, and environmental applications. Webster's Dictionary defines a biodegradable system as one capable of being broken down, especially into innocuous products by the action of living things (i.e., micro-organisms) (Kamath and Park 1993). However, for biomedical and pharmaceutical applications, the definition of biodegradation has to be broad enough to include all kinds of degradation occurring *in vivo* either by simple hydrolysis or by metabolic processes. Formulation scientists are regularly using these biodegradable polymers for drug delivery purpose, such as covalently cross-linked polymer nanoparticles, microparticles, self-assembled polymer micelles, supramolecular hydrogels, liposomes and dendrimers (Armentano et al. 2010, Concheiro and Alvarez-Lorenzo 2013, Larionova et al. 1999). There are lots of significant challenges that still remain in drug delivery technology, i.e., loading capacity, poor bioavailability as small molecules and biologics often suffer from low plasma half-life due to metabolism, poor cell permeability, and rapid systemic clearance. Hydrogels have received considerable attention in last decades as one of the prognosticating drug delivery systems owing to their unique potentials. In the early 1960s Wichterle and Lim developed a unique type of hydrophobic gel for biological uses (Wichterle and Lím 1960). Subsequently a large number of studies have been devoted to boosting and increasing the potential of hydrogels. The development of an ever-increasing scope of functional monomers and macromers continue to extend the versatility of hydrogel applications (Baker et al. 1984, Khutoryanskiy 2007, Misra and Siegel 2002, Ulbrich et al. 1995). Hydrogels can protect drugs from inimical environment, e.g., enzymes and low pH present in stomach and can also be formulated in various physical forms including nanoparticles, microparticles, slabs, coatings, and films (Alhaique et al. 2016, Oh et al. 2008, Sakthivel et al. 2016). It is utilized in clinical practice and experimental medicine, diagnostics, biosensors, cellular immobilization, tissue engineering and regenerative medicine, separation of biomolecules or cells and barrier materials to regulate biological adhesions (Calo and Khutoryanskiy 2015, Fleige et al. 2012, Koetting et al. 2015, Sivashanmugam et al. 2015).

Encapsulation of the active drug in an inert delivery system and control of drug activity through conversion into a stimuli responsive prodrug are the basic approach to reduce the systemic toxicity and increase the half-life of drugs. The cross-linked three dimensional polymeric networks having high number of hydrophilic groups or domains that can absorb large amount of water or biological fluid and spectacularly gain the volume are known as Hydrogels (Peppas et al. 2000). The prodrug-hydrogel transformation could be beneficial in three different ways, i.e., the bioactive become "self-deliverable" in the form of hydrogels, self-assembly of hydrogelators of bioactive might confer new and useful properties such as multivalency or high local densities and the exploration of molecular hydrogels of bioactive may ultimately lead to bioactive molecules that have dual or multiple roles (Chen et al. 2016, Wang et al. 2015). This chapter provides an overview of current research in the fields of hydrogels especially prodrug and bioconjugated hydrogels in the pharmaceutical and biomedical field, and their use as an intelligent carrier for prolonged and controlled drug delivery techniques.

2. Classification of Hydrogels

The hydrogel can be classified on different basses, i.e., origin of polymer, polymeric composition, configuration, type of cross linking, physical appearance and network electric charge (Fig. 1). It can also be classified on the basis of source: Natural and Synthetic. Polymeric composition is another way to classify, i.e., homopolymeric, copolymeric and multipolymer interpenetrating polymeric hydrogel (IPN). Classification based on configuration (physical, structural, chemical composition): (a) amorphous, semicrystalline and crystalline. Based on physical appearance, hydrogel can be divided as matrix, film, microsphere or nanogel, depending on the technique of polymerization involved in the preparation process. The network electrical charges located on the cross-linked chains give different classification: ionic, nonionic, amphoteric electrolyte and zwitterionic (polybetaines). Chemical and physical cross linking is another way of hydrogels classification. The hydrogels used for pharmaceutical applications can be classified on the basis of route of administration: oral hydrogels, topical, transdermal and implantable hydrogels, hydrogel devices for gastrointestinal (GI) drug delivery and ocular hydrogels (Montoro et al. 2014, Peppas and Sahlin 1996, Ullah et al. 2015).

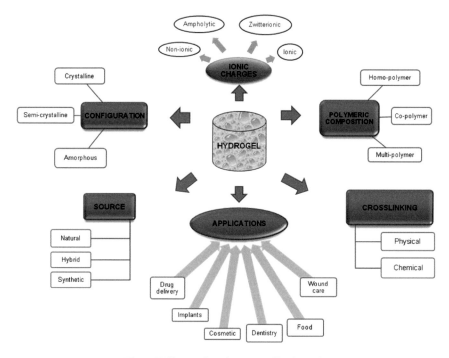

Fig. 1. Different classifications of hydrogels.

3. Chemical and Physical Gels

The preparation of hydrogel basically depends on the cross linking of polymers (Fig. 2) which is either physical (e.g., ionic interaction, crystallization) or chemical (e.g., chemical reaction, radical polymerization, enzyme induced) (Hamidi et al. 2008). In the last few decades, many advances in the development of novel hydrogels for drug delivery applications have focused on several aspects related to synthesis, characterization and behaviour.

Covalent or chemical cross linking hydrogel is achieved by chemical reaction, radical polymerization, and enzyme induction. It is permanent and irreversible as a result of configurational changes. Approaches: (a) simultaneous polymerization crosslinking (b) post-crosslinking.

Non-covalent or physical cross linking hydrogel is achieved by—ionic interaction, crystallization, association, aggregation, complexation, and hydrogen bonding. It is reversible due to the conformational changes. Approaches: (a) ion–polymer complexation (b) polymer–polymer complexation (c) hydrophobic association (d) chain aggregation and (e) hydrogen bonding (Alvarez-Lorenzo et al. 2013, Concheiro and Alvarez-Lorenzo, Montoro et al., Ullah et al.).

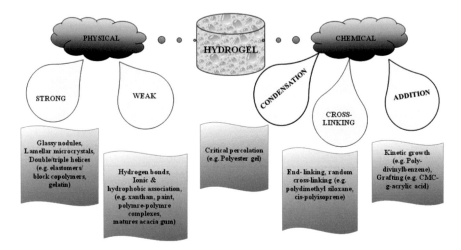

Fig. 2. Cross linking methods for hydrogels.

4. Prodrug-Based Hydrogel

Formulation scientists have done a lot of research to reduce the systemic toxicity and increase the half-life of the drugs, and have developed several approaches, including physical drug loading in an inert carrier and control of drug activity by prodrug approach. Prodrugs are usually pharmacologically inert form of the parent drug (active drug) and require a stimulus (i.e., pH, temperature, enzyme, microbes, etc.) to be transformed into its active form. Bioactive or drug can be loaded into pre-formed gels or mixed during the self-assembly process without causing detrimental effects to their structure (Cohn and Younes 1988). Prodrug-based self-assembled hydrogels signify a new class of active biomaterials that can be used for biomedical applications, specifically the design of stimuli responsive drug delivery systems (Akiyoshi et al. 1998, Nemani et al. 2015). A promoiety or polymer is chemically conjugated with a drug molecule to generate an amphiphilic prodrug and develop prodrug based self assembled hydrogel. It has various advantages namely, altered solubility, enhanced drug loading, eliminates the use of harmful excipients and can be designed to undergo controlled drug release. The development of prodrug based self-assembled hydrogels as an emerging class of biomaterials could overcome several common limitations encountered in conventional drug delivery systems (CalÃ³ and Khutoryanskiy, Koetting et al., Saboktakin and Tabatabaei 2015). A huge number of work related to prodrug hydrogel approaches has been carried out by formulation scientists, discussed in next sections in stimuli responsive hydrogels of the chapter.

5. Bioconjugated Hydrogels

A covalent coupling of two or more distinct biological molecules to attain a specific functionality is known as bioconjugation, which could be utilized to obtain reliable, controllable, and functional combinations of various biomolecules for extensive biomedical applications (Jensen et al. 2015). Hydrogels played a vital role as scaffolds for cells, as carriers for various bioactives (e.g., drugs, genes, and soluble factors), and as injectable biomaterials in tissue engineering and regenerative medicine (Anjum et al. 2016, Kamath and Park 1993, Nguyen et al. 2015). The performance of hydrogels using cell-responsive components, such as proteins and peptides, which have high affinity to regulate cellular behaviours and tissue morphogenesis, is known as bioconjugation hydrogels approach. Microparticulate and nanoparticulate techniques have been utilized to manipulate bioconjugated hydrogels to regulate cell functioning (Kapoor and Kundu 2016, Sivashanmugam et al. 2015). Biomolecules can be conjugated to hydrogels and produce a cell-responsive matrix and has been discussed in next section.

6. Biomedical Applications of Stimuli-Responsive Hydrogels

Stimuli responsive hydrogels (SRHs), so called 'Intelligent' or 'Smart' hydrogels, are reported to cover a number of applications based on the most common stimuli in the body, i.e., low pH and elevated temperature in inflammatory conditions or at intracellular site (Fleige et al. 2012, Jain and Jain 2015c). These anomalous characteristics offer targeted controlled drug delivery (Jain et al. 2013a). Chemical stimuli like glucose or antigens have also been employed as biosensors and triggers for drug delivery to a specific site. Moreover, physical stimuli such as light, pressure and electric current have also been used to facilitate drug delivery (Jain and Jain 2016). SRHs can provide protection to the drug from hostile gastric milieu, i.e., enzymes and low pH (Jain and Jain 2015a). They possess potential to control drug release by means of transforming gel structure with reversible volume phase transitions or gel–sol phase transitions in response to external stimulus lasting for few minutes (Jain and Jain 2015b). SRHs can be suitable candidates to devise self-regulated systems for drug delivery provided they should be biocompatible and biodegradable in nature (Perche et al. 2015). Figure 3 represents schematic picture showing stimuli responsive behaviour of SRH. Figure 4 depicts various regions in polymer chains responsible for stimuli responsiveness in SRH. Different types of SRHs are discussed under separate subheadings.

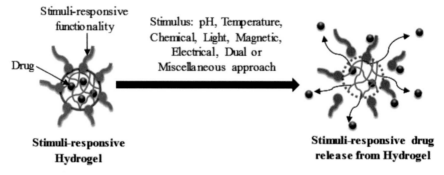

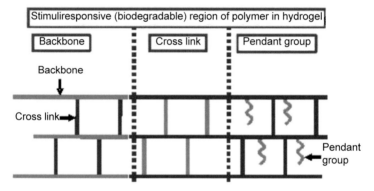

Fig. 3. Schematic picture showing stimuli responsive behaviour of SRH.

Fig. 4. Various regions in polymer chains responsible for stimuli responsiveness in SRH.

6.1 Thermo-responsive hydrogels

Thermo-responsive hydrogels (TRHs) are one of the most exploited SRHs in drug delivery (Drapala et al. 2014, Qiu and Park 2012). Phase transition characteristics in different polymers provide thermo-responsiveness owing to presence of hydrophobic groups like methyl, ethyl and propyl groups. Most exploited exemplary polymer in this category is Poly(N,N-diethylacrylamide) (PDEAAm). Other polymers and copolymers include Poly(N,N-diethylacrylamide (PDEAAm) and butyl methacrylate (BMA). PEO–PPO block copolymers are used to render thermosensitivity, e.g., Pluronics® (or Poloxamers®) and Tetronics® (Bae et al. 1987, Jain and Jain 2015b, Qiu and Park 2012).

Polymers with LCST, however, decrease their water-solubility as the temperature increases. Hydrogels made of LCST polymers shrink as the temperature increases above the LCST, so it is called inverse (or negative) temperature-dependent swelling. In such cases, the hydrogels are made of polymer chains with reasonable hydrophobic groups or having a mixture of hydrophilic and hydrophobic groups (Censi et al. 2015, Klouda 2015). The LCST can be modulated by changing the ratio of hydrophilic and hydrophobic segment of the polymer, e.g., use of copolymers made of hydrophobic (e.g., NIPAM) and hydrophilic (e.g., acrylic acid) monomers (Irie 1993, Wei et al. 2009). Various copolymers are reported with NIPAM resulting in temperature-sensitive hydrogels and thermally reversible gels. The hydrogel underwent temperature-induced collapse due to the cooperative conformational transition. Thermo-sensitive hydrogels have been widely explored owing to their unique applications (Jeong et al. 2002, Lin and Metters 2006, Ruel-Gariepy and Leroux 2004, Zhang and Zhuo 2000). These hydrogels are broadly categorized as negatively thermosensitive, positively thermosensitive, and thermally reversible gels. In a controlled manner, thermo-responsive "On–Off" drug release profile can be obtained using monolithic hydrogels which generally include crosslinked P(NIPAAm–co-BMA) hydrogels (Bae et al. 1991, He et al. 2008, Yoshida et al. 1994), and interpenetrating polymer networks (IPNs) of P(NIPAAm) and poly(tetramethyleneether glycol) (PTMEG). Thermo-responsive hydrogels can be placed inside a rigid capsule having perforations or orifice to obtain on–off release profile (squeezing hydrogel) upon reversible volume change (Fig. 5) (Gutowska et al. 1997). Similarly, NIPAM hydrogel microparticles can be dispersed in a gelatin matrix to provide micro-channels for drug release or a reservoir type microcapsule bearing hydrogel nanoparticles have also been reported (Ichikawa and Fukumori 2000). Some IPN based hydrogels reveals swelling at high temperature and shrinking at low temperature, e.g., IPNs of poly(acrylic acid) and polyacrylamide (PAAm) or P(AAm–co-BMA) (Katono et al. 1991, Owens et al. 2007).

The thermoreversible gels which are commonly used include Pluronics® and Tetronics®. Poly(L-lactic acid) is generally used to enhance

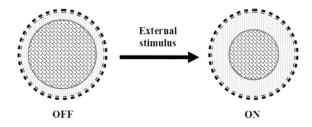

Fig. 5. Schematic showing of "On–Off" release.

the biodegradability of the co-polymer (Jeong et al. 2000, Yu and Ding 2008). Clinical applications of thermosensitive NIPAM based hydrogels are limited because of issues with biocompatibility and biodegradability (Hoare and Kohane 2008). To overcome this problem, it is the need of the time to explore copolymers like PEO–PLA block copolymers for developing thermoreversible hydrogels (Agrawal et al. 2006, Cohn and Younes 1988).

6.2 pH-responsive hydrogels

The polymers having number of ionizable groups are called as polyelectrolytes. pH-responsive polymers respond to pH changes in surrounding because of presence of pendant acidic groups (e.g., carboxylic and sulfonic acids) that release protons or basic (e.g., ammonium salts) groups that accept protons. For example, poly(acrylic acid) (PAA) becomes ionized at high pH as it is polyanionic and dissolves more at high pH while poly(N,N'-diethylaminoethyl methacrylate) (PDEAEM) gets ionized at low pH as it polycationic and dissolves more at this pH (Yang et al. 2005). This pH-responsive behaviour of polyelectrolytes renders hydrogels a dynamic capability to swell and respond to desired conditions. This swelling in polyelectrolyte hydrogels is accounted to the electrostatic repulsion among similar charges present over the polymer chain and the extent of swelling is affected by any factor (like pH, ionic strength, and type of counter ions) that influences this repulsion (Firestone and Siegel 1991). For instance, the swelling and pH-responsiveness in such cases can be controlled by employing neutral comonomers that renders hydrophobicity to the polymer chain, e.g., 2-hydroxyethyl methacrylate, methyl methacrylate and maleic anhydride (Brannon-Peppas and Peppas 1990, Falamarzian and Varshosaz 1998).

pH-responsive hydrogels are widely explored for oral drug delivery owing to large variation in pH of gastrointestinal tract (Karim et al. 2016). Polycationic hydrogels showed minimal swelling at neutral pH avoiding release of bitter taste drugs in the mouth and more swelling at gastric acidic milieu leading to local delivery of drugs like antibiotics (Risbud et al. 2000, Siegel et al. 1988). On the other hand, PAA or PMA based polyanions hydrogels can release drugs at neutral pH conditions (Brannon-Peppas and Peppas 1990). Such hydrogels when crosslinked with azoaromatic crosslinkers have been prepared for colon-specific drug delivery as they swell very less in the stomach but swelling increases upon passing down to intestinal region because of ionization of the carboxylic groups with increasing pH. Moreover, the azoaromatic cross-links are degraded by azoreductase enzyme found in the colon resulting in more pronounced drug release in that region. In this way, the kinetics of hydrogel swelling can be regulated by controlling the polymer composition (Chourasia and

Jain 2003, Ghandehari et al. 1997, Subudhi et al. 2015). pH-responsive hydrogels can also be placed inside capsules or silicone matrices to regulate the release kinetics (Carelli et al. 1999). When poly(ethylene glycol) (PEG) is grafted to poly(methacrylic acid) (PMA) the resulting hydrogels show dual characteristics in pH-responsiveness. At low pH, hydrogen bonding occurs between the acidic protons of the carboxyl groups of PMA and the ether oxygen of PEG leading to complexation followed by shrinkage of the hydrogels, whereas at high pH, the carboxyl groups of PMA get ionized and results in swelling of the hydrogels because of decomplexation (Peppas and Klier 1991, Serra et al. 2006). Similar fundamentals are also applied to IPN systems in which two different types of polymer chain interact by means of pH-dependent hydrogen bonding. The major issue with synthetic pH-sensitive polymers is of non-biodegradability and it poses the problem of elimination from the body after use as in the case of implants. Therefore, great attention has been paid to develop biodegradable, pH-responsive hydrogels based on polypeptides, proteins and polysaccharides. Synthetic polypeptides with biodegradability have also been used to prepare hydrogels, e.g., poly(hydroxyl-L-glutamate), poly(L-ornithine), poly(aspartic acid), poly(L-lysine) and poly(L-glutamic acid). The pH-responsive swelling can be controlled by varying hydrophobicity and degree of ionization of polypeptide (Jeong and Gutowska 2002, Markland et al. 1999, Rodríguez-Hernández and Lecommandoux 2005).

6.3 Glucose-responsive hydrogels (GRHs)

One of the most challenging problems in controlled drug delivery area is the development of self-regulated (modulated) insulin delivery systems. Delivery of insulin is different from delivery of other drugs, since insulin has to be delivered in an exact amount at the exact time of need. Thus, self-regulated insulin delivery systems require the glucose sensing ability and an automatic shut-off mechanism. Many hydrogel systems have been developed for modulating insulin delivery, and all of them have a glucose sensor built into the system. Glucose oxidase (GOX) oxidizes glucose to gluconic acid that lowers the pH of the environment resulting in the collapse of chain upon protonation of the carboxyl groups of the polymer. Consequently, the pores get open to allow diffusion of insulin. This concept offers the modulated delivery of insulin (Ehrick et al. 2009, Ito et al. 1989). Similarly, Concanavalin A (Con A, a glucose-binding protein) has also been reported for the modulated delivery of insulin, e.g., the glycosylated insulin-Con A system by means of competitive binding of Con A with glucose and glycosylated insulin. In another approach, glucose responsive reversible sol-gel based hydrogels have also been developed using glucose—Con A crosslinks (non-covalent). Free glucose molecules after diffusing into the hydrogel from external medium compete with the polymer-attached glucose molecules and are exchanged with them (Han et al. 2002, Kim and Park 2001, Obaidat and Park 1996). Table 1 summarizes various types of GRHs.

Although a number of glucose-responsive insulin delivery systems have been developed, there are still some drawbacks to implement them at clinical level viz. slow response to change in glucose concentration of environment, insufficient reversibility to original position changing glucose concentration and an issue to reduce size of the hydrogel to keep reproducibility of results. Moreover, biocompatible and biodegradable characteristics of polymer are also of due consideration to avoid undesirable immune response (Kost and Langer 2012).

Table 1. Various types of GRHs.

Type of GRHs	Examples	Reference
pH-sensitive membrane systems	Hydrogel of polycations like PDEAEM swells at lower pH which is caused by gluconic acid leading more release of insulin.	(Ishihara et al. 1984)
	Insulin loaded hydrogel matrix collapsed (or shrunken) in response to lowering pH leading to release of insulin in as 'squeezing' pattern.	(Hassan et al. 1997)
Con A-immobilized systems	Different glycosylated insulins with varying binding affinities to Con A have been prepared to facilitate insulin release at different glucose levels in a controlled manner.	(Makino et al. 1991, Seminoff et al. 1989)
Sol–gel phase reversible hydrogel systems	Glucose responsive controlled release of insulin has been studied with different polymer systems, e.g., poly(glucosyloxye thylmethacrylate)–Con A complexes and polysaccharide, e.g., polysucrose, dextran, glycogen)–Con A gel membranes.	(Nakamae et al. 1995, Taylor et al. 1995)
	Glucose-responsive-reversible hydrogels lacking Con A have also been reported with polymers having phenylboronic groups, e.g., poly[3-(acrylamido) phenylboronic acid] and its copolymers and polyol polymers (e.g., PVA). Glucose, having pendant hydroxyl groups, competes with polyol polymers for the borate cross-linkages.	(Hisamitsu et al. 1997)

6.4 *Miscellaneous approaches*

Stimuli responsive hydrogels are widely explored using various stimuli. Apart from aforementioned approaches, there are number approaches which involve stimulus such as electric-signal, light, pressure, etc. (Bawa et al. 2009, Lee et al. 1990). Electric current can also be used as an environmental signal to induce responses of hydrogels. Hydrogels sensitive to electric current are usually made of polyelectrolytes, as are pH-sensitive hydrogels. Electro-sensitive hydrogels undergo shrinking or swelling in the presence of an applied electric field. Sometimes, the hydrogels show swelling on one side and deswelling on the other side, resulting in bending of the hydrogels. The hydrogel shape change (including swelling, shrinking and bending) depends on a number of conditions (Li Hua et al. 2004, Qiu and Park 2012). Table 2 discusses miscellaneous approaches of stimuli-responsive hydrogels.

Stimuli-responsive hydrogels cover an area of biomedical applications based on various stimuli *viz.* pH and temperatures, etc. The most widely explored hydrogels belong to thermo-responsive or pH-responsive category for site-specific controlled or modulated drug delivery. Other stimuli include glucose, antigen, light, pressure and electric signal which are well discussed above. However, significant improvements are needed in the hydrogels such as fast-response to stimulus, biocompatibility and biodegradability with use of newer or modified polymers and cross-linkers for a wide array of applications including drug delivery (Roy et al. 2010, Stuart et al. 2010, Weber et al. 2009).

7. Applications and Advances in Hydrogels

Bioconjugate hydrogel based nanocarriers (BHNs) have shown promising outcomes in drug delivery because of multipronged features of both hydrogel system (i.e., hydrophilic nature and large water content) and nanosized carrier. There are number of polymeric bioconjugate hydrogels that have been developed using natural (e.g., chitosan and alginate) and synthetic polymers (e.g., poly(vinyl alcohol), poly(ethylene oxide), poly(ethyleneimine), poly(vinyl pyrrolidone), and poly-N-isopropylacrylamide). These BHNs show complex release mechanism depending upon drug diffusion, hydrogel matrix swelling, and chemical reactivity of the drug/matrix (Omidian et al. 2007, Ulbrich et al. 1995). Emerging hydrogel technology has documented an arena of pharmaceutical and biomedical applications (Kashyap et al. 2005, Venkatesh et al. 2005). The pharmaceutical hydrogels are intended

Table 2. Miscellaneous approaches of stimuli-responsive hydrogels.

	Properties of electro-sensitive hydrogels	Applications	Limitations and improvements	Ref.
Electric signal-sensitive hydrogels	Upon a small change in electric potential across partially hydrolyzed polyacrylamide hydrogels, these undergo volume collapse because of forced migration of counter ions leading to loss of water. 'On–Off' based modulated drug delivery using hydrogel (in water without any salts) under the influence of the electric field show shrinkage (electroosmosis and electrophoresis) of the hydrogel.	Microparticles of PAA hydrogel showed 'on–off' release profiles under the effects of the electric field. Such pulsatile delivery has been reported for hydrocortisone and insulin using different polymers and copolymers.	It is easy to control the release rate in electrical influence but requires a controllable voltage source. Moreover, most of these hydrogels work in the absence of electrolytes that poses a hurdle to develop a suitable drug delivery device to function under physiological conditions.	(Li et al. 2004, Tanaka et al. 1982)
Light-sensitive hydrogels	Light-sensitive hydrogels are categorized into UV-sensitive and visible light-sensitive hydrogels. The UV-sensitive hydrogels can be prepared using bis(4-dimethylamino)phenylmethyl leucocyanide and triphenylmethane leuco derivatives comprised polymer network. The swelling in response to UV light accounts for an increase in osmotic pressure because of ions generated upon UV irradiation. Similarly, visible light-sensitive hydrogels are prepared using a light-sensitive chromophore, e.g., trisodium salt of copper chlorophyllin along with poly(N-isopropylacrylamide). The local increase in temperature increase swelling in poly(N-isopropylacrylamide) hydrogels in which increase in temperature is proportional	Light-sensitive hydrogels are used in photo-responsive artificial muscles, switches and memory devices. These are of great importance in temporal drug delivery.	They respond slowly even if the light is instantaneous and offers thermal energy to restructure the polymer chains. There are chances of leaching of chromophores if not attached covalently during swelling–deswelling process.	(Charati et al. 2010, Suzuki et al. 1996, Yui et al. 1993)

Light-sensitive hydrogels	to the light intensity and the chromophore concentration. If PAA is added to the light-sensitive hydrogels then it imparts pH sensitivity to the hydrogels.			
Pressure-sensitive hydrogels	In these hydrogels, pressure-induced volume phase transition which involves collapse at low pressure and expand at higher pressure. The pressure sensitivity of the temperature-sensitive gels was due to an increase in their LCST value with pressure.	Polymers such as poly(N-isopropylacrylamide), poly(N-n-propylacrylamide), poly(N,N-diethylacrylamide) and poly(N-isopropylacrylamide) based hydrogels are used in various sensor and drug delivery applications.	They also possess drawback of slow responding behaviour and demands great care to control stimuli-responsiveness.	(Feldstein et al. 2014, Garg et al. 2013, Zhong et al. 1996)
Specific ion-sensitive hydrogels	Nonionic NIPAM hydrogel responds to sodium chloride with volume phase transition [118]. The collapse is found to be dependent on water content of hydrogel, sodium chloride concentration and temperature. LCST of the hydrogel is reported to get lowered by increasing the chloride concentration.	Such type of hydrogels find applications in chloride ion-sensitive biosensors and modulated drug delivery [119].	A large hysteresis occurs in this transition. Other salts are not found to begin collapse phenomenon that follows an ion pair and multiplet theory.	
Specific antigen-responsive hydrogels	Sol–gel phase-reversible hydrogels which involved antigen–antibody interactions have been developed. Triggered swelling in response to free antigens occurs with a competition to the polymer-bound antigen resulting in decrease of the crosslinking density.	Semi-IPN hydrogel with grafted antigen directed to specific antibody has been reported in biotech applications.	Safety concerns are needed to resolve in these systems.	(Lu et al. 2015, Miyata et al. 1999)

to improve bioavailability in case of nasal and vaginal routes (D'Cruz and Uckun 2001, Wu et al. 2007). Recently, hydrogel nanoparticles (NPs) which are also called Nanogels™ are being explored for improved drug delivery potential in terms of better hydrophilicity, flexibility, versatility, high water absorptivity, biocompatibility and flexibility of chemical modifications for targeting the specific sites (Oh et al. 2008). Chitosan being water-soluble and cationic charged can interact with polyanions in aqueous medium. Mucoadhesive property in chitosan offers applications to open tight junctions between epithelial cells of different parts of the body. These amiable properties of chitosan, chitosan hydrogel NPs have been developed by different methods such as ionotropic gelation, precipitation, emulsion-droplet coalescence method, reverse micellization, and emulsion polymerization method (Jain and Jain 2013, Jain et al. 2013b). Alginic acid is an anionic biopolymer that shows good aqueous solubility, gelation capacity, biocompatibility, and low bio-toxicity (Jain and Bar-Shalom 2014). Different methods of preparation are reported to control the gelification process to obtain required size ranges with considerations of affecting factors such as alginate concentration/viscosity, and counter-ion concentration, etc. Similarly, PVA hydrogel NPs have been developed to deliver protein/peptide using a w/o emulsion/cyclic freezing–thawing method (Li Jia Kui et al. 1998). Other methods for PVA hydrogel NPs include salting-out, emulsification diffusion, and nanoprecipitation for the delivery of ibuprofen (Galindo-Rodríguez et al. 2005). Such polymeric nanogels show great promise in various biomedical applications. For instance, temperature-sensitive N-isopropylacrylamide hydrogels crosslinked with ethylene glycol dimethacrylate, tetraethylene glycol dimethacrylate, and poly(ethylene glycol) 400 dimethacrylate (PEG400DMA) were developed using UV free radical polymerization method. Iron oxide magnetic NPs were incorporated into this system to study the thermoresponsive behaviour of the developed hydrogels. Poly(methacrylic acid-grafted-poly(ethylene glycol)) (P(MA-g-PEG)) hydrogel NPs were prepared by a thermally-initiated free radical polymerization method (Deng et al. 2007, Yanfeng and Min 2001). These hydrogel NPs showed pH-responsive swelling which was found to be influenced by concentration of crosslinker. Table 3 summarizes applications of different polymeric Nano-hydrogels.

8. Conclusion

While the prodrug-based self-assembled hydrogels showed distinct advantages, i.e., maximum drug loading, controlled drug release, minimum burst release, and multiple drugs delivery, some limitations remain, i.e., weak mechanical properties, which limit the use of these materials in tissue engineering. Recent developments of hydrogels as prodrug and

Table 3. Applications of different polymeric Nano-hydrogels.

Polymer	NP type in hydrogel	Remarks	Reference
Chitosan	Unmodified NPs	These NP hydrogels have found applications in various bioactive entrapment/encapsulation. Chitosan based NP hydrogels have also been exploited in the delivery of macromolecular compounds such as peptides, proteins, antigens, oligonucleotides, and genes.	(Bhattarai et al. 2010, Fan et al. 2006, Pandey et al. 2005)
	NPs with covalent crosslinks	For example, w/o emulsion method with glutaraldehyde crosslinking for preparation of nanospheres has been reported for 5-fluorouracil (5-FU) delivery.	(Liu et al. 2007)
	NPs with ionic crosslinks	Chitosan NPs hydrogel system was developed using ionotropic gelation method with the use of tripolyphosphate (TPP) for encapsulation of insulin and other drugs. Hydrogel NPs showed improved oral bioavailability of peptide and proteins, and better bioadhesion with intestinal mucosa.	(Dung et al. 2007)
	NPs prepared by desolvation method	Controlled delivery of antineoplastic proteoglycans for immunostimulation was studied with these hydrogel NPs. These hydrogel NPs were also found effective in protecting plasmid DNA from nuclease degradation.	(Bhattarai et al. 2010, Ray et al. 1999)
	NPs prepared by emulsion-droplet coalescence method	Gadopentetic acid-loaded chitosan hydrogel NPs were developed using 100% deacetylated chitosan. These showed improved drug loading efficiency of around 45%.	(Tokumitsu et al. 1999)
	NPs prepared by reverse micellar method	Using this technique, doxorubicin-dextran conjugate was entrapped within chitosan hydrogel NPs. These hydrogel NPs showed controlled delivery of conjugate and improved efficacy of drug.	(Mitra et al. 2001)

Table 3 contd. ...

...Table 3 contd.

Polymer	NP type in hydrogel	Remarks	Reference
	NPs prepared by self-assembly *via* chemical modification	Palmitic acid tethered glycol chitosan nanovesicles loaded with bleomycin showed good biocompatibility, and serum stability in serum. Chitosan conjugated with deoxycholic acid self-assembled and associated with DNA for gene delivery using this method.	(Mao et al. 2010, UCHEGBU et al. 1998)
Alginate	Alginate-based hydrogel NPs	Alginate-based hydrogel NPs have been used to deliver insulin, antitubercular and antifungal drugs, etc. Anti-tubercular drugs *viz.* isoniazid, rifampin, pyrazinamide, and ethambutol were studied for their pharmacokinetic parameters after encapsulating in hydrogel NPs and there was improved bioavailability of drugs in case of hydrogel NPs as compared to free drugs.	(Rajaonarivony et al. 1993, Reis et al. 2007)
Poly(vinyl alcohol)	Poly(vinyl alcohol)-based hydrogel NPs	Poly(lactone) chains grafted PVA and charge-modified sulfobutyl-PVA were synthesized to improve water solubility and they self-assemble to produce hydrogel NPs which were used to deliver proteins like human serum albumin, tetanus toxoid and cytochrom C. Paclitaxel was loaded in PVA-g-PLGA hydrogel NPs for the treatment of restenosis and showed better therapeutic effects as compared to free drug.	(Soppimath et al. 2001, Westedt et al. 2007)
Poly(ethylene oxide) and poly(ethyleneimine)	Poly(ethylene oxide) and poly(ethyleneimine)-based hydrogel NPs	Networks of crosslinked poly(ethylene oxide) (PEO), poly(ethyleneimine) (PEI), and PEO-cl-PEI were used to developed hydrogel NPs bearing oligonucleotides. These systems were also found capable to immobilize anionic drugs such as retinoic acid and indomethacin.	(Bronich et al. 2001)
Poly(vinyl pyrrolidone), PVP	PVP-based hydrogel NPs	PVP hydrogel magnetic nanospheres enhanced therapeutic efficacy because of magnetically guided chemotherapeutic drug delivery.	(Guowei et al. 2007)

Poly-N-isopropylacrylamide (NIPAM)	PNIPAM-based hydrogel NPs	PNIPAM-co-allylamine NP networks and PNIPAM-co-acrylic acid NP networks are formed by covalent crosslinking. These thermoresponsive core-shell PNIPAM NPs were studied for phase transition and thermodynamic behaviour.	(Elsaeed et al. 2012)
Pullulan	Pullulan-based hydrogel NPs	Self-assembled hydrogel NPs of cholesterol-pullulan were complexed with insulin and these hydrogel NPs decreased thermal denaturation/aggregation of insulin. These hydrogels also enhanced the delivery of nucleic acid and plasmids.	(Akiyoshi et al. 1998, Gupta and Gupta 2004)
Dextran and PEG	Self-assembled dextran-PEG nanogels	These nanogels were prepared using glycidyl methacrylate dextran (GMD) and dimethyl methacrylate poly(ethylene glycol) (DMP) *via* radical polymerization for effective delivery of doxorubicin.	(Chacko et al. 2012, Missirlis et al. 2006)

bioconjugations for biological and biomedical applications were reviewed in this chapter. A huge number of bioactives or biomolecules including drugs, proteins, short peptides, polysaccharides, antibodies, and DNA molecules have been conjugated with hydrogels for therapeutic, diagnostic, controlling cell survival, adhesion, matrix degradation and organization, migration, differentiation, and apoptosis. The recent studies clearly demonstrate that bioactive and biomolecules maintain their therapeutic activity after conjugation with hydrogel, so the future research objectives should be focused on the unsolved issues such as synergistic effect of conjugating several biomolecules to a hydrogel on cell function, study the bioconjugated hydrogels *in vivo* in animal models and human clinical trials. Researchers need to enlighten the specific interactions of bioactive or biomolecules with cellular integral receptors and should design novel hydrogels to present these proteins or antibodies on the surface of the novel hydrogels for site specific targeting. In similar fashion, deliberate control over stability, size, biodegradability, and functionality for bioconjugation will manoeuvre the design of the next generation of novel hydrogels.

References

Agrawal, S.K., N. Sanabria-DeLong, J.M. Coburn, G.N. Tew and S.R. Bhatia. 2006. Novel drug release profiles from micellar solutions of PLA–PEO–PLA triblock copolymers. Journal of Controlled Release. 112: 64–71.

Akiyoshi, K., S. Kobayashi, S. Shichibe, D. Mix, M. Baudys, S.W. Kim et al. 1998. Self-assembled hydrogel nanoparticle of cholesterol-bearing pullulan as a carrier of protein drugs: complexation and stabilization of insulin. Journal of Controlled Release. 54: 313–320.

Alhaique, F., M.A. Casadei, C. Cencetti, T. Coviello, C. Di Meo, P. Matricardi et al. 2016. From macro to nano polysaccharide hydrogels: An opportunity for the delivery of drugs. Journal of Drug Delivery Science and Technology.

Alvarez-Lorenzo, C., B. Blanco-Fernandez, A.M. Puga and A. Concheiro. 2013. Crosslinked ionic polysaccharides for stimuli-sensitive drug delivery. Advanced Drug Delivery Reviews. 65: 1148–1171.

Anjum, F., P.S. Lienemann, S. Metzger, J. Biernaskie, M.S. Kallos and M. Ehrbar. 2016. Enzyme responsive GAG-based natural-synthetic hybrid hydrogel for tunable growth factor delivery and stem cell differentiation. Biomaterials. 87: 104–117.

Armentano, I., M. Dottori, E. Fortunati, S. Mattioli and J.M. Kenny. 2010. Biodegradable polymer matrix nanocomposites for tissue engineering: A review. Polymer Degradation and Stability. 95: 2126–2146.

Bae, Y.H., T. Okano, R. Hsu and S.W. Kim. 1987. Thermo-sensitive polymers as on-off switches for drug release. Die Makromolekulare Chemie, Rapid Communications. 8: 481–485.

Bae, Y.H., T. Okano and S.W. Kim. 1991. "On–Off" thermocontrol of solute transport. I. Temperature dependence of swelling of N-isopropylacrylamide networks modified with hydrophobic components in water. Pharmaceutical Research. 8: 531–537.

Baker, R., M. Tuttle and R. Helwing. 1984. Novel erodible polymers for the delivery of macromolecules. Pharm. Technol. 8: 26–28.

Bawa, P., V. Pillay, Y.E. Choonara and L.C. du Toit. 2009. Stimuli-responsive polymers and their applications in drug delivery. Biomedical Materials. 4: 022001.

Bhattarai, N., J. Gunn and M. Zhang. 2010. Chitosan-based hydrogels for controlled, localized drug delivery. Advanced Drug Delivery Reviews. 62: 83–99.

Brannon-Peppas, L. and N.A. Peppas. 1990. Dynamic and equilibrium swelling behaviour of pH-sensitive hydrogels containing 2-hydroxyethyl methacrylate. Biomaterials. 11: 635–644.

Bronich, T.K., S.V. Vinogradov and A.V. Kabanov. 2001. Interaction of nanosized copolymer networks with oppositely charged amphiphilic molecules. Nano Letters. 1: 535–540.

Caló, E. and V.V. Khutoryanskiy. 2015. Biomedical applications of hydrogels: A review of patents and commercial products. European Polymer Journal. 65: 252–267.

Carelli, V., S. Coltelli, G. Di Colo, E. Nannipieri and M. Serafini. 1999. Silicone microspheres for pH-controlled gastrointestinal drug delivery. International Journal of Pharmaceutics. 179: 73–83.

Censi, R., A. Dubbini and P.D. Martino. 2015. *In situ* Gelling Thermosensitive Hydrogels for Protein Delivery Applications. Handbook of Polymers for Pharmaceutical Technologies: Processing and Applications, Volume 2: 95–120.

Chacko, R.T., J. Ventura, J. Zhuang and S. Thayumanavan. 2012. Polymer nanogels: a versatile nanoscopic drug delivery platform. Advanced Drug Delivery Reviews. 64: 836–851.

Charati, M.B., I. Lee, K.C. Hribar and J.A. Burdick. 2010. Light-Sensitive Polypeptide Hydrogel and Nanorod Composites. Small. 6: 1608–1611.

Chen, Y., T. Zahui, I. Alberti and Y.N. Kalia. 2016. Cutaneous biodistribution of ionizable, biolabile aciclovir prodrugs after short duration topical iontophoresis: Targeted intraepidermal drug delivery. European Journal of Pharmaceutics and Biopharmaceutics. 99: 94–102.

Chourasia, M.K. and S.K. Jain. 2003. Pharmaceutical approaches to colon targeted drug delivery systems. J. Pharm. Pharm. Sci. 6: 33–66.

Cohn, D. and H. Younes. 1988. Biodegradable PEO/PLA block copolymers. Journal of Biomedical Materials Research. 22: 993–1009.

Concheiro, A. and C. Alvarez-Lorenzo. Chemically cross-linked and grafted cyclodextrin hydrogels: From nanostructures to drug-eluting medical devices. Advanced Drug Delivery Reviews. 65: 1188–1203.

D'Cruz, O.J. and F.M. Uckun. 2001. Gel-microemulsions as vaginal spermicides and intravaginal drug delivery vehicles. Contraception. 64: 113–123.

Deng, L., X. He, A. Li, Q. Yang and A. Dong. 2007. Preparation of poly(MAA-g-EG) hydrogel nanoparticles by a thermally-initiated free radical dispersion polymerization. Journal of Nanoscience and Nanotechnology. 7: 626–633.

Drapala, P.W., B. Jiang, Y.-C. Chiu, W.F. Mieler, E.M. Brey, J.J. Kang-Mieler et al. 2014. The effect of glutathione as chain transfer agent in PNIPAAm-based thermo-responsive hydrogels for controlled release of proteins. Pharmaceutical Research. 31: 742–753.

Dung, T.H., S.-R. Lee, S.-D. Han, S.-J. Kim, Y.-M. Ju, M.-S. Kim et al. 2007. Chitosan-TPP nanoparticle as a release system of antisense oligonucleotide in the oral environment. Journal of Nanoscience and Nanotechnology. 7: 3695–3699.

Ehrick, J.D., M.R. Luckett, S. Khatwani, Y. Wei, S.K. Deo, L.G. Bachas et al. 2009. Glucose responsive hydrogel networks based on protein recognition. Macromolecular Bioscience. 9: 864–868.

Elsaeed, S.M., R.K. Farag and N.S. Maysour. 2012. Synthesis and characterization of pH-sensitive crosslinked (NIPA-co-AAC) nanohydrogels copolymer. Journal of Applied Polymer Science. 124: 1947–1955.

Falamarzian, M. and J. Varshosaz. 1998. The effect of structural changes on swelling kinetics of polybasic/hydrophobic pH-sensitive hydrogels. Drug Development and Industrial Pharmacy. 24: 667–669.

Fan, Y., Y. Wang, Y. Fan and J. Ma. 2006. Preparation of insulin nanoparticles and their encapsulation with biodegradable polyelectrolytes *via* the layer-by-layer adsorption. International Journal of Pharmaceutics. 324: 158–167.

Feldstein, M.M., K.A. Bovaldinova, E.V. Bermesheva, A.P. Moscalets, E.E. Dormidontova, V.Y. Grinberg et al. 2014. Thermo-switchable pressure-sensitive adhesives based on poly(N-vinyl caprolactam) non-covalently cross-linked by poly(ethylene glycol). Macromolecules. 47: 5759–5767.

Firestone, B. and R. Siegel. 1991. Kinetics and mechanisms of water sorption in hydrophobic, ionizable copolymer gels. Journal of Applied Polymer Science. 43: 901–914.

Fleige, E., M.A. Quadir and R. Haag. 2012. Stimuli-responsive polymeric nanocarriers for the controlled transport of active compounds: Concepts and applications. Advanced Drug Delivery Reviews. 64: 866–884.

Galindo-Rodríguez, S.A., F. Puel, S. Briançon, E. Allémann, E. Doelker and H. Fessi. 2005. Comparative scale-up of three methods for producing ibuprofen-loaded nanoparticles. European Journal of Pharmaceutical Sciences. 25: 357–367.

Garg, T., S. Singh and A.K. Goyal. 2013. Stimuli-sensitive hydrogels: an excellent carrier for drug and cell delivery. Critical Reviews™ in Therapeutic Drug Carrier Systems 30.

Ghandehari, H., P. Kope-ková and J. Kopecek. 1997. *In vitro* degradation of pH-sensitive hydrogels containing aromatic azo bonds. Biomaterials. 18: 861–872.

Guowei, D., K. Adriane, X. Chen, C. Jie and L. Yinfeng. 2007. PVP magnetic nanospheres: Biocompatibility, *in vitro* and *in vivo* bleomycin release. International Journal of Pharmaceutics. 328: 78–85.

Gupta, M. and A.K. Gupta. 2004. Hydrogel pullulan nanoparticles encapsulating pBUDLacZ plasmid as an efficient gene delivery carrier. Journal of Controlled Release. 99: 157–166.

Gutowska, A., J.S. Bark, I.C. Kwon, Y.H. Bae, Y. Cha and S.W. Kim. 1997. Squeezing hydrogels for controlled oral drug delivery. Journal of Controlled Release. 48: 141–148.

Hamidi, M., A. Azadi and P. Rafiei. 2008. Hydrogel nanoparticles in drug delivery. Advanced Drug Delivery Reviews. 60: 1638–1649.

Han, I.S., Y.H. Bae and J.J. Magda. 2002. Glucose biosensor: Google Patents.

Hassan, C.M., F.J. Doyle and N.A. Peppas. 1997. Dynamic behavior of glucose-responsive poly(methacrylic acid-g-ethylene glycol) hydrogels. Macromolecules. 30: 6166–6173.

He, C., S.W. Kim and D.S. Lee. 2008. *In situ* gelling stimuli-sensitive block copolymer hydrogels for drug delivery. Journal of Controlled Release. 127: 189–207.

Hisamitsu, I., K. Kataoka, T. Okano and Y. Sakurai. 1997. Glucose-responsive gel from phenylborate polymer and poly(vinyl alcohol): prompt response at physiological pH through the interaction of borate with amino group in the gel. Pharmaceutical Research. 14: 289–293.

Hoare, T.R. and D.S. Kohane. 2008. Hydrogels in drug delivery: progress and challenges. Polymer. 49: 1993–2007.

Ichikawa, H. and Y. Fukumori. 2000. A novel positively thermosensitive controlled-release microcapsule with membrane of nano-sized poly(N-isopropylacrylamide) gel dispersed in ethylcellulose matrix. Journal of Controlled Release. 63: 107–119.

Irie, M. 1993. Stimuli-responsive poly(N-isopropylacrylamide). Photo-and chemical-induced phase transitions. pp. 49–65. Responsive Gels: Volume Transitions II, Springer.

Ishihara, K., M. Kobayashi, N. Ishimaru and I. Shinohara. 1984. Glucose induced permeation control of insulin through a complex membrane consisting of immobilized glucose oxidase and a poly(amine). Polymer Journal. 16: 625–631.

Ito, Y., M. Casolaro, K. Kono and Y. Imanishi. 1989. An insulin-releasing system that is responsive to glucose. Journal of Controlled Release. 10: 195–203.

Jain, A. and S.K. Jain. 2013. Engineered chitosan: A potential tool in biomedical applications. International Journal of Biotechnology and Bioengineering Research. 4: 1–4.

Jain, A., A. Gulbake, A. Jain, S. Shilpi, P. Hurkat and S.K. Jain. 2013a. Dual drug delivery using "smart" liposomes for triggered release of anticancer agents. Journal of Nanoparticle Research. 15: 1–12.

Jain, A., A. Gulbake, S. Shilpi, A. Jain, P. Hurkat and S.K. Jain. 2013b. A new horizon in modifications of chitosan: syntheses and applications. Crit. Rev. Ther. Drug Carrier. Syst. 30: 91–181.

Jain, A. and S.K. Jain. 2015a. Colon Targeted Liposomal Systems (CTLS): Theranostic Potential. Curr. Mol. Med. 15: 621–633.

Jain, A. and S.K. Jain. 2015b. Environmentally Responsive Chitosan-based Nanocarriers (CBNs). Handbook of Polymers for Pharmaceutical Technologies, Biodegradable Polymers. 3: 105.

Jain, A. and S.K. Jain. 2015c. Multipronged, strategic delivery of paclitaxel-topotecan using engineered liposomes to ovarian cancer. Drug Dev. Ind. Pharm. 1–14.

Jain, A. and S.K. Jain. 2016. Stimuli-responsive smart liposomes in cancer targeting. Curr. Drug Targets 17 DOI: 10.2174/1389450117666160208144143.

Jain, D. and D. Bar-Shalom. 2014. Alginate drug delivery systems: application in context of pharmaceutical and biomedical research. Drug Development and Industrial Pharmacy. 40: 1576–1584.

Jensen, B.E.B., K. Edlund and A.N. Zelikin. 2015. Micro-structured, spontaneously eroding hydrogels accelerate endothelialization through presentation of conjugated growth factors. Biomaterials. 49: 113–124.

Jeong, B., Y.H. Bae and S.W. Kim. 2000. Drug release from biodegradable injectable thermosensitive hydrogel of PEG–PLGA–PEG triblock copolymers. Journal of Controlled Release. 63: 155–163.

Jeong, B. and A. Gutowska. 2002. Lessons from nature: stimuli-responsive polymers and their biomedical applications. Trends in Biotechnology. 20: 305–311.

Jeong, B., S.W. Kim and Y.H. Bae. 2002. Thermosensitive sol–gel reversible hydrogels. Advanced Drug Delivery Reviews. 54: 37–51.

Kamath, K.R. and K. Park. 1993. Biodegradable hydrogels in drug delivery. Advanced Drug Delivery Reviews. 11: 59–84.

Kapoor, S. and S.C. Kundu. 2016. Silk protein-based hydrogels: Promising advanced materials for biomedical applications. Acta Biomaterialia. 31: 17–32.

Karim, R., C. Palazzo, B. Evrard and G. Piel. 2016. Nanocarriers for the treatment of glioblastoma multiforme: Current state-of-the-art. Journal of Controlled Release. 227: 23–37.

Kashyap, N., N. Kumar and M.R. Kumar. 2005. Hydrogels for pharmaceutical and biomedical applications. Critical Reviews™ in Therapeutic Drug Carrier Systems. 22.

Katono, H., A. Maruyama, K. Sanui, N. Ogata, T. Okano and Y. Sakurai. 1991. Thermo-responsive swelling and drug release switching of interpenetrating polymer networks composed of poly(acrylamide-co-butyl methacrylate) and poly(acrylic acid). Journal of Controlled Release. 16: 215–227.

Khutoryanskiy, V.V. 2007. Hydrogen-bonded interpolymer complexes as materials for pharmaceutical applications. International Journal of Pharmaceutics. 334: 15–26.

Kim, J.J. and K. Park. 2001. Modulated insulin delivery from glucose-sensitive hydrogel dosage forms. Journal of Controlled Release. 77: 39–47.

Klouda, L. 2015. Thermoresponsive hydrogels in biomedical applications. European Journal of Pharmaceutics and Biopharmaceutics. 338–349.

Koetting, M.C., J.T. Peters, S.D. Steichen and N.A. Peppas. 2015. Stimulus-responsive hydrogels: Theory, modern advances, and applications. Materials Science and Engineering: R: Reports 93: 1–49.

Kost, J. and R. Langer. 2012. Responsive polymeric delivery systems. Advanced drug delivery Reviews. 64: 327–341.

Larionova, N.V., G. Ponchel, D. Duchêne and N.I. Larionova. 1999. Biodegradable cross-linked starch/protein microcapsules containing proteinase inhibitor for oral protein administration. International Journal of Pharmaceutics. 189: 171–178.

Lee, K., E. Cussler, M. Marchetti and M. McHugh. 1990. Pressure-dependent phase transitions in hydrogels. Chemical Engineering Science. 45: 766–767.

Li, H., J. Chen and K. Lam. 2004. Multiphysical modeling and meshless simulation of electric-sensitive hydrogels. Journal of Polymer Science Part B: Polymer Physics. 42: 1514–1531.

Li, J.K., N. Wang and X.S. Wu. 1998. Poly(vinyl alcohol) nanoparticles prepared by freezing–thawing process for protein/peptide drug delivery. Journal of Controlled Release. 56: 117–126.

Lin, C.-C. and A.T. Metters. 2006. Hydrogels in controlled release formulations: network design and mathematical modeling. Advanced Drug Delivery Reviews. 58: 1379–1408.

Liu, C., Y. Tan, C. Liu, X. Chen and L. Yu. 2007. Preparations, characterizations and applications of chitosan-based nanoparticles. Journal of Ocean University of China. 6: 237–243.

Lu, C.-H., X.-J. Qi, J. Li and H.-H. Yang. 2015. Aptamer-Based Hydrogels and Their Applications. pp. 163–195. Aptamers Selected by Cell-SELEX for Theranostics, Springer.

Makino, K., E.J. Mack, T. Okano and S.W. Kim. 1991. Self-regulated delivery of insulin from microcapsules. Biomaterials, Artificial Cells and Immobilization Biotechnology. 19: 219–228.

Mao, S., W. Sun and T. Kissel. 2010. Chitosan-based formulations for delivery of DNA and siRNA. Advanced Drug Delivery Reviews. 62: 12–27.

Markland, P., Y. Zhang, G.L. Amidon and V.C. Yang. 1999. A pH- and Ionic Strength-Responsive Polypeptide Hydrogel: Synthesis, Characterization, and Preliminary Protein Release Studies.

Misra, G.P. and R.A. Siegel. 2002. New mode of drug delivery: long term autonomous rhythmic hormone release across a hydrogel membrane. Journal of Controlled Release. 81: 1–6.

Missirlis, D., R. Kawamura, N. Tirelli and J.A. Hubbell. 2006. Doxorubicin encapsulation and diffusional release from stable, polymeric, hydrogel nanoparticles. European Journal of Pharmaceutical Sciences. 29: 120–129.

Mitra, S., U. Gaur, P. Ghosh and A. Maitra. 2001. Tumour targeted delivery of encapsulated dextran–doxorubicin conjugate using chitosan nanoparticles as carrier. Journal of Controlled Release. 74: 317–323.

Miyata, T., N. Asami and T. Uragami. 1999. A reversibly antigen-responsive hydrogel. Nature. 399: 766–769.

Montoro, S.r.R., S.d.F.t. Medeiros, G.M. Alves, R. Shanks and S. Chandrasekharakurup. 2014. Nanostructured Hydrogels A2—Thomas, Sabu. pp. 325–355. Nanostructured Polymer Blends. Oxford: William Andrew Publishing.

Nakamae, K., T. Miyata, A. Jikihara and A.S. Hoffman. 1995. Formation of poly(glucosyloxyethyl methacrylate)-concanavalin A complex and its glucose-sensitivity. Journal of Biomaterials Science, Polymer Edition. 6: 79–90.

Nemani, K.V., R.C. Ennis, K.E. Griswold and B. Gimi. 2015. Magnetic nanoparticle hyperthermia induced cytosine deaminase expression in microencapsulated *E. coli* for enzyme–prodrug therapy. Journal of Biotechnology. 203: 32–40.

Nguyen, Q.V., D.P. Huynh, J.H. Park and D.S. Lee. 2015. Injectable polymeric hydrogels for the delivery of therapeutic agents: A review. European Polymer Journal. 72: 602–619.

Obaidat, A.A. and K. Park. 1996. Characterization of glucose dependent gel-sol phase transition of the polymeric glucose-concanavalin A hydrogel system. Pharmaceutical Research. 13: 989–995.

Oh, J.K., R. Drumright, D.J. Siegwart and K. Matyjaszewski. 2008. The development of microgels/nanogels for drug delivery applications. Progress in Polymer Science. 33: 448–477.

Omidian, H., K. Park and J.G. Rocca. 2007. Recent developments in superporous hydrogels. Journal of Pharmacy and Pharmacology. 59: 317–327.

Owens, D.E., Y. Jian, J.E. Fang, B.V. Slaughter, Y.-H. Chen and N.A. Peppas. 2007. Thermally responsive swelling properties of polyacrylamide/poly(acrylic acid) interpenetrating polymer network nanoparticles. Macromolecules. 40: 7306–7310.

Pandey, R., Z. Ahmad, S. Sharma and G. Khuller. 2005. Nano-encapsulation of azole antifungals: potential applications to improve oral drug delivery. International Journal of Pharmaceutics. 301: 268–276.

Peppas, N.A. and J. Klier. 1991. Controlled release by using poly(methacrylic acid-g-ethylene glycol) hydrogels. Journal of Controlled Release. 16: 203–214.

Peppas, N.A. and J.J. Sahlin. 1996. Hydrogels as mucoadhesive and bioadhesive materials: a review. Biomaterials. 17: 1553–1561.

Peppas, N.A., P. Bures, W. Leobandung and H. Ichikawa. 2000. Hydrogels in pharmaceutical formulations. European Journal of Pharmaceutics and Biopharmaceutics. 50: 27–46.

Perche, F., S. Biswas and V. Torchilin. 2015. Stimuli-Sensitive Polymeric Nanomedicines for Cancer Imaging and Therapy. Handbook of Polymers for Pharmaceutical Technologies: Processing and Applications, Volume. 2: 311–344.

Qiu, Y. and K. Park. 2012. Environment-sensitive hydrogels for drug delivery. Advanced Drug Delivery Reviews. 64: 49–60.

Rajaonarivony, M., C. Vauthier, G. Couarraze, F. Puisieux and P. Couvreur. 1993. Development of a new drug carrier made from alginate. Journal of Pharmaceutical Sciences. 82: 912–917.

Ray, K., H. Mao, K. Lin, S. Huang and K. Leong. 1999. Oral immunization with DNA chitosan nanoparticles. pp. 348–349. Proc. Int. Symp. Control. Release Mater.

Reis, C.P., A.J. Ribeiro, S. Houng, F. Veiga and R.J. Neufeld. 2007. Nanoparticulate delivery system for insulin: design, characterization and *in vitro/in vivo* bioactivity. European Journal of Pharmaceutical Sciences. 30: 392–397.

Risbud, M.V., A.A. Hardikar, S.V. Bhat and R.R. Bhonde. 2000. pH-sensitive freeze-dried chitosan–polyvinyl pyrrolidone hydrogels as controlled release system for antibiotic delivery. Journal of Controlled Release. 68: 23–30.

Rodríguez-Hernández, J. and S. Lecommandoux. 2005. Reversible inside-out micellization of pH-responsive and water-soluble vesicles based on polypeptide diblock copolymers. Journal of the American Chemical Society. 127: 2026–2027.

Roy, D., J.N. Cambre and B.S. Sumerlin. 2010. Future perspectives and recent advances in stimuli-responsive materials. Progress in Polymer Science. 35: 278–301.

Ruel-Gariepy, E. and J.-C. Leroux. 2004. *In situ*-forming hydrogels—review of temperature-sensitive systems. European Journal of Pharmaceutics and Biopharmaceutics. 58: 409–426.

Saboktakin, M.r. and R.M. Tabatabaei. 2015. Supramolecular hydrogels as drug delivery systems. International Journal of Biological Macromolecules. 75: 426–436.

Sakthivel, M., D.S. Franklin and S. Guhanathan. 2016. pH-sensitive itaconic acid based polymeric hydrogels for dye removal applications. Ecotoxicology and Environmental Safety. 134: 427–432.

Seminoff, L.A., J.M. Gleeson, J. Zheng, G.B. Olsen, D. Holmberg, S.F. Mohammad et al. 1989. A self-regulating insulin delivery system. II. *In vivo* characteristics of a synthetic glycosylated insulin. International Journal of Pharmaceutics. 54: 251–257.

Serra, L., J. Doménech and N.A. Peppas. 2006. Drug transport mechanisms and release kinetics from molecularly designed poly(acrylic acid-g-ethylene glycol) hydrogels. Biomaterials. 27: 5440–5451.

Siegel, R.A., M. Falamarzian, B.A. Firestone and B.C. Moxley. 1988. pH-controlled release from hydrophobic/polyelectrolyte copolymer hydrogels. Journal of Controlled Release. 8: 179–182.

Sivashanmugam, A., R. Arun Kumar, M. Vishnu Priya, S.V. Nair and R. Jayakumar. 2015. An overview of injectable polymeric hydrogels for tissue engineering. European Polymer Journal. 72: 543–565.

Soppimath, K.S., T.M. Aminabhavi, A.R. Kulkarni and W.E. Rudzinski. 2001. Biodegradable polymeric nanoparticles as drug delivery devices. Journal of Controlled Release. 70: 1–20.

Stuart, M.A.C., W.T. Huck, J. Genzer, M. Müller, C. Ober, M. Stamm et al. 2010. Emerging applications of stimuli-responsive polymer materials. Nature Materials. 9: 101–113.

Subudhi, M., A. Jain, A. Jain, P. Hurkat, S. Shilpi, A. Gulbake et al. 2015. Eudragit S100 Coated Citrus Pectin Nanoparticles for Colon Targeting of 5-Fluorouracil. Materials. 8: 832–849.

Suzuki, A., T. Ishii and Y. Maruyama. 1996. Optical switching in polymer gels. Journal of Applied Physics. 80: 131–136.

Tanaka, T., I. Nishio, S.-T. Sun and S. Ueno-Nishio. 1982. Collapse of gels in an electric field. Science. 218: 467–469.

Taylor, M., S. Tanna, P. Taylor and G. Adams. 1995. The delivery of insulin from aqueous and non-aqueous reservoirs governed by a glucose sensitive gel membrane. Journal of Drug Targeting. 3: 209–216.

Tokumitsu, H., H. Ichikawa and Y. Fukumori. 1999. Chitosan-gadopentetic acid complex nanoparticles for gadolinium neutron-capture therapy of cancer: preparation by novel emulsion-droplet coalescence technique and characterization. Pharmaceutical Research. 16: 1830–1835.

Uchegbu, I.F., A.G. Schätzlein, L. Tetley, A.I. Gray, J. Sludden, S. Siddique et al. 1998. Polymeric chitosan-based vsicles for drug delivery. Journal of Pharmacy and Pharmacology. 50: 453–458.

Ulbrich, K., V. Subr, P. Podpěrová and M. Burešová. 1995. Synthesis of novel hydrolytically degradable hydrogels for controlled drug release. Journal of Controlled Release. 34: 155–165.

Ullah, F., M.B.H. Othman, F. Javed, Z. Ahmad and H.M. Akil. 2015. Classification, processing and application of hydrogels: A review. Materials Science and Engineering: C. 57: 414–433.

Venkatesh, S., M.E. Byrne, N.A. Peppas and J.Z. Hilt. 2005. Applications of biomimetic systems in drug delivery. Expert Opinion on Drug Delivery. 2: 1085–1096.

Wang, Z., Y. Lu, K. Qin, Y. Wu, Y. Tian, J. Wang, J. Zhang, J. Hou, Y. Cui, K. Wang and J. Shen. 2015. Enzyme-functionalized vascular grafts catalyze *in-situ* release of nitric oxide from exogenous NO prodrug. Journal of Controlled Release. 210: 179–188.

Weber, W., M. Fussenegger and R. Schoenmakers. 2009. Stimuli-responsive hydrogel: Google Patents.

Wei, H., S.-X. Cheng, X.-Z. Zhang and R.-X. Zhuo. 2009. Thermo-sensitive polymeric micelles based on poly(N-isopropylacrylamide) as drug carriers. Progress in Polymer Science. 34: 893–910.

Westedt, U., M. Kalinowski, M. Wittmar, T. Merdan, F. Unger, J. Fuchs et al. 2007. Poly(vinyl alcohol)-graft-poly(lactide-co-glycolide) nanoparticles for local delivery of paclitaxel for restenosis treatment. Journal of Controlled Release. 119: 41–51.

Wichterle, O. and D. Lím. 1960. Hydrophilic gels for biological use. Nature. 185: 117–118.

Wu, J., W. Wei, L.-Y. Wang, Z.-G. Su and G.-H. Ma. 2007. A thermosensitive hydrogel based on quaternized chitosan and poly(ethylene glycol) for nasal drug delivery system. Biomaterials. 28: 2220–2232.

Yanfeng, C. and Y. Min. 2001. Swelling kinetics and stimuli-responsiveness of poly(DMAEMA) hydrogels prepared by UV-irradiation. Radiation Physics and Chemistry. 61: 65–68.

Yang, Q., S. Wang, P. Fan, L. Wang, Y. Di, K. Lin et al. 2005. pH-responsive carrier system based on carboxylic acid modified mesoporous silica and polyelectrolyte for drug delivery. Chemistry of Materials. 17: 5999–6003.

Yoshida, R., Y. Okuyama, K. Sakai, T. Okano and Y. Sakurai. 1994. Sigmoidal swelling profiles for temperature-responsive poly(N-isopropylacrylamide-co-butyl methacrylate) hydrogels. Journal of Membrane Science. 89: 267–277.

Yu, L. and J. Ding. 2008. Injectable hydrogels as unique biomedical materials. Chemical Society Reviews. 37: 1473–1481.

Yui, N., T. Okano and Y. Sakurai. 1993. Photo-responsive degradation of heterogeneous hydrogels comprising crosslinked hyaluronic acid and lipid microspheres for temporal drug delivery. Journal of Controlled Release. 26: 141–145.

Zhang, X.-Z. and R.-X. Zhuo. 2000. Novel synthesis of temperature-sensitive poly(N-isopropylacrylamide) hydrogel with fast deswelling rate. European Polymer Journal 36: 643–645.

Zhong, X., Y.-X. Wang and S.-C. Wang. 1996. Pressure dependence of the volume phase-transition of temperature-sensitive gels. Chemical Engineering Science. 51: 3235–3239.

Carbohydrate based Hydrogels for Controlled Release of Cancer Therapeutics

S. Eswaramma,[1] *K.S.V. Krishna Rao,*[1,2,*] *Qian Zhong*[2] and *K. Madhusudana Rao*[3]

ABSTRACT

Hydrogels, which are three dimensional water swellable polymer networks, existing with many advantageous polymer characteristics, have been attracting many researchers due to their unique methods of preparation to achieve inimitable properties such as high water absorbability, biocompatibility, permeability, soft and rubber consistency. Carbohydrates are widely used in drug delivery applications as they are natural, non-toxic, and biocompatible and have various desirable functional groups along the polymer chains which can readily form network structures with other polymers offering desirable properties. These properties could make carbohydrate-based hydrogels a first class biodegradable material for several biomedical and pharmaceutical applications. The present review prominently focuses on recent advances in the development of carbohydrate-based hydrogels, their advantageous features, applications

[1] Polymer Biomaterial Design and Synthesis Laboratory, Department of Chemistry, Yogi Vemana University, Kadapa. Andhra Pradesh, India, 516003.
[2] Department of Chemical Engineering and Material Science, Wayne State University, Detroit, MI, USA.
[3] Nano Information Materials Laboratory, Department of Polymer Science and Engineering, Pusan National University, Busan, South Korea-609735.
* Corresponding author

and subsequent future perspectives, particularly in drug delivery systems. Indeed, this chapter has been arranged in four separate sections including defining hydrogels and their beneficial properties; exploration of a wide range of carbohydrates employed in different hydrogel architectures and their developing methods; illustration of stimuli-responsive behaviour of hydrogels towards different environmental stimuli; and description of applications of carbohydrate-based hydrogels, particularly in the area of cancer drug delivery. The chapter ends with a look at some of the features and future trends for the utilization of natural polysaccharides based hydrogels in diverse applications.

Keywords: hydrogels, polymer matrices, carbohydrates, swelling, controlled release, cancer therapeutics

1. Introduction

Since the past 50 years, many researchers have paid a great attention to hydrogels. Hydrogels are usually defined as hydrophilic three-dimensional crosslinking networks constructed by either a single chain of polymers (monomers) or chains of polymers through physical and chemical interactions. Hydrogels are able to swell in water rather than dissolve. Due to the presence of hydrophilic groups, ionic and hydrogen bond interactions hydrogels can imbibe huge amount of water or other biological fluids. Because of large water content, soft and rubbery consistency, structural integrity and degree of flexibility, they resemble natural living tissues more than any other type of synthetic biomaterials (Marija et al. 2012, Okay 2009). The hydrophilic behaviour is attained by the presence of specific chemical groups such as hydroxylic (–OH), carboxylic (–COOH), amidic (–CONH), $1°$ amide (–CONH$_2$), sulphonic (–SO$_3$H). However the hydrophilic nature can be tuned by introducing hydrophobic segments into the network through blending or copolymerization (Fariba et al. 2010). This hydrophilic/hydrophobic ratio of the networks, extent of crosslinking, and degree of ionization may affect the water uptake capacity, change in the dimensions and release profiles of biological molecules.

2. Methods Involved in Hydrogel Preparation

Hydrogels are three-dimensional polymer networks which have hydrophilic behaviour, since they are mainly constructed with hydrophilic monomers. Sometimes, hydrophobic monomers are also used to synthesize hydrogels in order to enhance their properties. These hydrophobic hydrogels are mainly derived from synthetic polymers and the preparation methods involve optimal design as they are having both slow degradation rate and durability because of their mechanical strength (Wu and Chu 2008).

The following ways are commonly employed to produce a crosslinked polymeric network.

1. **Chemical crosslinking** of polymer chains
2. **Physical crosslinking** of polymer chains

The chemical crosslinking is usually achieved by radical polymerization, chemical reactions taking place between complementary functional groups, photo polymerization and crosslinking polymerization using enzymes whereas physical crosslinked gels can be prepared by ionic interactions, crystallization and protein interactions through hydrogen bonds (Witthayaprapakorn 2011, Kobayashi et al. 2001).

3. Classification

Hydrogels can be designed and classified based on various criteria by considering their methodology of preparation and physicochemical properties (Omidian and Park 2012, Das 2013).

Hydrogels are primarily categorized into **natural** and **synthetic** hydrogels based on the origin of the polymeric material. Natural hydrogels generally consist of natural polymers such as polysaccharides (Ahmadi et al. 2015), proteins (Anika et al. 2012) and nucleic acids (Peng et al. 2012) whereas synthetic hydrogels are constructed by polymerization of synthetic monomers (Gibas and Janik 2010). Since the past two decades, natural hydrogels have been interestingly replaced by synthetic hydrogels as they have excellent water absorption capacity, high gel strength with long service life and well-defined structures which favour the modification of networks to get degradable and multifunctional hydrogels. Also, synthetic hydrogels are more stable at sharp and strong temperature fluctuations (Ahmed 2015).

Based on the crosslinking forces present between the polymeric chains of both natural and synthetic networks, hydrogels can be grouped into two categories. **Reversible/physical hydrogels** are formed due to the molecular entanglements, and/or physical interactions such as ionic, H-bonding and hydrophobic interactions between the polymeric chains. But the **permanent/chemical hydrogels** are covalently crosslinked networks and the usually employed crosslinking methods are free-radical polymerization, chemical reactions between reactive functional groups, high energy irradiation and the use of enzymes. Chemical gels are highly strong and stable compared to physical gels since covalent interactions are much stronger than non-covalent interactions.

Besides, hydrogels can be classified into 4 types depending on the nature of pendant groups that exist in the network.

i) **Non-ionic hydrogels** (neutral)
ii) **Ionic hydrogels** (cationic & anionic)

iii) **Ampholytic hydrogels** (electrolytes containing both acidic and basic groups)

iv) **Zwitterionic hydrogels** (containing both cationic & anionic groups)

Depending on method of preparation, hydrogels can classified into the following classes:

a) **Homopolymeric hydrogels** are formed when the basic structural unit of the network derived from a single polymer, which is resulted from the polymerization of single hydrophilic monomer species.

b) **Copolymeric hydrogels** are constructed by crosslinking of two or more monomer species, in which atleast one hydrophilic monomer must be present to allow the gel to be swellable. These are having random, block or alternative configuration of arrangement along the polymer chain.

c) **Multi polymer interpenetrating hydrogel**, plays an important role now-a-days, as they comprise of two independent crosslinked networks of synthetic and or natural polymers. If the network consists of both crosslinked polymer and non crosslinked polymer, it is defined as **semi-IPN hydrogel**.

It has also been observed that the performance of hydrogels, like diffusion of water molecules and release mechanism of drugs, is greatly affected by the porosity and pore size distribution of the network. Considering the porosity of the network, hydrogels are significantly classified as **nonporous, microporous, macroporous** and **superporous** hydrogels. In the case of microporous, and macroporous hydrogels, the slow swelling is observed due to normal diffusion mechanism, but a rapid swelling rate is observed for superporous hydrogels due to absorption of water by capillary mechanism instead of normal diffusion method (Chen and Park 1999).

Apart from the above classification, hydrogels can also be divided into two groups based on the existence of functional groups present in the network.

i) **Conventional hydrogels:** The hydrogels which do not exhibit any considerable changes in the physicochemical properties with the change in the environmental conditions.

ii) **Stimuli-responsive hydrogels (or) Smart (or) Intelligent hydrogels:** They have similar structures to that of conventional hydrogels but consist of specific functional groups, hence they are able to perform abrupt volume changes in response to small changes in the external environmental conditions such as pH, temperature, electric charge, light, ionic strength and so on (Qiu and Park 2012).

4. Properties of Hydrogels

Over the years, researchers have been showing a great interest towards the applications of hydrogels in various fields of pharmaceutical and biomedical areas, because of their excellent and unique combination of inevitable properties such as swelling, mechanical stability, biocompatibility, permeability and surface properties. All of these properties render them as wonderful and promising biomaterials. Thus it has a great significance to evaluate the characteristic properties of hydrogels before they are employed in the application, so that they could be effectively useful in numerous fields of applications. Here we have discussed the following properties of hydrogels in order to understand the importance of hydrogels during the studies.

4.1 Swelling and absorption behaviour

The swelling and absorption properties of a hydrogel play a crucial role in biomedical and pharmaceutical applications. Since hydrogels are hydrophilic in nature, they can interact with the surrounding solvent molecules (water) and are able to expand the network until they reach fully solvates state, while the crosslinking network also tends to retract its structure. Therefore, the equilibrium is attained due to counterbalance of expanding and retracting forces of the network.

Structural factors such as composition of monomers and crosslinking density, and environmental parameters like pH, temperature, ionic strength, electric signal and enzymes seriously affect the physical structure of the network which further influences different swelling characteristics such as solute diffusion coefficient, surface wettability, and mobility, and also optical and mechanical properties of the hydrogel network (Fariba et al. 2010).

4.2 Mechanical properties

The mechanical properties of crosslinked gels are superior to incorporate them as a challenging material into the pharmaceutical and biomedical fields. The mechanical stability of the hydrogel network was extremely tuned by its chemical composition like monomers proportions, extent of crosslinking, various polymerization conditions and degree of swelling and also the physical texture and structural integrity (porosity and pore size distribution). However, since many factors can exist, the mechanical properties are greatly influenced by degree of crosslinking of the network. The optimum amount of crosslinker can be used to produce a hydrogel network with good strength and relative elasticity (Naficy et al. 2013).

4.3 Biocompatibility

Biocompatibility is one of the favourable properties of hydrogels which enables their applications in biomedical field. Before employing hydrogels in biomedical applications, one should confirm that it should be specifically biocompatible and non toxic. Biocompatibility is mainly defined as the ability of a material to reside in the body without causing any damage to the host living cells. The high water absorption capacity of hydrogels allows them as excellent biocompatible materials. Generally, the toxicity may arise due to the involvement of toxic chemicals in the form of initiators, solvents, stabilizers, emulsifiers, crosslinkers and unreacted monomers during the polymerization processes. Hence, it should be necessary to eliminate toxic materials using various processes such as solvent washing or dialysis. In general, natural polymeric hydrogels are more compatible over synthetic hydrogels (Uday 2010).

4.4 Surface properties

The biocompatibility of hydrogel is generally governed by the surface properties of the same network as the surface structure, predominantly responses by the tissues. Commonly, the surfaces are highly crystalline and inhomogeneous in nature. Many studies have been carried out to know the importance of various surface characteristics such as roughness, wettability, surface mobility, chemical composition, crystallinity and heterogeneity but no reports have been made to evaluate the significant surface parameter which is important during the biomedical applications (Sirkecioglu et al. 2013).

4.5 Permeability

Permeability is the ability of hydrogel network to transport another material like solvents, cells and proteins. Based on this property, various types of bioartificial organ transplantations have been developed. The permeability behaviour of hydrogel can be controlled by the degree of crosslinking or by the ratio of hydrophilic and hydrophobic monomers used in the copolymerization process (Hoch et al. 2003).

5. Carbohydrate Based Hydrogels

During the past few decades, wide-spread use of synthetic materials has been limited due to the lack of biodegradability even though they are attributed with excellent biocompatibility. In order to impart biodegradability, tremendous research has been ongoing in the design, production and use of new materials from renewable and biodegradable sources. To accomplish the same, natural carbohydrate polymers have emerged into the field as highly promising and exciting materials, since they are replacing synthetic polymers in different areas (Vieira et al. 2008). Carbohydrates are one of the four major classes of organic molecules found in the living systems. These are commonly known as hydrates of carbon usually followed the empirical formula of simple sugars $C_m(H_2O)_n$ (where m could be different from n), where the carbon atoms are generally combined with water. These natural polymers are considered as a large untapped reservoir of valuable materials over synthetic ones as they are highly and easily abundant organic molecules in nature, in-expensive, non-toxic, biodegradable, biocompatible, having various desirable functional groups along the polymer chains which can readily form network structures with other polymers offering desirable properties and can be easily modified into other advanced forms in order to increase their effective properties (Shukla and Tiwari 2012, Paterson et al. 2011). Carbohydrates comprise a wide range of compounds ranging from monosaccharides to polysaccharides. The well known monosaccharide units are glucose, galactose, arabinose, etc. Furthermore, numerous monosaccharide repeating units are together linked *via* glycoside linkages to form a wide variety of other macromolecules called as polysaccharides. Cellulose, for example, comprising of glucose moieties, is connected through β-1,4 glycoside linkages, whereas the glycoside bonds of starch are α-1,4. On the other hand, the glucose units in glycogen are bonded through α-1,4 and α-1,6-linkages. Based on the repeating units present in the polysaccharides, they are simply categorized into two groups: (1) Homopolysaccharides, also known as homoglycans in which single type of monomer repeating units are present, (2) Heteropolysaccharides, also termed as heteroglycans or hemicelluloses, having more than one type of monosaccharide repeating units. These polysaccharides may also contain sugar moieties either in the form of deoxy sugars, amino sugars and sulfate/ sulfonate sugars. The complexity of various carbohydrates is mainly derived from their characteristics such as: (i) the availability of glycoside bonds, (ii) the structural properties of the molecules, (iii) the configuration of anomeric linkage, and (iv) the absence or presence of branching at a given position (Garner and Park 2014). Plants are the main origins for many of the polysaccharides such as pectin, konjac glucomannan, gum arabic, guargum, xanthan gum and so on, while others have been largely extracted from marine organisms. Seaweeds are the prominent abundant source for polysaccharide such as chitin, chitosan, alginates, agar, agarose, carrageenan, etc. (Laurienzo 2010). Various carbohydrate polymers are listed in Table 1 along with their source and structural units. Traditionally, the polysaccharides were employed as such alone, but the usage is not much effective, hence they have been chemically or physically modified

Table 1. Types of Polysaccharides—Their Sources and Structures of backbone.

Linear Homoglycans

S. No.	Example	Source	Structural Discription	Structure	Reference
1.	Amylose	Plants	α(1→4) linked D-glucopyranosyl units		Kadokawa 2012
2.	Cellulose	Plants and Bacteria	Assembly of glucose units through 1,4-β-glucosidic linkages		Sannino et al. 2009
3.	Chrysolaminarin	Marine diatoms	β-D-1,3- and 1,6-linked glucose residues		Xia et al. 2014

4.	Curdlan	Microorganisms	β-1,3-linked glucose residues		Zheng et al. 2014
5.	Pullulan	Fungi	α-(1,6)-linked maltotriose units		Karim et al. 2009
Branched Homoglycans					
6.	Amylo pectin	Plants	α(1→4) linked D-glucopyranosyl units with α(1→6) branching sites		Sarkar et al. 2013

Table 1 contd. ....

...Table 1 contd.

S. No.	Example	Source	Structural Discription	Structure	Reference
7.	Dextran	Sucrose, Microorga-nisms	α-D-1,6-glucose-linked glucan with 1–3 linked side-chains		Sun et al. 2011
8.	Schizophyllan	Fungi	β-(1→3)- D-glucose residues substituted with a â-β (1→6)-D-glucose side chain for every three backbone residues		Zhang et al. 2013
9.	Scleroglucan	Fungi	(1→3)-linked β-D-glucopyranosyl units; every third unit bears a single β-D-glucopyranosyl unit by (1→6) linkage		Coviello et al. 2005

No.	Name	Source	Structure		Reference
10.	Chitin	Aquatic organisms, Terrestrial organisms and some micro organisms	β-(1,4)- 2-acetamido-2-deoxy-β-D-glucopyranose units		Rinaudo 2006
11.	Chitosan	Aquatic organisms, Terrestrial organisms and some micro organisms	β-(1,4)-2-amino -2-deoxy-β-D-glucopyranose units		Rinaudo 2006
12.	Alginate (or) Alginic acid	Brown algae	Repeating (1,4)-linked β-D-mannuronic and α-L-guluronic acid residues		Sachan et al. 2009
13.	Gellan	Micro organisms	Tetrasaccharide repeat units containing β-D-glucose, β-D-glucuronic acid and α-L-rhamnose monomers in the molar ratio 2:1:1		Ferris et al. 2013

Table 1 contd. ...

...Table 1 contd.

S. No.	Example	Source	Structural Discription	Structure	Reference
14.	Laminarin	Brown algae	β(1→3)-glucan with β(1→6)-branches		Kadam et al. 2015
15.	Welan	Micro organisms	Tetrasaccharide units with single branches of L-mannose or L-rhamnose		Kaur et al. 2014
16.	Xylan	Plants and seaweed	D-xylopyranoside units connected by β-(1→4)-linkages along with acetyl-, glucuronic acid and species dependent side groups		Pahimanolis et al. 2014

17.	Carrageenan	Seaweed	Repeating units of (1,3)-D galactopyranose and (1,4)-3,6-anhidro-α-D-galactopyranose with sulfate groups		Distantina et al. 2013
18.	Chondroitin sulfate	Animal cartilage and bovine (cow)	Copolymer of the D-glucuronic acid and sulfated N-acetyl-D-galactosamine in C4 or C6		Oprea et al. 2010
Branched Heteroglycans					
19.	Galactomannan	Plants	β-(1-4)-D-mannan backbone with single D-galactose branches linked α-(1-6)		Cerqueira et al. 2009

Table 1 contd. ...

...Table 1 contd.

S. No.	Example	Source	Structural Discription	Structure	Reference
20.	Guargum	Plants	(1→4)-linked β-D mannopyranosyl units with (1→6)-linked α-D-galactopyranosyl residues as side chains with mannose: galactose ratio is approximately 2:1		Patel et al. 2014
21.	Locust bean gum	Plants	(1-4) linked beta-D mannose residues and the side chain of (1-6) linked alpha-D galactose		Dionísio and Grenha 2012
22.	Xanthn gum	Microorga-nisms	β-D-glucose units linked at 1 and 4 positions		Bueno et al. 2013

into their derivatives and sometimes they can be associated with other polysaccharides or their modified forms. The presence of specific functional groups such as carboxyl (–COOH), hydroxyl (–OH), amine (–NH$_2$), sulfate and sulfonate (–SO$_3$H) groups permit for chemical modification of polysaccharides (Gulrez et al. 2011).

In recent years, carbohydrate based natural polymers such as chitosan, alginate, Guargum, pectin, chitin, hyaluronic acid, cellulose derivatives, carrageenan, xanthan, etc. have been exploited in the development of various types of hydrogel networks, which have been significantly applied in numerous biomedical fields including controlled/sustained drug delivery, bio-engineering, tissue engineering as well as in typical environmental applications. In general, hydrogels have been developed from polysaccharides alone, however they may not be sufficient for hydrogel synthesis due to their poor mechanical strength and chemical stability (Sekhar et al. 2011). In order to improve those properties, it is necessary to modify the polysaccharide using widely accepted techniques such as blending, grafting and other means. Modification of polysaccharides is necessary to synthesize better polymeric materials. It is very difficult to get desired properties from the newly prepared materials in order to meet various challenges. In other words, modification technique can improve the surface and bulk properties of polymers such as enhanced thermal stability, multi-phase physical responses, compatibility, flexibility and rigidity. Moreover, many polysaccharide modifications were developed since there is a great demand for environmentally friendly, biocompatible and biodegradable hydrogels. This chapter mainly aims at highlighting the recent modification techniques of carbohydrate polymers. Recent literature has been cited to discuss the modification methods including blending, grafting and others.

5.1 *Grafting of natural polysaccharides*

Among various polymer modification methods, graft copolymerization is the most versatile technique, where the chemical and physical properties of natural polymers are readily modified into required desirable properties. Grafting is an irreversible process and is achieved by the covalent attachment of functionalized monomer units on the polymer backbone by either "grafting to" or "grafting from" pathways (Bhattacharya et al. 2009). According to literature, a wide range of natural polysaccharides such as chitosan, pectin, Guargum, alginate, gelatin, etc. have been successively modified with different monomers through grafting technique and the resulting materials have been used for developing hydrogel networks.

Peng et al. reported the graft copolymerization of acrylic acid on xylan-rich hemicelluloses. Furthermore, the graft polymer was used to prepare hemicelluloses based hydrogels. The introduction of carboxylic acid groups on hemicelluloses back bone can improve the mechanical and chemical properties of developed hydrogels (Peng et al. 2011). Kulkarni and Sa developed electro responsive hydrogels using poly(acrylamide-*g*-Xanthan gum). In this study, the grafted copolymer easily converted into polyanionic copolymer by the hydrolysis of amide groups into acid groups, which are highly responsive to electrical stimulus (Kulkarni and Sa 2009). Pankaj Kumar et al. performed the grafting of methy methacrylate on natural polymer starch, where they combined the useful properties of MMA viz bioadhesion and chemical stability with those of starch like swelling behaviour and biodegradability. Advantageously, the acrylate group also serves as crosslinker, therefore, the bioadhesion property of starch will be enhanced (Kumar et al. 2014). Geethanjali et al. modified the natural polymer pectin by graft copolymerization with poly acrylic acid and poly acrylamide. Since the grafting involved hetero atom containing monomers such as acrylic acid and acrylamide, the obtained products are greatly suitable for environment friendly corrosion inhibitors. The grafting certainly provided enhanced inhibition efficiency compared to their homopolymers (Geethanjali et al. 2014). Rao et al. attempted the grafting of poly(acrylamidoglycolic acid) onto chitosan backbone which led to the exploration of desirable properties for creating polyelectrolyte complex with hydroxyl apatite. The presence of both amino and acid functional groups in the graft copolymer result in complexation of HA and chelation of Ca^{2+} (Rao et al. 2008). Grafting of poly(N-vinyl imidazole) onto carboxy methyl chitosan was achieved by Sabaa et al. (2010). The chemical modification of chitosan with imidazole ring or its derivatives enlarges its potential applications in the field of anti bacterial and metal binding studies. Agar and sodium alginate blend was successfully grafted with polyacrylo nitrile, which was first reported by Mahesh U. Chhatbar (Chhatbar et al. 2009). The resulting graft copolymer showed improved swelling properties and chemical stability. Similar to the above, numerous studies have been performed on graft copolymerization of vinyl monomers like acrylamide, polyacrylamide and methacrylamide on carboxy methyl cellulose (Tame et al. 2011, Eldin et al. 2011, Sadeghi et al. 2012). The natural polymer, Guargum has been grafted with versatile vinylic monomers such as acrylamide (Kajjari et al. 2011), N-vinyl-2-pyrrolidone (Srivastava and Behari 2006), N-vinylformamide (Behari et al. 2005), acrylic acid (Sullad et al. 2010), etc. It has been observed that the grafting of vinyl monomers on to Guargum backbone can improve the biodegradability, avoid the rapid hydration and microbial contamination of polymer, hence offering a considerable attention towards its applications.

5.2 Blending of natural polysaccharides

Now a days, polymer blends are interestingly being developed, which are highly useful in the preparation of hydrogels. Blending may be defined as the process whereby two or more different polymers are together mixed to form a homogenous mixture at macroscopic level and in such process, the mixture is defined as polymer blend. The blending of standard polymers combines the essential properties of all the constituents present in the blend mixture, which provides considerable attention to the development of new materials with desirable and unique characteristics including predominant phase, no phase separation, unaltered dispersed phase, ability to provide modifications, enhanced processing capability and uniformity of the product. This chapter introduces recent advances in carbohydrate based polymeric blends and their potential applications, particularly biomedical applications.

The usage of petroleum-based polymers has been rapidly decreasing due to their non-ecofriendly nature and scarce availability. Hence, there is a significant need to find out environment friendly and widely available materials. The discovery of natural polymers from renewable sources could enhance their advantages over petroleum based products. As carbohydrate polymers are renewable resources, they provide new opportunities to produce powerful materials for new potential applications with an environmental concern (Moore 2008). In fact, the inherent biodegradability and hydrophilic behaviour of these polymers are important to understand the effect of control polymers on environment, to avoid premature degradation. The applications of many natural polymers are effectively limited by their moisture sensitive behaviour, lower softening temperature and lower modulus as well. In principle, these unsatisfactory properties of natural polymers is drastically enhanced by a well-employed technique, polymer blending. The usual polymer blending involves the combination of natural polymer with synthetic polymers. However, the blending of two or more dissimilar natural polymers has also been used to overcome the above difficulties. Numerous polymeric blends have been studied interestingly by many researchers.

Chitosan is a versatile natural polymer having unique properties, and hence exhibits diversity in wide range of applications. Many reports have been found in literature regarding blending of chitosan with both synthetic and natural polymers and such blends offer applications ranging from biomedical to environmental fields (El-Hefian et al. 2014). Studies on different blends of chitosan/agar (El-Hefian et al. 2012), chitosan/agar/PVA (El-Hefian et al. 2011), chitosan/silk fibroin (Ramya et al. 2012), chitosan/poly caprolactone (Sarasam and Madihally 2005), chitosan/cellulose (Shih et al. 2009) have been reported for various occasions. The production of scaffolds using chitosan has been limited by its poor mechanical properties. But these characteristics can be improved by blending such natural polymer chitosan with synthetic poly(L-Lactic acid), which is highly useful in biomedical applications. Duarte et al. fabricated the polymeric blend of chitosan and poly(L-Lactic acid) using super critical assisted phase inversion process, a new, clean and environmentally processing technique. Furthermore, this polymeric blend was used to develop 3D porous scaffolds for tissue engineering applications (Duarte et al. 2010). Now a days, the production and consumption of plastics has increased in the modern world, which causes serious environmental pollution. Since plastics cannot be recycled effectively, therefore, there is a necessity to recycle them involving biological methods over traditional procedures. Parra et al. prepared edible films of cassava starch. These edible films were further blended with glycerol and poly ethylene glycol as plasticizers in order to get the enhanced mechanical properties and water vapor transmission. As these edible films are made from polysaccharides, which are naturally available at low cost, in large scale and have no plasticity, they can be readily returned to biological cycle after their usage. These advantageous features of starch edible films have shown a great impact on the packaging of pharmaceutical and food products (Parra et al. 2004).

In general, the use of single polymer is not much suitable for controlled drug release due to its weak mechanical properties. Consequently, heterogeneous hydrogels were developed from natural polymers and biopolymers using blending procedure. Jianhong Liu et al. reported three types of blend hydrogels and one is by physical blending of a pair of three natural polymers, gelatin, agar and k-carrageenan. These blended hydrogels were further immobilized with the drug Theophylline. The release studies were investigated and the results showed that the blending of gelatin with other two polymers exhibits controlled release of drug when the blend ratio is 1:1 (Liu et al. 2005). Soares et al. reported the successful use of blended amylase starch and pectin microparticles for pharmaceutical controlled release of diclofenac. The blending of different natural polymers results in different and desired properties to the polymer networks, which results therapeutic benefits (Soares et al. 2013).

5.3 Development of carbohydrate based hydrogels

As earlier defined, hydrogels are crosslinked polymer networks, swell by imbibing water but do not dissolve at all. Carbohydrates are readily converted into hydrogels since the polysaccharides are polymeric in nature and have a variety of nucleophilic moieties in the form of hydroxyl and amine units along the backbone. The hydrogel networks can form either through physical crosslinking or by chemical crosslinking between the functional groups. Generally, the chemical crosslinking can be done either in one-step process or two-step process. In one-step process, the polysaccharide can be crosslinked by direct addition of crosslinked agent to form hydrogel network while in the case of two-step process, the polysaccharide is initially modified into an activated form (such as olefinic form) which can subsequently be crosslinked in the second step. The first explained method is robust and simple whereas the second one is effective which may offer more flexibility to the network as well provide versatile properties (Chen et al. 2004).

5.4 Stimuli-responsive carbohydrate based hydrogels

A variety of biological processes fundamentally rely on the feedback that many of the important substances in living systems dramatically respond to external stimuli such as pH, temperature, ionic strength, light, magnetic field, electric field, biological molecules, chemicals and so on. The designing of stimuli-responsive polysaccharide hydrogels has been paid a great attention during the past few decades. These are also referred to as Smart or Intelligent or environmentally sensitive hydrogels which exhibit a phase transition behaviour which results in abrupt changes in the volume of polymeric chains relative to specific external stimuli (Roy et al. 2010, Maeda et al. 2009) (see Fig. 1).

The pH-sensitive behaviour of carbohydrate based hydrogels is mainly due to the bearing of weak acidic or basic groups in the structure, which are ready either to accept or release protons with respect to changes

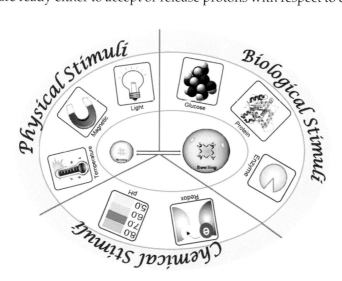

Fig. 1. Types of hydrogels based on external stimuli.

in environmental pH. The difference in the pKa values of the ionizable polymers is highly responsible for change in the hydrodynamic volume of the polymer. The pH-responsive behaviour of these hydrogels not only depends on the nature of ionizable moieties, but also on the polymer composition, hydrophobicity of polymer network and the percentage of crosslinking density. The degradation behaviour of such hydrogels can be achieved by dramatic alterations such as reversible or irreversible bond breakage in the polymeric backbone or pendent crosslinking groups (Aguilar et al. 2007). Many researchers have designed such sophisticated pH-responsive hydrogels using versatile polysaccharides in order to provide promising applications in both the environmental and biomedical applications.

Wang and Wang attempted to prepare pH-responsive superabsorbent semi-IPN hydrogels composed of sodium alginate-g-poly(sodium acrylate) and poly vinyl pyrrolidone (Wang and Wang 2010). Subsequently, Soleimani and Sadeghi synthesized acrylic acid and 2-hydroxy ethyl methacrylate grafted starch based superabsorbent hydrogels (Soleimani and Sadeghi 2012). The pH-responsive behaviour of genipin crosslinked chitosan-poly vinyl pyrrolidone hydrogels was studied by Chinyelumndu Jennifer Nwosu et al. The developed hydrogels were used to examine the pH-response in pH 2 buffer. The poly(acrylic acid) hydrogels were reinforced with cellulose nanocrystals (CNC) which were extracted from kenaf fiber cellulose through acid hydrolysis. The presence of CNC results in excellent thermal stability of the hydrogel (Lim et al. 2015). Apart from the development, most of the pH-responsive carbohydrate based hydrogels have found extensive applications in drug delivery, wherein a wide range of model drugs were used to investigate the release studies under various biological pH conditions. These hydrogels exhibit thermodynamic compatibility with water or other biological fluids having different pH able to swell or deswell. This admirable property of pH-responsive hydrogels makes them a potential carrier for release of bioactive molecules (Singh et al. 2007).

Ibrahim M.El. Sherbiny investigated the oral delivery of protein drugs using pH-responsive alginate and sodium acrylate grafted carboxy methyl chitosan hydrogel microspheres. The main objective of author's attempt is protection of protein and peptide drugs from the harsh acidity of the stomach and some protease enzymes such as tripsin and chymotripsin as well as enhanced and sustained release of proteins. In addition, the mucoadhesive properties of these polymers prolong the oral administered forms and consequently the absorption is increased at the epithelial surface of the intestinal tract (Sherbiny 2010). The protein release studies were also successively achieved by other polysaccharides such as alginate (Yang et al. 2013) and pachyman (Xiao et al. 2009) also. In addition to the release of proteins, a wide variety of drugs have also been encapsulated and released consequently, involving potential pH-responsive systems comprising a broad range of carbohydrate based polymers including gelatin (Sekhar et al. 2014), chitosan (Rao et al. 2013, Das and Subuddhi 2013), Guargum (George and Abraham 2007, Huang et al. 2007, Chandrika et al. 2014), sodium alginate (Ghaffar et al. 2012), carrageenan (Mohamadnia et al. 2007), etc.

Since temperature is another important stimulus, temperature responsive hydrogels are in development. These thermo-responsive hydrogels exhibit phase transition behaviour in aqueous solutions at a specific transition temperature are known as lower critical solution temperature (LCST). When the temperature is increased above the LCST, a sharp change is observed in the salvation state of the network which results in the transition of the polymeric chains from coiled state to dehydrated globular state as a consequence of large reversible change in the hydrophilicity. The change in hydrophilicity is due to the presence of intra and inter molecular forces such as H-bonding and hydrophobic interactions that exist between hydrogel network and water molecules surrounded the network. The thermo responsive behaviour is because of the existence of hydrophobic groups or mixture of hydrophilic and hydrophobic groups that appear in the hydrogel. At low temperatures, the hydrophilic groups exhibit hydrogen bond interactions with water molecules, hence swelling or dissolution is predominant. But at high temperatures, the hydrophobic groups show relative hydrophobic interaction. Consequently, hydrophobic interactions become stronger and hydrogen bond interactions become weaker, which results in contraction of the network (Ward and Georgiou 2011, Sanna 2013). The most well known thermo responsive polymers are PNIPAAm (LCST = 32°C), PNVCL (LCST = 32–34°C). The incorporation of these synthetic polymers provides thermal sensitivity to carbohydrate based hydrogels. Many researchers have investigated the fast response of thermo-sensitive hydrogels in response to change in the surrounding thermal environment. To obtain thermo responsive hydrogels, different polysaccharides are in usage, such as chitosan (Fan et al. 2009, Lee et al. 2004), ethyl cellulose (Yu et al. 2012), Guargum (Li et al. 2008), carboxy methyl cellulose (Ma et al. 2007, Ekic 2011), hydroxyl methyl cellulose (Peng and Chen 2010), hyaluronic acid (Fang et al. 2008). The invention of these thermo responsive hydrogels has led to limited applications in different areas.

Hence, in this connection, many studies have been carried out to focus on the combination of both the pH and temperature responsive behaviour to achieve various applications from biomedical (Schmaljohann 2006) to environmental regions (Jocic et al. 2009). These dual pH and temperature responsive hydrogels have wide range of applications in controlled drug delivery since these two factors can be easily controlled and are applicable for physiological conditions to perform both *in vitro* and *in vivo* evaluations.

So, researchers have found lot of applications in drug delivery (Guo and Gao 2007, Amin et al. 2012, Fundueanu et al. 2008). On the other hand, the other stilmuli responsive such as ioinic responsive (Zhang et al. 2005), glucose-responsive (Tan et al. 2010), electro responsive (Li et al. 2007), light responsive (Luo et al. 2014) and chemo responsive (Haldorai and Shim 2014) carbohydrate based hydrogels have also become attractive to recent applications.

5.5 Biomedical applications of carbohydrate based hydrogels

Owing to the fascinating properties of carbohydrates, these hydrogels have been arising tremendous interest in biomedical fields including drug delivery, gene delivery, wound healing, tissue engineering and especially pharmaceutical fields, where the bioavailability of the drug needs to be enhanced. Many of these biodegradable carbohydrate based polymers have been used to design different types of suture matrices for pharmaceutical applications, all of which support survival of patient through controlled release of therapeutics. The present chapter reviews the recent studies involving the state of art on current research of polysaccharide based hydrogels for biomedical applications (Table 2).

Pectin-poly(NaAA-co-AAm) superabsorbent hydrogel networks were produced through green synthetic process. These superabsorbent hydrogels are highly sensitive to pH, which makes them suitable candidates for controlled release of ibuprofen (Sadeghi 2011). The polysaccharide based superabsorbent hydrogels are attributed to high ratio of ionic moieties, flexibility of the network and high porosity ratio which allows them to be ecologically and economically viable alternative sources for soil conditioning, water purification and waste water treatment. The excellent water uptake and consequent diffusion of solutes into the polymer networks or flow of fluids inwards and outwards, hydrogels support their usage as absorbents or releasers of many inorganic and organic species from the water or soil. Macros R. Geilherme et al. reported pectin based polymer hydrogels helps to conserve water for horticultural plants, to remove heavy metals like Cu^{+2} and Pb^{+2} either from industrial waste water or contaminated river water and are also used to release agricultural nutrients and fertilizers for agricultural plants (Guilherme et al. 2010). The layer-by-layer deposition of pectin and lysozyme on the surface of cellulose nanofibrous mats was successively achieved by Zhang et al. by self assembly technique. These bilayer nanofibrous mats improve the bacterial inhibition activity compared to pure cellulose fibers, since the lysozyme and pectin are natural antibacterial agents themselves, hence the antibacterial activity is enhanced (Zhang et al. 2015).

Table 2. Environmental and Biomedical applications of carbohydrate based hydrogels.

Application	Example	Carbohydrate involved in the hydrogel	Reference
Environmental Applications			
Water treatment	Removal of metals	Pectin	Guilherme et al. 2010
	Removal of dyes	Chitosan	Xu et al. 2011
Soil treatment	Removal of dyes	Chitosan	Xu et al. 2011
	Removal of plastics	Sodium alginate and pectin	Solak and Dyankova 2014
Agriculture	Releasing of fertilizers, pesticides and agricultural nutrients	Alginate & Starch Pectin	Singh et al. 2009, Guilherme et al. 2010
	Seed coating & seed encapsulation	Calcium alginate Chitosan	Sarrocco et al. 2004, Zeng et al. 2012
Food	Packaging	Cassava Starch Chitosan	Parra et al. 2004, Saiz et al. 2013
	Food processing	Carrageenan, CMC, Alginate	Ye 2008
Industries	Removal of industrial waste	Gellan Chitosan	Hellriegel et al. 2014, Sorby 2015
Biomedical Applications			
Medical	Drug delivery	Chitosan Pectin	Rao et al. 2013, Sadeghi 2011
	Protein delivery	Pullulan Chitosan	Jung et al. 2014, Sherbiny 2010
	Gene delivery	Chitosan alginate	Raftery et al. 2013, Nitta and Numata 2013

Table 2 contd. ...

...*Table 2 contd.*

Application	Example	Carbohydrate involved in the hydrogel	Reference
Medical	Controlled drug release	Chitosan Pectin sodium alginate	Rao et al. 2010, Sadeghi 2011, Reddy et al. 2014
	Wound healing	Hyaluronic acid Hydroxyl ethyl starch	Fahmy et al. 2015, Kenawy et al. 2014
	Artificial skins	Chitosan & Gelatin	Rahman et al. 2013
	Anti microbial studies	Cellulose Sodium alginate	Zhang et al. 2015, Reddy et al. 2014
Tissue engineering	Tissue regeneration	Chitosan Hyaluronic acid	Duarte et al. 2010, Camponeschi et al. 2015
	Artificial bones, cartilage repair	Carboxy methyl cellulose	Zakharov et al. 2005
	Vascular treatment	Pullulan & Fucoidan,	Thebaud et al. 2007
Biotechnology	Enzyme Immobilization	Alginate	Srivastava et al. 2005
	Protein separation	Alginate & Dextran	Susanto et al. 2008

The delivery of probiotics has become popular during the last decade, since it reduces the loss of sensitive bacteria which are induced by oxidative or acid stress during the process of storage and digestion. These probiotics should be viable and proper in function until they reach their destination and they must survive through the human GIT to reach the colon, wherein they facilitate colonization, thus they exert beneficial effects to the host. Li et al. encapsulate the probiotics, *Lactobacillus casei* ATCC 393 within the microcapsules composed of alginate, chitosan and carboxy mehyl cellulose *via* extrusion method. These encapsulated cells of *L. casei* have extended survival even after drying and are stable in strong acidic and bile conditions, hence they might be useful for release of probiotics in the human gastro intestinal tract (Li et al. 2011). A great deal of interest has been focused on the designing of biological constructs which support cell proliferation. These domains show specific interactions with the cell receptors to mimic the physiological conditions. In the last few years, hydrogel-like natural extra cellular matrices comprising of polysaccharides have been increasing in biomedical fields, particularly in tissue regeneration. The use of carbohydrate based polysaccharides, especially the ones of seaweed source, including alginate, k-carrageenan, agarose, etc., contributes to their applications for the regeneration of cartilage tissue due to their intrinsic properties such as chemical similarity with the surrounding tissues, non-harsh processing, excellent biocompatibility, large range of hydrophilic groups and finally they are readily fabricated into desired hydrogel networks (Popa et al. 2015).

During the protein bioactivity, the use of proteins as therapeutic molecules is generally limited because of their low physiological stability. To overcome those limitations of protein delivery systems, several researchers have reported various effective methods including microspheres and nanoparticles. To achieve the same, Jung et al. developed thermo-sensitive poly electrostatic (TPE) complex, used to enhance the physical stability of proteins by changing their structure more rigid, which results in controlled environment surrounding the protein. Hence, no functional group modifications were to take place on the polymer backbone. In this work, the TPE complex was designed from thermo-sensitive modified polymer, succinylated pullulan, which is a non-toxic and non-immunogenic polysaccharide. The developed TPE complex is more stable at physiological conditions, hence it may protect the encapsulated protein rather than a conventional PE complex because of their combined electrostatic and hydrophobic interactions between the polymer and protein (Jung et al. 2014).

The industrial revolution led to serious environmental and human health issues by releasing mutagenic and carcinogenic dyes and heavy metals into the environment. In order to eliminate these effluents from waste water, different conventional methods such as activated carbons, reverse osmosis, coagulation, flocculation, membrane filtration and electrochemical techniques, etc. are in use. But in reality, these conventional methods are either costly or not very effective. In this regard, polysaccharides have emerged as an alternative source of adsorbents for the removal of dyes and heavy metals with high adsorption capacity, ease of method, good recycling ability and at low cost (Xu et al. 2011). Hyaluronan based hydrogels have been successively used for regeneration of damaged cartilages during the treatment of osteoarthritis where it maintains the proper structural and functional features of the joints by reducing the viscoelasticity of the synovial fluid and by increasing the susceptibility of cartilages to breakdown (Camponeschi et al. 2015). Bone tissue engineering is another advanced strategy which involves emerging applications of hydrogels. Therefore, micro or nano hydrogel composites incorporated with inorganic components offer suitable mechanical properties and rough surface to increase cell adhesion and bioactivity. The incorporation of Hydroxy apatite nanocrystals into the hydrogel matrix of carboxy methyl cellulose (CMC) results in better control of the degree of crosslinking and therefore the mechanical properties. The interaction of inorganic Ca^{2+} ions with carboxylate groups of CMC favors the formation of composite hydrogel network which exhibits good mechanical properties. The function of adhesion of osteoblast cells increases with increase in the roughness of the surface of hydrogel which is attributed to the presence of hydroxyl apatite crystals on the surface of CMC comprising hydrogels (Zakharov et al. 2005).

Since the past decade, physically crosslinked gels have been potentially employed for various biomedical applications to avoid chemical crosslinking agents which are often toxic and must be removed from the gel, before its application. By considering the same, Kenawy et al. blended hydroxyl ethyl starch (HES) with poly(vinyl alcohol) (PVA) to get hydrogel membranes *via* physical crosslinking using freeze-thaw cycle method. The developed physically crosslinked PVA-HES hydrogel membranes results in high swelling, good flexibility and elasticity as well as higher protein adsorption. In addition to that, the thermal stability of PVA-HES hydrogels was greatly improved by the incorporation of HES to PVA hydrogel. The prepared hydrogel membranes were loaded with ampicillin in order to investigate the biomedical applications and the release profiles showed that the release of ampicillin increased with increasing the amount of HES in the formulation. At last, they concluded that the enormous characteristics of physically crosslinked hydrogel membranes are extremely suitable for biomedical applications, particularly for wound dressings (Kenawy et al. 2014). Similar to the above, Fahmy et al. prepared physically crosslinked poly(vinyl alcohol)-Hyaluronic acid (HA) hydrogel membranes loaded with ampicillin to evaluate wound dressing applications. The antimicrobial activities were also investigated in the same work, and it was found that the hydrogel membranes without ampicillin showed better anti-microbial activity against *Candida albicans* due to the presence of HA whereas the ampicillin loaded PVA-HA membranes showed similar activity towards *Staphylococcus aureus* (Fahmy et al. 2015).

The agrochemicals such as pesticides, herbicides, fungicides, etc. are essential to protect the crop and also to control the pest. The wide usage of these hazardous substances enters into the biological cycle through various natural processes, hence cause severe environmental, ecological and economic problems. In addition to that, the agrochemicals also create health risks to humans since they cause carcinogenic, mutagenic and reproductive effects. To achieve an ideal pesticide formulation, the agrochemicals to be encapsulated in the polymer matrix which furnish enhanced activity, decrease in the evaporative and degradation losses, minimizing leaching and dermal toxicity. Singh et al. developed starch and alginate hydrogel beads to deliver thiram fungicide through controlled and sustained release. The obtained results concluded that the percentage release of fungicide has increased with increase in starch content but has decreased with increase in alginate content and amount of crosslinker. Based on this, the polymeric beads are to be considered as safe handling alternative methods for releasing of agrochemicals to control the environment, ecosystem and health hazards *via* controlled and sustained release patterns (Singh et al. 2009).

The administration of protein and peptide drugs is generally carried out by injection, which is an expensive and low-patient acceptable way. The oral administration route is greatly limited by acidic denaturation and enzymatic degradation of these administered drugs in the upper GIT. In this connection, various approaches have been designed to sustain these drugs under acidic and enzymatic conditions. pH-sensitive alginate/N-α-glutaric acid chitosan hydrogel beads were crosslinked by Ca^{2+} ions and $SO4^{-2}$ ions. These dual crosslinked beads were used to load and release Bovine serum albumin, a protein drug in a sustained manner (Gong et al. 2011). In the tissue engineering, the artificial blood vessels can be constructed through the seeding of endothelial cells (EC). With this purpose, biocompatible and biodegradable polysaccharide based hydrogel was developed from natural polymers pullulan and fucoidan and semi-synthetic dextran to culture the ECs on the gels. The results revealed that the pullulan based hydrogels greatly support the high level of adhesion on gel network which is a pre-requisite for vascular tissue engineering (Thebaud et al. 2007).

The biomimitic hybrid hydrogels developed from the native extra cellular matrix (ECM) have showed an interest towards tissue engineering and regenerative medicine. Unal et al. generated such biomimitic hydrogels derived from hyaluronic acid (HA) and gelatin, since these natural polymers are major constituents of the ECM in most of the tissues such as cardiovascular, cartilage, neural, etc. It was found that significant mechanical properties were enhanced rather than their single component analogues due to the addition of methacrylated gelatin to methacrylated HA. Furthermore, the bioadhesive properties of Gel-MA allow the spreading and seeding of cells either on the surface or within the 3D structure (Unal et al. 2013).

6. Carbohydrate Based Hydrogels in Drug Delivery

6.1 Conventional vs. controlled drug release systems

During the treatment of drugs, only a specific and small portion of drug will reach the desired and affected area due to the loss in biological functions. In general, the drug molecule itself has a therapeutic region, wherein it is effective and has selective therapeutic activity, above this region the drug reaches toxic level where it can damage both the affected and healthy cells as well, but below this region, the drug is ineffective to attribute its performance. The conventional drug release also works on the same scenario, which results in irregular delivery of drug molecules which may further lead to poor patient compliance and painful side effects (Singh et al. 2008). Indeed there is a need for frequent cycling of drugs between the toxic and ineffective levels according to their administration.

To overcome the issues involved in the conventional release of drugs, controlled release systems were introduced as one of the most advanced techniques being used in the drug therapy. The field of controlled drug delivery has grown and diversified since past decades, as it mainly focuses on improving therapeutic activity, minimizing the intensity of side effects, and reducing the repeated drug administration during the treatment. In controlled release systems, the drug molecule is slowly released over time which results in no concentration fluctuations of the drug administered. Patient compliance is one of the advantages of these controlled systems. During the treatment of severe diseases, the patient requires regular dosage of drugs for a much longer time, but it results in drug resistant forms due to a lapse in the drug availability. However, this could be achieved by controlled release systems, where one can reduce the drug resistant forms of the disease, and even the drug administration is once for every few weeks or months (Duncan 2006).

Targeted drug delivery is another type of system, that has gained lot of attention in drug therapy, in which the drug molecules specifically move towards desired or targeted sites. Such systems are obvious for cancer treatment, where the chemotherapy and radiotherapy attributed to kill both the cancer cells and healthy cells, which led to painful side effects. If the developed delivery device is selected to deliver the drug molecules at tumour sites, then the drug efficacy will be increased and toxicity may be minimized. The device must destroy tumour cells selectively, but is not harmful to healthy cells. In order to achieve such a controlled and targeted drug delivery, the pharmaceutical agent can be encapsulated within the polymer, lipid or surfactant (Byrne et al. 2008). Hence, the innovative polymer chemistry has been introduced to a wide variety of polymers and polymeric matrices involved in drug therapeutic systems. Among those, carbohydrates based hydrogels have gained a sincere attention in this area, as they are associated with several advantages as mentioned previously.

6.2 Cancer

Cancer is one of the most wide spread and dreaded diseases of 21st century, even though it has been in existence since long, still it instills fear in the hearts of a large portion of the world's population. Cancer is a major cause of death in the western world today, since effective treatment has not yet been developed. It leads to more than 11 million cancer afflictions worldwide and this number is expected to increase up to 16 million by 2020. Cancer results from unconstrained multiplication of abnormal or modified human cells, known as cancer cells, which can destroy the healthy cells and consequently the tissue and finally the host (Hu and Jing 2009, Narang and Desai 2009).

6.2.1 Therapeutic treatment of cancer

Typically, four major types of treatment methods are employed in the cancer therapy (Johnson 2005, Jacques 2009).

A. **Surgery:** It is the oldest cancer therapeutic method and is effectively used to treat solid tumours, localized primary tumours and associated regional lymphatics by physical removing of affected tissue.

B. **Radiotherapy:** It is another modality method of cancer treatment, used specifically to treat benign and malignant tumours using ionizing radiation of X-rays.

C. **Photodynamic Therapy (PDT) (Immunotherapy):** It is an emerging therapeutic approach used to treat neoplastic and non-neoplastic diseases using the drugs, called photosensitizers, which are activated by the light of a specific wavelength. When the photosensitizer is exposed to a particular wavelength of light, it produces active form of oxygen that destroys nearby cancer cells. Since the photosensitizers can also activate the immune system of the body, which helps to fight cancer, therefore PDT is also known as immunotherapy.

D. **Chemotherapy:** It is the modality of cancer treatment where various chemical substances are used to kill the tumour tissue. Such chemical substances are called chemotherapeutic agents. The effectiveness of chemotherapy predominantly depends on the type and the stage of cancer.

Of these methods, radiotherapy and chemotherapy are more preferred, since they are least invasive. However, chemotherapy has gained great attention for long term adjuvant therapy following surgery or radiotherapy. Indeed, there is a need to develop chemotherapeutic agents with good efficacy. At present, numerous chemotherapeutic agents are in use to treat cancer. Based on mode of action, these are classified into alkylating agents, antimetabolites and antibiotics (Praetorius and Mandal 2007). The commonly employed chemotherapeutic agents in conventional chemotherapy are 5-Fluorouracil, Doxorubicin, Paclitaxel, Camptothecin, etc. These conventional chemotherapeutic agents are limited by their low therapeutic index which results from its non-specific distribution throughout the body. This may lead to unwanted toxicity to the normal healthy cells which promotes uncontrolled cell division. In order to prevent the toxic side effects to healthy cells and also to enhance the therapeutic index, new therapeutic system was developed, i.e., targeted therapy. In this, targeting of tumour cells can be performed either by passive targeting or active targeting. The passive targeting can be achieved by using macromolecular drug delivery systems while the active targeting involves anti bodies, receptors or oligo nucleotides (Savitri 2010).

6.2.2 Carbohydrate based hydrogel systems in cancer drug delivery

Since the past few decades, different types of carbohydrate based hydrogel networks such as hydrogels, microgels, nanogels, composites and polymer-drug complexes have been effectively produced as promising drug delivery carriers to release a wide range of cancer chemotherapeutic agents. In this connection, the present chapter addresses the passive targeting involving macromolecular drug delivery systems, constructed by the carbohydrate based polymers. The ultimate goal of cancer therapeutics is to enhance the survival time, the quality of life of the patient with increase in site specificity and decrease in serious side effects. Carbohydrate based hydrogel systems offer such desired improvements through their site specific behaviour and multi-drug resistance.

6.2.2.1 Hydrogels as controlled drug delivery devices

The sustained release of Capecitabine was reported by Davoudi et al. They designed Capecitabine floating tablets using hydroxyl propyl methyl cellulose and sodium alginate using granulation method. The release studies revealed that HPMC and K_4M could affect the drug release pattern. These floating tablets have been used to treat advanced breast cancers (Davoudi et al. 2013). Chitosan based thermo-sensitive hydrogels and hydrogel composites were developed as controlled release devices of 5-FU. Heping Li et al. prepared pure N-carboxy ethylchitosan (ACS) hydrogel, 5-FU-ACS hydrogel and their composite hydrogels. The incorporation of drug molecules into the hydrogel network results in composite hydrogel. In this work, 5-FU-ACS composite hydrogel has excellent drug loading and release behaviours rather than the regular networks and are expected to prove as best carriers in order to meet the clinical requirements (Li et al. 2012). Reddy et al. carried out the *in vitro* release of 5-FU using dual pH and temperature responsive hydrogels from sodium alginate. In addition to the hydrogel preparation, silver nanocomposites were also developed in order to investigate the effect of silver nano particles both in the release profile of 5-FU and other biomedical application (Reddy et al. 2014). Konjac glucomannan (KGM) based semi IPN hydrogel networks were developed in combination with poly(aspartic acid) (Liu et al. 2010) and poly(methacrylic acid) (Xu et al. 2013) and these are pH-responsive. These KGM networks can serve as excellent biocompatible drug delivery carriers for colon targeting systems since KGM is undegradable by digestive enzymes present in the stomach while it can be degraded by the activity of colonic enzymes such as β-mannase or other β-glucosidases. To achieve *in vitro* release experiments, the degradation studies were carried out Mannaway 25L, which repot that the appreciable enhancement is observed under the influence of enzyme, Mannaway 25L.

6.2.2.2 Microgels as controlled drug delivery devices

Rao et al. reported 5-FU loaded pH-sensitive micro networks from acrylamidoglycolic acid grafted chitosan to investigate release of 5-FU in both pH 1.2 and 7.4 and observed that the release profiles were controlled due to the penetration of drug with the matrix or by diffusion of drug into the pores of the network or by both the processes (Rao et al. 2010). The encapsulation of Doxorubicin in pectin hydrogel microspheres was achieved by Bosio et al. The encapsulation of Doxorubicin was enhanced due to the ionotropic gelation of pectins. The hydrophobic methyl groups of pectin can interact with the hydrophilic groups present in Doxorubicin, therefore result in hydrophobic/hydrophilic pec-Dox clusters in the structure. The encapsulation and release of Doxorubicin was strongly affected by the esterification degree of pectin and found that 55% pectin showed the encapsulation of Doxorubicin as 66% with excellent stability even after 6 mon storage (Bosio et al. 2012). Cellulose acetate phthalate was blended with poly(3-hydroxy butyrate) in order to prepare hydrogel microspheres by solvent evaporation technique. These pH-sensitive blend microspheres were utilized to carry out the release of 5-FU, for targeted delivery of colon cancers (Chaturvedi et al. 2011). The semi IPN microspheres composed of Chitosan/Guargum-g-AAm were examined to study the release of 5-FU and was found that the developed microspheres were attributed to high stability to improve the bioavailability of 5-FU (Sekhar et al. 2011). Poly ethylene glycol crosslinked chitosan microspheres were able to swell significantly in both the stomach and intestine. Consequently, the release of drugs is also achieved in both the areas, but the release of drug in the stomach is not much useful, hence it was overcome by entering coating of microspheres using cellulose acetate phthalate (CAP). These CAP coated microspheres are expected to be more preferable for the delivery of 5-FU to treat colon cancers with prolong release in a protective environment (Ganguly et al. 2011). Reddy et al. prepared chitosan-hydroxy propyl methyl cellulose (CS-HPMC) blend microspheres for 5-FU release and indicated that the release studies greatly depended on the blend ration of polymers taken. The high 5-FU release was observed for the formulation having high amount of HPMC (80%) (Reddy et al. 2013). Olukman et al. fabricated crosslinked alginate beads using different ions such as Fe^{3+}, Al^{3+}, Zn^{2+}, and Ca^{2+} as crosslinking agents. These ionic crosslinked alginate beads were used to evaluate the effect of ionic crosslinking during the release of 5-FU and it was reported that the Fe^{3+} crosslinked alginate beads exhibit highest release of 5-FU compared to other crosslinked beads (Olukman et al. 2012). Swamy et al. worked on alginate based thermo responsive hydrogel beads, wherein the sodium alginate was associated with PNVCL *via* grafting method to modify the mechanical properties of sodium alginate, which has been used to make them attractive drug delivery carriers during the therapeutic release of anti cancer agents (Swamy et al. 2013).

6.2.2.3 Nanogels as controlled drug delivery devices

The targeting ability of the treatment can decide the degree of the change in the patient's quality of life and eventual life. Unfortunately, all other treatment methods involved are not much effective to kill the cancer cells before it kills the patient. In order to gain progress, nanoformulations have shown new therapeutic options for delivering both old and new chemotherapeutics to target tumours with high specificity, hence the survival time and quality of life of cancer patients is increased (Peppas and Blanchette 2012, Vinogradov 2010). The advantageous properties of nanoformulations such as size, longer circulation time and hydrophilic surface can allow them to be taken up by the different parts of the body like liver, spleen, lungs, etc. and hence are able to target the site of interest (Lim et al. 2013, Soni and Yadav 2016). The dispersion of Curcumin in gelatin and acrylamidoglycolic acid based IPN nanogels could improve the stability of curcumin which, furthermore, is used to prevent the environmental degradation of curcumin and hence the bioavailability is enhanced (Rao et al. 2015). R. Seda Tigli Algin et al. suggested promising targeted and localized delivery of 5-FU using chitosan nanoparticles which are pH-sensitive and effectively released the drug in a sustained and controlled manner with reduced side effects (Aydın and Pulat 2012).

Acknowledgements

The author Mrs. S. Eswaramma would like to acknowledge for the financial support of Department of Science and Technology-INSPIRE Program Division, New Delhi, India (DST/INSPIRE/IF120344/2012). Also author Dr. K.S.V. Krishna Rao would like to acknowledge for the financial support of University Grants Commission (UGC), New Delhi, India under RAMAN Fellowship (No. F 5-84/2014 (IC)).

References

Aguilar, M.R., C. Elvira, A. Gallardo, B. Vázquez and J.S. Román. 2007. Smart Polymers and Their Applications as Biomaterials. Topics in Tissue Engineering. 3.

Ahmadi, F., Z. Oveisi, S.M. Samani and Z. Amoozgar. 2015. Chitosan based hydrogels: Characteristics and pharmaceutical applications. Res. Pharm. Sci. 10(1): 1–16.

Ahmed, E.M. 2015. Hydrogel: Preparation, characterization and applications: A review. J. Adv. Res. 6: 105–121.

Amin, M.C.I.M., N. Ahmad, N. Halib and I. Ahmad. 2012. Synthesis and characterization of thermo- and pH-responsive bacterial cellulose/acrylic acid hydrogels for drug delivery. Carbohydr. Polym. 88: 465–473.

Anika, M.J., W.P.M.L. Dennis and C.M.V.H. Jan. 2012. Peptide- and protein-based hydrogels. Chem. Mater. 24: 759–773.

Aydın, R.S.T. and M. Pulat. 2012. 5-fluorouracil encapsulated chitosan nanoparticles for pH-stimulated drug delivery: Evaluation of controlled release kinetics. J. Nanomater. 2012: 1–10.

Behari, K., J. Banerjee, A. Srivastava and D.K. Mishra. 2005. Studies on graft copolymerization of N-vinyl formamide onto Guargum initiated by bromated/ascorbic acid redox pair. Ind. J. Chem. Technol. 12: 664–670.

Bhattacharya, A., J.W. Rawlins and P. Ray. 2009. Polymer grafting and crosslinking. A John Wiley & Sons. Inc. Publication.

Bosio, V.E., V. Machain, A.G. López, I.O.P.D. Berti, S.G. Marchetti, M. Mechetti et al. 2012. Binding and encapsulation of doxorubicin on smart pectin hydrogels for oral delivery. Appl. Biochem. Biotechnol. 167: 1365–1376.

Bueno, V.B., R. Bentini, L.H. Catalani and D.F.S. Petri. 2013. Synthesis and swelling behavior of xanthan-based hydrogels. Carbohydr. Polym. 92(2): 1091–1099.

Byrne, J.D., T. Betancourt and L.B. Peppas. 2008. Active targeting schemes for nanoparticle systems in cancer therapeutics. Adv. Drug Deliver. Rev. 60: 1615–1626.

Camponeschi, F., A. Atrei, G. Rocchigiani, L. Mencuccini, M. Uva and R. Barbucci. 2015. New formulations of polysaccharide-based hydrogels for drug release and tissue engineering. Gels. 1: 3–23.

Cerqueira, M.A., A.C. Pinheiro, B.W.S. Souza, Á.M.P. Lima, C. Ribeiro, C. Miranda et al. 2009. Extraction, purification and characterization of galactomannans from non-traditional sources. Carbohydr. Polym. 75: 408–414.

Chandrika, K.S.V.P., A. Singh, D.J. Sarkar, A. Rathore and A. Kumar. 2014. pH-sensitive crosslinked guar gum-based superabsorbent hydrogels: Swelling response in simulated environments and water retention behavior in plant growth media. J. Appl. Polym. Sci. 131(22): 1–12.

Chaturvedi, K., A.R. Kulkarni and T.M. Aminabhavi. 2011. Blend microspheres of poly(3-hydroxybutyrate) and cellulose acetate phthalate for colon delivery of 5-fluorouracil. Ind. Eng. Chem. Res. 50: 10414–10423.

Chen, J. and K. Park. 1999. Superporous hydrogels: fast responsive hydrogel systems. J. Macromol. Sci. Pure Appl. Chem. A36(7-8): 917–930.

Chen, S.C., Y.C. Wu, F.L. Mi, Y.H. Lin, L.C. Yu and H.W. Sung. 2004. A novel pH-sensitive hydrogel composed of N,O-carboxymethyl chitosan and alginate cross-linked by genipin for protein drug delivery. J. Control. Release. 96(2): 285–300.

Chhatbar, M.U., R. Meena, K. Prasad and A.K. Siddhanta. 2009. Agar/sodium alginate-graft-polyacrylonitrile, a stable hydrogel system. Ind. J. Chem. 48A: 1085–1090.

Coviello, T., A. Palleschi, M. Grassi, P. Matricardi, G. Bocchinfuso and F. Alhaique. 2005. Scleroglucan: A versatile polysaccharide for modified drug delivery. Molecules. 10: 6–33.

Das, N. 2013. Preparation methods and properties of hydrogel: a review. Int. J. Pharm. Pharm. Sci. 5(3): 112–117.

Das, S. and U. Subuddhi. 2013. Cyclodextrin mediated controlled release of naproxen from pH sensitive chitosan/poly(vinyl alcohol) hydrogels for colon targeted delivery. Ind. Eng. Chem. Res. 52: 14192–14200.

Davoudi, E.T., M.I. Noordin, A. Kadivar, B. Kamalidehghan, A.S. Farjam and H.A. Javar. 2013. Preparation and characterization of a gastric floating dosage form of capecitabine. BioMed. Res. Int. 2013: 1–8.

Dionísio, M. and A. Grenha. 2012. Locust bean gum: Exploring its potential for biopharmaceutical applications. J. Pharm. Bioallied. Sci. 4(3): 175–185.

Distantina, S., Rochmadi, M. Fahrurrozi and Wiratni. 2013. Hydrogels based on carrageenan extracted from Kappaphycus alvarezii. Int. J. Med. Heal. Biomed. Bioeng. Pharm. Eng. 7(6): 244–247.

Duarte, A.R., J.F. Mano and R.L. Reisa. 2010. Novel 3D scaffolds of chitosan–PLLA blends for tissue engineering applications: Preparation and characterization. J. of Supercrit. Fluids. 54: 282–289.

Duncan, R. 2006. Polymer conjugates as anticancer Nanomedicines. Nature Reviews-Cancer. 6: 688–701.

Ekic, S. 2011. Intelligent poly(N-isopropylacrylamide)-carboxymethyl cellulose full interpenetrating polymeric networks for protein adsorption studies. J. Mater. Sci. 46(9): 2843–2850.

Eldin, M.S.M., H.M.E. Sherif, E.A. Soliman, A.A. Elzatahry and A.M. Omer. 2011. Polyacrylamide-grafted carboxymethyl cellulose: Smart pH-sensitive hydrogel for protein concentration. 122(1): 469–479.

El-Hefian, E.A., M.M. Nasef and A.H. Yahaya. 2011. Mechanical, thermal and surface investigations of chitosan/Agar/PVA ternary blended films. E-J. Chem. 8(S1): S105–S112.

El-Hefian, E.A., M.M. Nasef and A.H. Yahaya. 2012. Preparation and characterization of chitosan/agar blended films: Part 1. Chemical Structure and Morphology. E-J. Chem. 9(3): 1431–1439.

El-Hefian, E.A., M.M. Nasef and A.H. Yahaya. 2014. Chitosan-based polymer blends: Current status and applications. J. Chem. Soc. Pak. 36(1): 11–28.

Fahmy, A., E.A. Kamoun, R.E. Eisawy, E.M.E. Fakharany, T.H. Taha, B.K.E. Damhougy et al. 2015. Poly(vinyl alcohol)-hyaluronic acid membranes for wound dressing Applications: synthesis and *in vitro* bio-evaluations. J. Braz. Chem. Soc. 26(7): 1466–1474.

Fan, J., J. Chen, L. Yang, H. Lin and F. Cao. 2009. Preparation of dual-sensitive graft copolymer hydrogel based on N-maleoyl-chitosan and poly(N-isopropylacrylamide) by electron beam radiation. Bull. Mater. Sci. 32(5): 521–526.

Fang, J.Y., J.P. Chen, Y.L. Leu and J.W. Hu. 2008. Temperature-sensitive hydrogels composed of chitosan and hyaluronic acid as injectable carriers for drug delivery. Eur. J. Pharm. Biopharm. 68(3): 626–636.

Fariba, G., V.F. Samira and V.F. Ebrahim. 2010. Theoretical description of hydrogel swelling: A review. Iran. Polym. J. 19 (5): 375–398.

Ferris, C.J., K.J. Gilmore, G.G. Wallace and M.I.H. Panhuis. 2013. Modified gellan gum hydrogels for tissue engineering applications. Soft Matter. 9(14): 3705–3711.

Fundueanu, G., M. Constantin and P. Ascenzi. 2008. Preparation and characterization of pH- and temperature-sensitive pullulan microspheres for controlled release of drugs. Biomaterials. 29(18): 2767–2775.

Ganguly, K., T.M. Aminabhavi and A.R. Kulkarni. 2011. Colon targeting of 5-fluorouracil Using polyethylene glycol cross-linked chitosan microspheres enteric coated with cellulose acetate phthalate. Ind. Eng. Chem. Res. 50: 11797–11807.

Garner, J. and K. Park. 2014. Chemically modified natural polysaccharides to form gels. Polysaccharides. 1555–1582.

Geethanjali, R., A.A.F. Sabirneeza and S. Subhashini. 2014. Water-Soluble and Biodegradable Pectin-Grafted Polyacrylamide and Pectin-Grafted Polyacrylic Acid: Electrochemical Investigation of Corrosion-Inhibition Behaviour on Mild Steel in 3.5% NaCl Media. Ind. J. Mat. Sci. 2014: 1–9.

George, M. and T.E. Abraham. 2007. pH sensitive alginate–guar gum hydrogel for the controlled delivery of protein drugs. Int. J. Pharm. 335(1-2): 123–129.

Ghaffar, M.A.A.E., M.S. Hashem, M.K.El. Awady and A.M. Rabie. 2012. pH-sensitive sodium alginate hydrogels for riboflavin controlled release. Carbohydr. Polym. 89(2): 667–675.

Gibas, I. and H. Janik. 2010. Review: Synthetic polymer hydrogels for biomedical applications. Ch. & Ch. T. 4(4): 297–304.

Gong, R., C. Li, S. Zhu, Y. Zhang, Y. Du and J. Jiang. 2011. A novel pH-sensitive hydrogel based on dual crosslinked alginate/N-α-glutaric acid chitosan for oral delivery of protein. Carbohydr. Polym. 85: 869–874.

Guilherme, M.R., A.V. Reis, A.T. Paulino, T.A. Moia, L.H.C. Mattoso and E.B. Tambourgi. 2010. Pectin-based polymer hydrogel as a carrier for release of agricultural nutrients and removal of heavy metals from wastewater. J. Appl. Polym. Sci. 117: 3146–3154.

Gulrez, S.K.H., S.A. Assaf and G.O. Phillips. 2011. Hydrogels: Methods of Preparation, Characterisation and Applications, Progress in Molecular and Environmental Bioengineering—From Analysis and Modeling to Technology Applications, Prof. Angelo Carpi (Ed.). 117–150.

Guo, B.L. and Q.Y. Gao. 2007. Preparation and properties of a pH/temperature-responsive carboxymethyl chitosan/poly(N-isopropylacrylamide)semi-IPN hydrogel for oral delivery of drugs. Carbohydr. Res. 342: 2416–2422.

Haldorai, Y. and J.J. Shim. 2014. Chemo-responsive bilayer actuator film: fabrication, characterization and actuator response. New J. Chem. 38: 2653–2659.

Hellriegel, J., S. Günther, I. Kampen, A.B. Albero, A. Kwade, M. Böl et al. 2014. A biomimetic gellan-based hydrogel as a physicochemical biofilm model. J. Biomater. Nanobiotechnol. 5: 83–97.

Hoch, G., A. Chauhan and C.J. Radke. 2003. Permeability and diffusivity for water transport through hydrogel membranes. J. Membr. Sci. 214: 199–209.

Hu, X. and X. Jing. 2009. Biodegradable amphiphilic polymer–drug conjugate micelles. Expert Opin. Drug Deliv. 6(10): 1079–90.

Huang, Y., H. Yu and C. Xiao. 2007. pH-sensitive cationic guar gum/poly(acrylic acid) polyelectrolyte, hydrogels: Swelling and *in vitro* drug release. Carbohydr. Polym. 69: 774–783.

Jacques, D.K. 2009. Design and synthesis of polymeric anticancer agents. Diss. 2009.

Jocic, D., A. Tourrette, P. Glampedaki and M.M.C.G. Warmoeskerken. 2009. Application of temperature and pH responsive microhydrogels for functional finishing of cotton fabric. Mater. Technol. 24(1): 14–23.

Johnson, M.T. 2005. Synthesis of water soluble polymer bound antiproliferative agents. Dissertation to University of Witwatersrand, Johannesburg, South Africa.

Jung, Y.S., W. Park and K. Na. 2014. Succinylated polysaccharide-based thermosensitive polyelectrostatic complex for protein drug delivery. J. Bioact. Compat. Polym. 29(1): 81–92.

Kadam, S.U., C.P. O'Donnell, D.K. Rai, M.B. Hossain, C.M. Burgess, D. Walsh et al. 2015. Laminarin from Irish Brown seaweeds Ascophyllum nodosum and Laminaria hyperborea: Ultrasound assisted extraction, characterization and bioactivity. Mar. Drugs. 13: 4270–4280.

Kadokawa, J.I. 2012. Preparation and applications of amylose supramolecules by means of phosphorylase-catalyzed enzymatic polymerization. Polymers. 4: 116–133.

Kajjari, P.B., L.S. Manjeshwar and T.M. Aminabhavi. 2011. Novel interpenetrating polymer network hydrogel microspheres of chitosan and poly(acrylamide)-grafted-guar gum for controlled release of ciprofloxacin. Ind. Eng. Chem. Res. 50: 13280–13287.

Karim, M.R., H.W. Lee, R. Kim, B.C. Ji, J.W. Cho, T.W. Son et al. 2009. Preparation and characterization of electrospun pullulan/montmorillonite nanofiber mats in aqueous solution. Carbohydr. Polym. 78(2): 336–342.

Kaur, V., M.B. Bera, P.S. Panesar, H. Kumar and J.F. Kennedy. 2014. Welan gum: microbial production, characterization, and applications. Int. J. Biol. Macromol. 65: 454–61.

Kenawy, E.R., E.A. Kamoun, M.S.M. Eldin and M.A.E. Meligy. 2014. Physically crosslinked poly(vinyl alcohol)-hydroxyethyl starch blend hydrogel membranes: Synthesis and characterization for biomedical applications. Arabian J. Chem. 7: 372–380.

Kobayashi, S., H. Uyama and S. Kimura. 2001. Enzymatic polymerization. Chem. Rev. 101(12): 3793–3818.

Kulkarni, R.V. and B. Sa. 2009. Electroresponsive Polyacrylamide-grafted-xanthan hydrogels for drug. J. Bioact. Compat. Polym. 24: 368–384.

Kumar, P., A.L. Ganure, B.B. Subudhi and S. Shukla. 2014. Synthesis and characterization of pH sensitive ampiphillic new copolymer of methyl methacrylate grafted on modified starch: Influences of reaction variables on grafting parameters. Int. J. Pharm. Pharm. Sci. 6(1): 868–880.

Laurienzo, P. 2010. Marine polysaccharides in pharmaceutical applications: An overview. Mar. Drugs. 8: 2435–2465.

Lee, S.B., D.I. Ha, S.K. Cho, S.J. Kim and Y.M. Lee. 2004. Temperature/pH-sensitive comb-type graft hydrogels composed of chitosan and poly(N-isopropylacrylamide). 92(4): 2612–2620.

Li, H., R. Luo and K.Y. Lam. 2007. Modeling of ionic transport in electric-stimulus-responsive hydrogels. J. Membr. Sci. 289: 284–296.

Li, H., T. Yu, S. Li, L. Qin and J. Ning. 2012. Preparation and drug-releasing properties of chitosan-based thermosensitive composite hydrogel. J. Korean Chem. Soc. 56(4): 473–477.

Li, X., W. Wu and W. Liu. 2008. Synthesis and properties of thermo-responsive guar gum/poly(N-isopropylacrylamide) interpenetrating polymer network hydrogels. Carbohydr. Polym. 71(3): 394–402.

Li, X.Y., X.G. Chen, Z.W. Sun, H.J. Park and D.S. Cha. 2011. Preparation of alginate/chitosan/carboxymethyl chitosan complex microcapsules and application in *Lactobacillus casei* ATCC 393. Carbohydr. Polym. 83: 1479–1485.

Lim, E.K., E. Jang, K. Lee, S. Haam and Y.M. Huh. 2013. Delivery of cancer therapeutics using nanotechnology. Pharmaceutics. 5: 294–317.

Lim, L.S., I. Ahmad and A.M. Lazim. 2015. pH Sensitive Hydrogel Based on Poly(Acrylic Acid) and Cellulose Nanocrystals. Sains Malays. 44(6): 779–785.

Liu, C., Y. Chen and J. Chen. 2010. Synthesis and characteristics of pH-sensitive semi-interpenetrating polymer network hydrogels based on konjac glucomannan and poly(aspartic acid) for *in vitro* drug delivery. Carbohydr. Polym. 79: 500–506.

Liu, J., S. Lin, L. Li and E. Liu. 2005. Release of theophylline from polymer blend hydrogels. Int. J. Pharm. 298: 117–125.

Luo, R., Y. Cao, P. Shi and C.H. Chen. 2014. Near-Infrared Light Responsive Multi-Compartmental Hydrogel Particles Synthesized Through Droplets Assembly Induced by Superhydrophobic Surface. Small 2014. 1–9.

Ma, J., Y. Xu, B. Fan and B. Lian. 2007. Preparation and characterization of sodium carboxymethylcellulose/poly(N-isopropylacrylamide)/clay semi-IPN nanocomposite hydrogels. Eur. Polym. J. 43(6): 2221–2228.

Maeda, T., M. Takenouchi, K. Yamamoto and T. Aoyagi. 2009. Coil-Globule Transition and/or Coacervation of Temperature and pH Dual-Responsive Carboxylated Poly(N-isopropylacrylamide). Polym. J. 41(3): 181–188.

Marija, M.B., S.J. Jovana, M.F. Jovanka and L.T. Simonida. 2012. Diffusion of drugs in hydrogels based on (meth)acrylates, poly(alkylene glycol) (meth)acrylates and itaconic acid. Hem. Ind. 66(6): 823–829.

Mohamadnia, Z., M.J.Z. Mehr, K. Kabiri, A. Jamshidi and H. Mobedi. 2007. pH-sensitive IPN hydrogel beads of carrageenan-alginate for controlled drug delivery. J. Bioact. Compat. Polym. 22(3): 342–356.

Moore, C.J. 2008. Synthetic polymers in the marine environment: A rapidly increasing, long-term threat. Environ. Res. 108(2): 131–139.

Naficy, S., S. Kawakami, S. Sadeghvaad, M. Wakisaka and G.M. Spinks. 2013. Mechanical properties of interpenetrating polymer network hydrogels based on hybrid ionically and covalently crosslinked networks. J. Appl. Polym. Sci. 130(4): 2504–2513.

Narang, A.S. and D.S. Desai. 2009. Anticancer Drug Development. Pharm. Perspect. Cancer Therap. 49–92.

Nitta, S.K. and K. Numata. 2013. Biopolymer-based nanoparticles for drug/gene delivery and tissue engineering. Int. J. Mol. Sci. 14: 1629–1654.

Okay, O. 2009. General Properties of Hydrogels, Hydrogel Sensors and Actuators. Springer Series on Chemical Sensors and Biosensors. 6: 1–14.

Olukman, M., O. Şanlı and E.K. Solak. 2012. Release of anticancer drug 5-fluorouracil from different ionically crosslinked alginate Beads. J. Biomater. Nanobiotechnol. 3: 469–479.

Omidian, H. and K. Park. 2012. Hydrogels. pp. 75–106. In: J. Siepmann et al. (eds.). Fundamentals and Applications of Controlled Release Drug Delivery. Springer. New York.

Oprea, A.M., D. Ciolacu, A. Neamtu, O.C. Mungiu, B. Stoica and C. Vasile. 2010. Cellulose/chondroitin sulfate hydrogels: synthesis, drug loading/release properties and biocompatibility. Cellulose Chem. Technol. 44(9): 369–378.

Pahimanolis, N., A. Sorvari, N.D. Luong and J. Seppälä. 2014. Thermoresponsive xylan hydrogels *via* copper-catalyzed azide-alkyne cycloaddition. Carbohydr. Polym. 102: 637–644.

Parra, D.F., C.C. Tadini, P. Ponce and A.B. Lugão. 2004. Mechanical properties and water vapor transmission in some blends of cassava starch edible films. Carbohydr. Polym. 58: 475–481.

Patel, J.J., M. Karve and N.K. Patel. 2014. Guar gum: a versatile material for pharmaceutical industries. Int. J. Pharm. Pharm. Sci. 6(8): 13–19.

Paterson, S.M., J. Clark, K.A. Stubbs, T.V. Chirila and M.V. Baker. 2011. Carbohydrate-based crosslinking agents: potential use in hydrogels. J. Polym. Sci. Polym. Chem. 49: 4312–4315.

Peng, S., J.B. Lee, D. Yang, Y.H. Roh, H. Funabashi, N. Park et al. 2012. A mechanical meta material made from a DNA hydrogel. Nat. Nanotechnol. 109: 816–820.

Peng, X.W., J.L Ren, L.X. Zhong, F. Peng and R.C. Sun. 2011. Xylan-rich hemicelluloses-graft-acrylic acid ionic hydrogels with rapid responses to pH, salt, and organic solvents. J. Agric. Food Chem. 59: 8208–8215.

Peng, Z. and F. Chen. 2010. Synthesis and properties of temperature-sensitive hydrogel based on hydroxyethyl cellulose. Int. J. Polym. Mater. Polym. Biomater. 59(6): 450–461.

Peppas, L.B. and J.O. Blanchette. 2012. Nanoparticle and targeted systems for cancer therapy. Adv. Drug Deliver. Rev. 64: 206–212.

Popa, E.G., R.L. Reis and M.E. Gomes. 2015. Seaweed polysaccharide-based hydrogels used for the regeneration of articular cartilage. Crit. Rev. Biotechnol. 35(3): 410–24.

Praetorius, N.P. and T.K. Mandal. 2007. Engineered Nanoparticles in Cancer Therapy. Recent Patents on Drug Delivery & Formulation. 1: 37–51.

Qiu, Y. and K. Park. 2012. Environment-sensitive hydrogels for drug delivery. Adv. Drug Deliv. Rev. 64: 49–60.

Raftery, R., F.J. O'Brien and S.A. Cryan. 2013. Chitosan for gene delivery and orthopedic tissue engineering applications. Molecules. 18: 5611–5647.

Rahman, M.M., S. Pervez, B. Nesa and M.A. Khan. 2013. Preparation and characterization of porous scaffold composite films by blending chitosan and gelatin solutions for skin tissue engineering. Polym. Int. 62(1): 79–86.

Ramya, R., P.N. Sudha and Dr. J. Mahalakshmi. 2012. Preparation and characterization of chitosan binary blend. Int. J. Sci. Res. Pub. 2(10): 1–9.

Rao, K.M., K.S.V.K. Rao, G. Ramanjaneyulu and C.S. Ha. 2015. Curcumin encapsulated pH sensitive gelatin based interpenetrating polymeric network nanogels for anti cancer drug delivery. Int. J. Pharm. 478: 788–795.

Rao, K.S.V.K., I. Chung and C.S. Ha. 2008. Synthesis and characterization of poly(acrylamidoglycolic acid) grafted onto chitosan and its polyelectrolyte complexes with hydroxyapatite. React. Funct. Polym. 68: 943–953.

Rao, K.S.V.K., K.M. Rao, P.V.N. Kumar and I.D. Chung. 2010. Novel chitosan-based pH sensitive micro-networks for the controlled release of 5-Fluorouracil. Iran. Polym. J. 19(4): 265–276.

Rao, K.S.V.K., B.V.K. Naidu, M.C.S. Subha, M. Sairam and T.M. Aminabhavi. 2013. Novel chitosan-based pH-sensitive interpenetrating network microgels for the controlled release of cefadroxil. Carbohydr. Polym. 66: 333–344.

Reddy, C.L.N., P.R.S. Reddy, K.S.V.K. Rao, M.C.S. Subha and K.C. Rao. 2013. Development of polymeric blend microspheres from chitosan-hydroxypropylmethyl cellulose for controlled release of an anti-cancer drug. J. Korean Chem. Soc. 57(4): 439–446.

Reddy, P.R.S., K.M. Rao, K.S.V.K. Rao, Y. Shchipunov and C.S. Ha. 2014. Synthesis of alginate based silver nanocomposite hydrogels for biomedical applications. Macromol. Res. 22(8): 832–842.

Rinaudo, M. 2006. Chitin and chitosan: properties and applications. Prog. Polym. Sci. 31(7): 603–632.

Roy, D., J.N. Cambre and B.S. Sumerlin. 2010. Future perspectives and recent advances in stimuli-responsive materials. Prog. Polym. Sci. 35: 278–301.

Sabaa, M.W., N.A. Mohamed, R.R. Mohamed, N.M. Khalil and S.M.A.E. Latif. 2010. Synthesis, characterization and antimicrobial activity of poly(N-vinyl imidazole) grafted carboxymethyl chitosan. Carbohydr. Polym. 79(4): 998–1005.

Sachan, N.K., S. Pushkar, A. Jha and A. Bhattcharya. 2009. Sodium alginate: the wonder polymer for controlled drug delivery. J. Pharm. Res. 2(8): 1191–1199.

Sadeghi, M. 2011. Pectin-based biodegradable hydrogels with potential biomedical applications as drug delivery systems. J. Biomater. Nanobiotechnol. 2: 36–40.

Sadeghi, M., N. Ghasemi and F. Soliemani. 2012. Graft copolymerization methacrylamide monomer onto carboxymethyl cellulose in homogeneous solution and optimization of effective parameters. World Appl. Sci. J. 16(1): 119–125.

Saiz, P.F., G. Sánchez, C. Soler, J.M. Lagaron and M.J. Ocio. 2013. Chitosan films for the microbiological preservation of refrigerated sole and hake fillets. Food Control. 34: 61–68.

Sanna, R. 2013. Synthesis and characterization of new polymeric materials for advanced applications.

Sannino, A., C. Demitri and M. Madaghiele. 2009. Biodegradable cellulose-based hydrogels: design and applications. Materials. 2: 353–373.

Sarasam, A. and S.V. Madihally. 2005. Characterization of chitosan–polycaprolactone blends for tissue engineering applications. Biomaterials. 26(27): 5500–5508.

Sarkar, A.K., N.R. Mandre, A.B. Panda and Sagar Pal. 2013. Amylopectin grafted with poly(acrylic acid): Development and application of a high performance flocculant. Carbohydr. Polym. 95: 753–759.

Sarrocco, S., R. Raeta and G. Vannacci. 2004. Seeds encapsulation in calcium alginate pellets. Seed Sci. Technol. 32: 649–661.

Savitri, M. 2010. Preparation and characterization of polymer-multi drug conjugate delivery system for efficient cancer therapy. Dissertation to Northeastern University Boston, Massachusetts.

Schmaljohann, D. 2006. Thermo- and pH-responsive polymers in drug delivery. Adv. Drug Deliv. Rev. 58: 1655–1670.

Sekhar, E.C., K.S.V.K. Rao and R.R. Raju. 2011. Chitosan/guargum-g-acrylamide semi IPN microspheres for controlled release studies of 5-Fluorouracil. J. Appl. Pharm. Sci. 01(08): 199–204.

Sekhar, E.C., K.S.V.K. Rao, K.M.S. Rao, S. Eswaramma and R.R. Raju. 2014. Development of gelatin-lignosulfonic acid blend microspheres for controlled release of an anti-malarial drug (pyronaridine). Ind. J. Adv. Chem. Sci. 3: 25–32.

Sherbiny, I.M.E. 2010. Enhanced pH-responsive carrier system based on alginate and chemically modified carboxymethyl chitosan for oral delivery of protein drugs: Preparation and *in vitro* assessment. Carbohydr. Polym. 80: 1125–1136.

Shih, C.M., Y.T. Shieh and Y.K. Twu. 2009. Preparation and characterization of cellulose/chitosan blend films. Carbohydr. Polym. 78(1): 169–174.

Shukla, R.K. and A. Tiwari. 2012. Carbohydrate polymers: Applications and recent advances in delivering drugs to the colon. Carbohydr. Polym. 88: 399–416.

Singh, B., G.S. Chauhan, S. Kumar and N. Chauhan. 2007. Synthesis, characterization and swelling responses of pH sensitive psyllium and polyacrylamide based hydrogels for the use in drug delivery (I). Carbohydr. Polym. 67: 190–200.

Singh, B., D.K. Sharma and A. Gupta. 2009. A study towards release dynamics of thiram fungicide from starch–alginate beads to control environmental and health hazards. J. Hazard. Mater. 161(1): 208–216.

Singh, Y., M. Palombo and P.J. Sinko. 2008. Recent trends in targeted anticancer prodrug and conjugate design. Curr. Med. Chem. 15(18): 1802–1826.

Sirkecioglu, A., H.B. Mutlu, C. Citak, A. Koc and F.S. Gёuner. 2013. Physical and surface properties of polyurethane hydrogels in relation with their chemical structure. Polym. Eng. Sci.

Soares, G.A., A.D.D. Castro, B.S.F. Cury and R.C. Evangelista. 2013. Blends of cross-linked high amylose starch/pectin loaded with diclofenac. Carbohydr. Polym. 91: 135–142.

Solak, A.O. and S.M. Dyankova. 2014. Composite films from sodium alginate and high methoxyl pectin—physicochemical properties and biodegradation in soil. Ecologia Balkanica. 6(2): 25–34.

Soleimani, F. and M. Sadeghi. 2012. Synthesis of pH-sensitive hydrogel based on starch-polyacrylate superabsorbent. J. Biomat. Nanobiotech. 3: 310–314.

Soni, G. and K.S. Yadav. 2016. Nanogels as potential nanomedicine carrier for treatment of cancer: A mini review of the state of the art. Saudi Pharmaceutical Journal. 24(2): 133–139.

Sørby, M. 2015. Removal of Phosphate from Wastewater by Adsorption onto Composite made from Chitosan and Calcium Carbonate. Master Thesis.

Srivastava, A. and K. Behari. 2006. Synthesis and characterization of graft copolymer (Guar Gum–g–N-vinyl-2-pyrrolidone) and investigation of metal ion sorption and swelling behavior. J. Appl. Polym. Sci. 100: 2480–2489.

Srivastava, R., J.Q. Brown, H. Zhu and M.J. McShan. 2005. Stable encapsulation of active enzyme by application of multilayer nanofilm coatings to alginate microspheres. Macromol. Biosci. 5(8): 717–727.

Sullad, A.G., L.S. Manjeshwar and T.M. Aminabhavi. 2010. Novel pH-sensitive hydrogels prepared from the blends of poly(vinyl alcohol) with acrylic acid-graft-guar gum matrixes for isoniazid delivery. Ind. Eng. Chem. Res. 49: 7323–7329.

Sun, G., X. Zhang, Y. Shen, R. Sebastian, L.E. Dickinson, K.F. Talbot et al. 2011. Dextran hydrogel scaffolds enhance angiogenic responses and promote complete skin regeneration during burn wound healing. Carbohydr. Polym. 84: 40–53.

Susanto, H., H. Arafat, E.M.L. Janssen and M. Ulbricht. 2008. Ultrafiltration of polysaccharide–protein mixtures: Elucidation of fouling mechanisms and fouling control by membrane surface modification. Sep. Purif. Technol. 63: 558–565.

Swamy, B.Y., J.H. Chang, H. Ahn, W.K. Lee and I. Chung. 2013. Thermoresponsive N-vinyl caprolactam grafted sodium alginate hydrogel beads for the controlled release of an anticancer drug. Cellulose. 20: 1261–1273.

Tame, A., M.K. Ndikontar, J.N. Ngamveng, H.N. Ntede, R. Mpon and E. Njungab. 2011. Graft copolymerisation of acrylamide on carboxymethyl cellulose (CMC). Rasayan J. Chem. 4(1): 1–7.

Tan, H., J.P. Rubin and K.G. Marra. 2010. Injectable *in situ* forming biodegradable chitosan-hyaluronic acid based hydrogels for adipose tissue regeneration. Organogenesis. 6(3): 173–180.

Thebaud, N.B., D.E. Pierron, R. Bareille, C.L. Visage, D. Letourneur and L. Bordenave. 2007. Human endothelial progenitor cell attachment to polysaccharide-based hydrogels: A pre-requisite for vascular tissue engineering. J. Mater. Sci. Mater. Med. 18: 339–345.

Uday, C. 2010. Non-intrusive Characterization of Properties of Hydrogels. Graduate School-New Brunswick Rutgers. The State University of New Jersey.

Unal, G.C., D. Cuttica, N. Annabi, D. Demarchi and A. Khademhosseini. 2013. Synthesis and characterization of hybrid hyaluronic acid-gelatin hydrogels. Biomacromolecules. 14(4): 1085–1092.

Vieira, E.F.S., A.R. Cestari, C. Airoldi and W. Loh. 2008. Polysaccharide-based hydrogels: Preparation, characterization, and drug interaction behaviour. Biomacromolecules. 9: 1195–1199.

Vinogradov, S.V. 2010. Nanogels in the race for drug delivery. Nanomedicine. 5(2): 165–168.

Wang, W. and A. Wang. 2010. Synthesis and swelling properties of pH-sensitive semi-IPN superabsorbent hydrogels based on sodium alginate-g-poly(sodium acrylate) and polyvinylpyrrolidone. Carbohydr. Polym. 80: 1028–1036.

Ward, M.A. and T.K. Georgiou. 2011. Thermoresponsive polymers for biomedical applications. Polymers. 3: 1215–1242.

Witthayaprapakorn, C. 2011. Design and preparation of synthetic hydrogels *via* photopolymerisation for biomedical use as wound dressings. Procedia Eng. 8: 286–291.

Wu, D.Q. and C.C. Chu. 2008. Biodegradable hydrophobic-hydrophilic hybrid hydrogels: swelling behavior and controlled drug release. J. Biomater. Sci. Polym. Ed. 19(4): 411–29.

Xia, S., B. Gao, A. Li, J. Xiong, Z. Ao and C. Zhang. 2014. Preliminary characterization, antioxidant properties and production of chrysolaminarin from marine diatom odontella aurita. Mar. Drugs. 12: 4883–4897.

Xiao, Y., W. Xu, Q. Zhu and X. Hu. 2009. Preparation and characterization of a novel pachyman-based pharmaceutical aid. II: A pH-sensitive, biodegradable and biocompatible hydrogel for controlled release of protein drugs. Carbohydr. Polym. 77: 612–620.

Xu, D., S. Hein, L.S. Loo and K. Wang. 2011. Modified chitosan hydrogels for the removal of acid dyes at high pH: Modification and regeneration. Ind. Eng. Chem. Res. 50: 6343–6346.

Xu, Q., W. Huang, L. Jiang, Z. Lei, X. Lid and H. Deng. 2013. KGM and PMAA based pH-sensitive interpenetrating polymer network hydrogel for controlled drug release. Carbohydr. Polym. 97: 565–570.

Yang, J., J. Chen, D. Pan, Y. Wan and Z. Wang. 2013. pH-sensitive interpenetrating network hydrogels based on chitosan derivatives and alginate for oral drug delivery. Carbohydr. Polym. 92: 719–725.

Ye, A. 2008. Complexation between milk proteins and polysaccharides via electrostatic interaction: principles and applications—a review. Int. J. Food Sci. Technol. 43: 406–415.

Yu, Y.L., M.J. Zhang, R. Xie, X.J. Ju, J.Y. Wang, S.W. Pi et al. 2012. Thermo-responsive monodisperse core-shell microspheres with PNIPAM core and biocompatible porous ethyl cellulose shell embedded with PNIPAM gates. J. Colloid Interface Sci. 376(1): 97–106.

Zakharov, N.A., A. Ezhova, E.M. Koval, V.T. Kalinnikov and A.E. Chalykh. 2005. Hydroxyapatite-carboxymethyl cellulose nanocomposite biomaterial. Inorg. Mater. 41: 509–515.

Zeng, D., X. Luo and R. Tu. 2012. Application of bioactive coatings based on chitosan for soybean seed protection. Int. J. Carbohydr. Chem. 2012: 1–5.

Zhang, R., M. Tang, A. Bowyer, R. Eisenthal and J. Hubble. 2005. A novel pH- and ionic-strength-sensitive carboxy methyl dextran hydrogel. Biomaterials. 26(22): 4677–4683.

Zhang, T., P. Zhou, Y. Zhan, X. Shi, J. Lin, Y. Du et al. 2015. Pectin/lysozyme bilayers layer-by-layer deposited cellulose nanofibrous mats for antibacterial application. Carbohydr. Polym. 117: 687–693.

Zhang, Y., H. Kong, Y. Fang, K. Nishinari and G.O. Phillips. 2013. Schizophyllan: A review on its structure, properties, bioactivities and recent developments. Bioact. Carbohydr. Diet. Fibre. 1(1): 53–71.

Zheng, Z.Y., Y. Jiang, X.B. Zhan, L.W. Ma, J.R. Wu, L.M. Zhang et al. 2014. An increase of curdlan productivity by integration of carbon/nitrogen sources control and sequencing dual fed-batch fermentors operation. Appl. Biochem. Micro. 50(1): 35–42.

7

Porous Hydrogels as Carrier for Delivery of Macromolecular Drugs

Ecaterina Stela Dragan,* *Ana Irina Cocarta* and
Maria Valentina Dinu

ABSTRACT

It is known that the therapeutic protein administration usually requires frequent doses due to the short residence times of protein in blood. Development of novel sustained drug release systems would help to overcome this drawback. Therefore, the interest in sustained release of macromolecular drugs, such as peptides and proteins has grown exponentially in the last decades. This review aims to give an overview of the recent design concepts of porous hydrogels and their applications as carriers in controlled delivery of macromolecular drugs. The main concern about the incorporation of proteins in such carriers relates to the biocompatibility of the gels and the preservation of protein activity. pH and temperature responsive hydrogels based mainly on polysaccharides, such as chitosan and alginate, and biocompatible synthetic polymers have attracted much of the attention. Synthesis parameters of the hydrogels, such as polymer concentration, synthesis strategy, cross-linker nature and concentration, which could influence the incorporation, sustained release, and activity of proteins, will be discussed in the chapter.

Keywords: cryogels, sustained release, protein delivery, release mechanism, bovine serum albumin, insulin, lysozyme, macroporous hydrogels, polyelectrolyte complexation

"Petru Poni" Institute of Macromolecular Chemistry, Aleea Grigore Ghica Voda 41A, 700487 Iasi, Romania.
* Corresponding author: sdragan@icmpp.ro

List of abbreviation at the end of the text.

1. Introduction

Among the macromolecular drugs, proteins, peptides, DNA-based constructs for gene therapy and growth factors are the most investigated (Censi et al. 2012, Moroz et al. 2016, Nguyen and Alsberg 2014, Tessmar and Göpferich 2007, Torchilin 2011, Vermonden et al. 2012). The design and production of protein and peptide drug formulations must take into account the mechanisms for stabilization and delivery of these drugs because each molecule has its own stability *in vitro* and *in vivo*, which is correlated with its physical and chemical properties such as molecular weight, isoelectric point (*iep*) and the amino acid composition (Cleland and Langer 1994). As found in literature, there are various routes for the administration of these drugs, such as direct injection, pulmonary route, oral, and transdermal delivery. The bioavailability, the extent and the rate at which a drug reaches the target tissue are connected with the route of administration (Bhattarai et al. 2010, Cleland and Langer 1994, Imren 2010, Moroz et al. 2016).

Advances in biotechnology have accelerated the large-scale production of therapeutic proteins, making them readily available for applications in medical practices and clinical studies. In addition, therapeutic proteins are capable of performing highly specific and complex functions that may not be achieved by other therapeutic moieties due to their exquisite specificity and bioactivity. Many therapeutic proteins are still administered parenterally, but the pain and discomfort associated with frequent injections often leads to low patient compliance and restricts the acceptance of proteins. The oral administration of proteins and peptides is preferred but the main drawback is that their delicate structure is subjected to proteolytic, chemical, and physical degradation, which may result in the loss of activity and elicit an immune response (Ahmad et al. 2014, LoPresti et al. 2011, Park et al. 2011). Therefore, the novel oral formulations of macromolecular drugs including peptides, proteins, and growth factors require overcoming the inconveniences such as low permeability, lack of lipophilicity, and rapid enzymatic degradation in the gastrointestinal tract (GIT) (Ahmad et al. 2014, Park et al. 2011).

It is known that the therapeutic protein administration usually asks for frequent doses due to the short residence times of protein in blood (Bocourt et al. 2011). Therefore, the development of novel sustained drug release systems would help to overcome this drawback (Bae et al. 2015, Bawa et al. 2009, Vermonden et al. 2012). An option for overcoming these problems is the use of delivery systems consisting of polymeric networks in which the proteins are loaded and from which they are gradually released (Dragan et al. 2016, Fundueanu et al. 2008, Imren et al. 2010, Kikuki and Okano 2002). Colon-specific protein delivery systems are of special interest because proteins are unstable in the upper GIT, the amount of digestive enzymes in the colon being significantly lower than in the upper GIT (Imren et al. 2010).

Many peptides and proteins possess biological activity that makes them potent and therapeutic, in particular, as anticancer agents. In certain circumstances, when the tumour delivery of such large molecules is of interest, Enhanced Permeability and Retention (EPR)–mediated drug delivery is currently seen as an effective way to bring macromolecular drugs and drug-loaded pharmaceutical nanocarriers into tumours (Bawa et al. 2009, Torchilin 2011).

Conjugation of polypeptides with water-soluble polymers reduces the renal filtration, thus increasing their residence in blood, allowing a better accumulation in tumours via the EPR effect. Polyethylene glycol (PEG) and poly(styrene-*co*-maleic acid anhydride) (SMA) are examples of water soluble polymers for the modification of peptides and proteins with therapeutic potential. It has also been found that the conjugation with SMA protects proteins from enzymatic degradation, and decreases immunogenicity of modified proteins (Torchilin 2011).

2. State-of-the-art in Hydrogels as Carrier for Proteins

2.1 Hydrogels for protein delivery

Controlled drug delivery systems (DDSs) constitute an alternative approach in which the bioactive compound is incorporated into a polymeric system to be released in a controlled manner (Bawa et al. 2009, Bhattarai et al. 2010, Byrne and Salian 2008, Lohani et al. 2014). Hydrogels as physical or chemical cross-linked hydrophylic polymers represent a class of DDSs largely used as vehicles for the storage or transport of active species. The polymer chain length, polymer composition, concentration of initiators, and cross-linker concentration are the factors which allow controlling the degree of network cross-linking and the hydrogel swelling properties. Among hydrogels, "smart" polymer gels, which undergo reversible phase transition in response to the external stimuli, have attracted much attention (Bhattarai et al. 2010, Peppas et al. 2006). These gels can change their volume and/or shape in response to a slight alteration of the external stimuli, such as pH, temperature, ionic strength, solvent composition, light, electric or magnetic field, etc. Temperature-responsive and pH-responsive hydrogels have been widely used to create intelligent DDSs. Furthermore, molecular recognition of the biologically significant target species has been lately developed in the field of controlled DDSs by the molecular imprinting (MIP) of hydrogels (Byrne and Salian 2008, Liu et al. 2016, Peppas et al. 2006, Peppas and Clegg 2016). Loading of therapeutics into the hydrogel could be performed either by preparation of the gel in the presence of drug, or synthesize the gel followed by loading of drug via equilibrium partitioning. Byrne and Salian explored the differences between the two strategies and clarified the role of imprinting in the mechanisms of drug release from hydrogel structures (Byrne and Salian 2008). The imprinting leads to delayed template transport because molecular imprinting can provide control of the drug release profile in swelling-controlled networks, and in responsive-swollen networks. Responsive hydrogels can be engineered to change network structure in response to a stimulus due to the presence of specific chemical/biological species along their polymer chains backbone.

Novel systems have been created by integrating biological molecules in synthetic hydrogels, which synergistically combine the biological mechanisms, such as high affinity and specificity of binding, with hydrogel properties (e.g., mechanical stability and environmental-responsive properties). By incorporating enzymes within environmentally responsive hydrogels, researchers have created DDSs that are responsive to biological analytes. Thus, activated glucose oxidase (GOD) has been incorporated into pH-sensitive cationic hydrogels to produce conjugated biomaterials, and pH-responsive hydrogels composed of PEG-containing ionic networks that have been applied for the oral delivery of proteins such as insulin (Bawa et al. 2009, Gil and Hudson 2004, Peppas et al. 2006). These systems exhibit release kinetics of insulin in response to changes in the glucose concentration making them useful as "smart" materials for diabetes applications.

Polysaccharide-based hydrogels typically exhibit valuable properties, such as biodegradability, biocompatibility, eco-friendliness, low cost, easy availability and biological functions. Various responsive hydrogels investigated for the *in vitro* release of proteins are based on natural polymers such as chitosan (CS), alginate, dextran, hyaluronic acid and their composites with synthetic biocompatible polymers (Bae et al. 2015, Bhattarai et al. 2010, Censi et al. 2012, Chen et al. 2004, Guo et al. 2007, Imren et al. 2010, Matricardi et al. 2013). Loading of protein into the hydrogel has been performed by two main ways: (1) preparation of protein loaded hydrogels by the incorporation of proteins after the formation of the hydrogel network by soaking (Chen et al. 2004, Imren et al. 2010); (2) incorporation of the proteins during the formation of cross-linked hydrogel (Guo et al. 2007, Imren et al. 2010). Loading of protein by the first method has several disadvantages, such as the toxic effects of the initiators, monomers and cross-linkers (Imren et al. 2010). *In vitro* release of protein from the discs of dextran hydrogels in simulated gastrointestinal fluids showed that bovine serum albumin (BSA) was mainly released by a Fickian diffusion, and this indicated that its hydrodynamic diameter (7.7 nm) was smaller than the hydrogel mesh size (~19 nm) (Imren et al. 2010). The incorporation of BSA after the hydrogel formation proportionally increased with the protein concentration, the release of BSA being much faster in pH 7.4 than in pH 1.2 (Chen et al. 2004).

Incorporation of separate release systems, such as micro- or nanocapsules containing proteins, into the hydrogels constitutes an efficient route to slow the release rate for long-term applications (Bhattarai et al. 2010, Ungaro et al. 2006). Injectable hydrogels as intelligent tools for delivery of biomolecules have attracted much attention (Bhattarai et al. 2005, Gilmore et al. 2016). Thus, injectable thermoreversible hydrogels based on PEG-grafted-CS have been used as systems for sustained release of BSA (Bhattarai et al. 2005). A steady linear release of protein has been achieved for a period of ~70 h, after an initial burst release in the first 5 h. *In situ* cross-linking of hydrogel with genipin led to a prolonged release of BSA up to 40 days with maintaining the injectability of the gel, the primary structure of protein released from the gel, either physically or genipin cross-linked, being generally preserved.

Finding carriers which should respond to the cancer immunotherapy used together with chemotherapy is an actual requirement, the differences between the biomolecules and a hydrophobic small molecule asking for novel strategies in drug delivery design. Thus, recent strategies are focused on the elaboration of dual drug release systems, able to simultaneously deliver more than one drug, for example small synthetic drugs and biomolecules such as proteins, peptides, growth factors and so on. This is much more difficult than the release of two synthetic small molecules because biological drugs have much higher molecular weights (20–70 kDa) and must be preserved in unmodified state (Gilmore et al. 2016). For example, the hydrophobic small drug is incorporated in a nano-carrier, and the biological therapeutic is mixed into a polymer matrix to prevent early degradation and to localize and confine the nanoparticle containing the small molecule drug. The synergetic effect of the two drugs occurs when the small molecule is released into the protein loaded polymer matrix (Gilmore et al. 2016).

Using the proteins as templates in the synthesis of MIP hydrogels present some limitations that contrast with MIP by small molecules connected with the diffusional aspects that limit bulk MIPs to much lower cross-linking densities (Peppas and Clegg 2016). Furthermore, to preserve the native protein structure, polymerizations must be carried out under low concentration of monomer, these requirements being in conflict with the conditions necessary to ensure the polymer-template specificity found for the MIP with small molecules (Peppas and Clegg 2016). However, Peppas and coworkers have succeeded in synthesizing recognitive networks for some proteins, such as Cytochrome C and lysozyme (LYS) (Bergman and Peppas 2008), and BSA (Kryscio and Peppas 2012) in hydrogels. Due to the structural similarities of proteins, the selectivity of some MIP hydrogel networks for families of proteins rather than for single proteins has been demonstrated (Bayer et al. 2011).

A known drawback of hydrogels is that due to their porosity, they present an inevitable burst release of the encapsulated proteins. To remove this disadvantage, Bae et al. have developed an effective approach to regulate the protein release kinetics by the generation of micrometer-sized domains into the hydrogels based on dextran (Bae et al. 2015). This system was endowed with sustained release of PEGylated interferon over 3 months, without compromising its bioavailability. As can be seen in Table 1, the main formulations containing proteins hosted in hydrogels are presented as: microgels, micro- and nanoparticles, beads, disks, monoliths, membranes, films, capsules.

Part of the systems used in the delivery of proteins, recently designed and characterized, will be discussed in more detail below.

2.2 Microgels, nanogels, and beads as formulations for protein delivery

Applications of the particulate forms of the hydrogels including micro- and nanogels, and beads are of continuous interest due to the enhanced control over their properties such as particle size and distribution, degradability and environmental responsiveness (Knipe et al. 2015, Kaygusuz and Erim 2013, Li et al. 2010, Shi et al. 2008, Yang et al. 2013). The gel carriers could be physically or covalently stabilized.

2.2.1 Physically stabilized gel carriers

CS-based nanoparticles have been used for oral delivery of insulin, either as blend of CS with poly-γ-glutamic acid ionically cross-linked with sodium tripolyphosphate (TPP) and $MgSO_4$ (Lin et al. 2008) or CS grafted with methyl methacrylate, N,N-dimethylaminoethyl methacrylate hydrochloride (DMAEMC) and N-trimethylaminoethylmethacrylate chloride (TMAEMC) (Qian et al. 2006). The insulin-loaded nanoparticles have been formed by the electrostatic interactions between the positively charged nanoparticles and the anionic protein. The *in vitro* insulin release study in phosphate buffered saline (PBS) solution, at 37°C, showed that, after an initial burst release, a slowly sustained release up to 90 h was found in the case of the nanoparticles formed with CS grafted with TMAEMC, the surface charge being the highest in the case of these nanoparticles. The effect of nanoparticles on the intestinal adsorption of protein has been investigated following the plasma glucose levels as a function of time after the oral administration. Usually, the most part of protein is destroyed by the conditions in the GIT (Qian et al. 2006). However, the results of *in vivo* tests indicated that the released insulin was in active form and that the bioavailability has been improved

Table 1. The main formulations containing proteins hosted in hydrogels.

Macromolecular drug	Carrier system	Physical status	Optimum pH and release place	References
Lysozyme	oxidized starch cross-linked with STMP	microgels	5–7; 0.2 M NaCl	Li et al. 2009, Li et al. 2010
Lysozyme	oxidized starch cross-linked with GDGE	microgels		Zhao et al. 2015a
Lysozyme	Poly(N-isopropylacrylamide-co-acrylamide) grafted onto pullulan microspheres	pH- and temperature-sensitive microspheres	7.4; 0.5 M NaCl	Fundueanu et al. 2008
Lysozyme	cyclodextrin anionic pullulan cross-linked with 3-(glycidoxypropyl)trimethoxysilan	microparticles	1.4; enzymatic activity preserved	Mocanu et al. 2009
Lysozyme	Anionic hydrogel confined in Daisogel silica	Composite microspheres	7.4; colon	Dragan and Bucatariu 2016
Bovine serum albumin	ionically cross-linked CS	microspheres	7.4	Ma and Liu 2010
Bovine serum albumin	m-PEG-g-CMCS	beads	7.4; colon	Yang et al. 2013
Insulin	DMAEMC or TMAEMC grafted on CSCS	nanoparticles	7.4; colon	Qian et al. 2006
Insulin	CS blended with poly(γ-glutamic acid)	nanoparticles	7.4; colon	Lin et al. 2008
Insulin	PDEAEM cross-linked with TEGDMA	microparticles	PBS	Marek and Peppas 2013
Insulin	P(MAA-co-N-vinylpyrrolidone)	microgels	6.8; small intestin	Knipe et al. 2015

by the nanoparticles, the protein being protected due to physicochemical interactions between enzymes and the hydrophilic chains of nanoparticles, the amount of free enzymes being thus reduced.

By the ionotropic gelation of CS with TPP, Ma and Liu prepared microspheres with sizes in the range of 100–450 μm, by adjusting the CS concentration from 0.5 to 1.2 g/L (Ma and Liu 2010). Using ethanol in the mixture with TPP, even larger microspheres have been prepared. The encapsulation efficiency of BSA into the CS microspheres decreased with the increase of the weight ratio between BSA and CS, and with the decrease of the concentration of the coagulation solution. The release of BSA from CS microspheres has been mainly controlled by the protein diffusion, which could be tailored by adjusting the concentration and pH of the coagulation solution. The primary mechanism for the release of BSA from the CS beads ionically cross-linked with TPP was Fickian diffusion, suggesting that the release of protein occurred without the alteration of the structural properties of the matrix (Ghanem and Skonberg 2002).

The efficiency of BSA entrapment and the diminution of the burst release of protein could be controlled by the preparation of composite matrices as beads, consisting of alginate/N,O-carboxymethyl chitosan (CMCS) (Lin et al. 2005) and alginate/methoxy poly(ethylene glycol) (mPEG) grafted CMCS (mPEG-g-CMCS) (Yang et al. 2013), ionically cross-linked with Ca^{2+}. Thus, the efficiency of the BSA entrapment in the ionically stabilized alginate/N,O-CMCS hydrogel beads increased up to 77% with the effective cross-linking density by Ca^{2+} (Lin et al. 2005). The amount of BSA released at pH 7.4 increased significantly as compared with the protein release at pH 1.2, because the swelling ratio of the beads was higher at this pH, the electrostatic repulsion between –COO⁻ groups being much higher. Retention of BSA in hydrogels could be further increased by rinsing the test beads with acetone, because more water molecules have been removed during the rinsing with acetone, resulting in a more compact morphology of the beads. Encapsulation of BSA into quaternary derivatives of CS ionically cross-linked with TPP showed that both the encapsulation efficiency and loading capacity increased with the increase of BSA concentration, at pH 5.0, i.e., above the isoelectric point of BSA (4.8) (Wan et al. 2009). The BSA release profiles showed a small burst release in the first 10 h, followed by a slow release up to several days. Beads of interpenetrating polymeric network (IPN), ionically cross-linked with Ca^{2+}, have been prepared from mPEG-g-CMC and alginate and compared with mPEG physically mixed with CMC hydrogel as vehicles for BSA (Yang et al. 2013). The loading capacity of the mPEG-g-CMC/alginate beads was enhanced in comparison with that of the hydrogel prepared by physically mixing mPEG. The cumulative protein release decreased at pH 1.2, while the release at pH 7.4 was enhanced, the swelling ratio also being much higher at this pH, suggesting that the mPEG-*g*-CMC/alginate pH-sensitive hydrogel could be promising for site-specific protein drug delivery in the intestine.

Formation of micro- and nanoparticles by the polyelectrolyte complexation (PEC) between two oppositely charged polyelectrolytes, either synthetic or natural, is well documented (Dragan and Schwarz 2004, George and Abraham 2006, Magnin et al. 2004), being exploited as a versatile way to encapsulate proteins (Bayat et al. 2008, George and Abraham 2006, Lin et al. 2007, Liu et al. 2007, Magnin et al. 2004, Sajeesh and Sharma 2006, Sarmento et al. 2007, Shi et al. 2006, Wan et al. 2009, Zhang et al. 2004). Due to the degradation by proteolytic enzymes, peptides and proteins have a low therapeutic activity when are orally administrated, their encapsulation in PEC nanoparticles as carrier being a very useful approach to protect them against degradation. The PEC nanoparticles have several valuable characteristics including suitable size and surface charge, spherical morphology and a low polydispersity index (Dragan and Schwarz 2004, Lin et al. 2007, Magnin et al. 2004). For example, for the oral delivery of insulin, PECs nanoparticles have been prepared either by the complex formation between insulin and quaternized derivatives of CS (Bayat et al. 2008) or by loading insulin in PEC nanoparticles formed by the electrostatic interaction between CS and various polyacids such as poly(γ-glutamic acid) (Lin et al. 2007), poly(methacrylic acid) (PMMA) (Sajeesh and Sharma 2006), dextran sulfate (Sarmento et al. 2007), alginate (George and Abraham 2006). By this approach, the bioavailability of protein has been improved, and the encapsulated proteins could preserve up to 100% of biological activity at neutral pH.

Liu et al. have reported the preparation of CS based microspheres consisting of the preparation first of CMCS followed by the ionic gelation in CaCl$_2$ solution (Liu et al. 2007). BSA has been loaded in both CMCS beads and CMCS-CS beads, ionically cross-linked. Entrapment efficiency is a critical issue when hydrogels are used as DDSs, because the bioactive compounds such as enzymes, peptides and proteins are expensive, and low entrapment efficiency would limit the applicability of these systems. In the above mentioned systems, it was found that only 44.4% BSA has been entrapped in the Ca^{2+}-CMCS beads, while 73.2% BSA has been retained in the Ca^{2+}-CMCS-CS beads, when the surface of beads was further coated with a PEC membrane formed through the ionic interactions between CMCS and CS. The entrapment efficiency has increased with the increase of the CS concentration. The PEC membrane also had a strong influence on the release profile of BSA, because it has limited the swelling of beads and reduced the protein cumulative release.

Depending on the nature and target of the encapsulated protein/peptide drugs, the release rate and duration should be controlled in order to achieve the best therapeutic effect. Beads composed of CS and alginate, stabilized by electrostatic interactions, have been used in the controlled release of BSA (Nam et al. 2011, Shi et al. 2006). A very low amount of protein left the beads in acidic range (pH 1.2), while the cumulative release has been consistent (up to 80%, in 24 h) in simulated intestinal fluid (SIF) (pH 7.4) (Shi et al. 2006). Nam et al. have correlated the stability of microspheres having a core-shell design with the protein release kinetics. It was found that both the alginate-coated CS beads and the CS-coated alginate beads displayed a linear profile of BSA release (up to 10 days), but the CS-coated alginate beads, which have been less stable, showed a faster release profile (Nam et al. 2011).

Pulsatile release of insulin is required to achieve an efficient therapeutic effect because the insulin secretion in the body has a pulsatile release profile, glucose sensitive hydrogels being an alternative approach. In this context, biodegradable *in situ* gelling and environment sensitive systems based on CS have been developed for pulsatile delivery of insulin (Kasyap et al. 2007). Such thermoresponsive "auto-gels" have been prepared by adding α, β-glycerol phosphate (GP) to CS solution, the obtained mixture being liquid at room temperature and gelled at 37°C. Biosensitive gels have been obtained by adding GOD and peroxidase to the cold CS-GP solution, which upon heating at 37°C resulted in gel. Insulin loaded biosensitive gels have been prepared by adding insulin to the cooled enzyme-loaded CS-GP sol, which has gelled when incubated at 37°C (Kasyap et al. 2007). The sol/gel transition has been attributed by the authors to physical interactions including: the increase in the CS interchain hydrogen bonding by the reduction of electrostatic repulsion due to the basic action of GP; the CS–GP electrostatic attractions via the remaining ammonium and phosphate groups; the CS–CS hydrophobic interactions which were enhanced by the structuring action of GP on water. These gels have been tested both *in vitro* and *in vivo*, the pulsatile release manner of insulin being demonstrated.

2.2.2 Covalently stabilized gel carriers

The physically cross-linked gels have the advantage of the absence of chemical cross-linker, but they exhibit some drawbacks in the control of the gel pore size, and dissolution kinetics. Therefore, chemical cross-linking is used to improve the physical properties of the gels such as porosity, mechanical strength, and the entrapment and controlled release of drugs. Uptake and release of globular proteins such as LYS on biocompatible microgels based on cross-linked oxidized starch (OS) have been investigated by Li et al. (Li et al. 2009, Li et al. 2010, Zhao et al. 2015a). When chemical cross-linking of OS has been carried out with sodium trimetaphosphate (Li et al. 2009, Li et al. 2010), the uptake of LYS increased with the degree of oxidation of OS. Highly charged microgels, having intermediate cross-linker content, have been found optimal for the encapsulation of LYS. The degree of protein release from the microgels increased with the increase of pH and ionic strength, a complete release occurred at 0.2 M NaCl, increasing pH from 4 to 7. The authors considered that their microgels could be used in biomedical applications of proteins or peptide drugs with charge properties comparable with LYS, encapsulated drug being protected in the upper GIT and released in the intestine, where the pH is 6.8–7.4. Biodegradable microgels based on 2,2,6,6-tetramethyl(piperidin-1-yl) oxyl (TEMPO)-oxidized potato starch cross-linked with glycerol-1,3-diglycidyl ether (GDGE) have been recently reported, their sorption and controlled release properties for LYS being evaluated (Zhao et al. 2015a). The average diameter of the OS microgels ranged between 1 and 100 µm, the most particles being distributed between 10 and 20 µm. The protein adsorption isotherm showed the initial part of the curve has risen steeply, indicating a high affinity for protein at low concentrations. The sorption of LYS at saturation increased with the increase of the degree of oxidation, the optimal microgel corresponding to the 100% degree of oxidation and the lower cross-linking density (GDGE/polymer, w/w = 0.025), the optimum conditions for protein adsorption being pH 7 and 0.05 M NaCl. The protein release increased with the decrease of pH, suggesting a stronger electrostatic interaction at high pH than at low pH. However, the protein release dramatically increased with the increase of ionic strength, being the highest at 0.5 M NaCl, at pH 7. Acid-labile poly(N-vinylformamide) nanogels, about 100 nm in size, have been synthesized by Shi et al. via inverse emulsion polymerization of N-vinylformamide. It was found that nanogels having a monomer:cross-linker ratio of 7 had a 90 min half-time at pH 5.8 compared to ~57 h at pH 7.4, the release of LYS being ~95% over 200 min at pH 5.8 and ~15% at pH 7.4. At least 50% of protein activity has been reported (Shi et al. 2008).

An interesting approach has been recently reported by Knipe et al., whose strategy consists of the enzymatic biodegradation by trypsin of oligopeptide cross-linked microgels for insulin delivery to the small intestine (Knipe et al. 2015). The microgels based on poly(methacrylic acid-*co*-N-vinylpyrrolidone) and the degradation products posed no cytotoxic effect toward two cell lines. Microparticles and nanoparticles of poly(diethylaminoethyl methacrylate) (PDEAEM) cross-linked with tetraethylene glycol dimethacrylate, decorated with GOD and catalase for the controlled release of insulin, have been developed by Marek and Peppas (Marek and Peppas 2013). The authors found that the cross-linking ratio had a strong influence on the release of protein, the gels having a nominal cross-linking ratio of 10% releasing a third of the insulin payload, compared to about 70% of insulin released from the microparticles with 3% of cross-linking. The release of insulin has been triggered by either pH or glucose concentration. PDEAEM microparticles with diameter of 150 µm have been considered promising components for a system able to intelligent delivery insulin for type I diabetics.

BSA has been intensively used as a model in the investigations of the protein delivery from various particulate hydrogels as nanoparticles (Wan et al. 2009), microspheres (Kaygusuz and Erim 2013, Wan et al. 2009, Yang et al. 2013, Yuan et al. 2007), or powder (Kono et al. 2013). Thus, BSA has been incorporated into the quaternary CS nanoparticles based on O-(2-hydroxy) propyl-3-trimethyl ammonium chitosan chloride (O-HTCC) prepared by the ionic gelation with TPP (Wan et al. 2009). The burst release of BSA from the O-HTCC nanoparticles has been significantly lower than that found in the case of CS nanoparticles, the release profile supporting a sustained release of protein. In the case of microspheres formed by the cross-linking of CS with genipin, the swelling ratio decreased with the increase of cross-linking duration or with the genipin concentration, the release of protein decreasing accordingly, suggesting that the release rate of BSA could be controlled by the degree of cross-linking (Yuan et al. 2007).

Albumin adsorption and release profiles from CS-based polyampholyte hydrogel, based on CS covalently cross-linked with 1,2,3,4-butanetetracarboxylic dianhydride, has been recently reported (Kono et al. 2013). The polyampholyte hydrogel exhibited the maximal adsorption capacity of BSA, in the absence of NaCl, at pH 4.5, consistent with the *iep* of BSA. A high desorption of protein has been achieved (89%) in aqueous solution at pH 2.0.

Novel anionic composites have been prepared by the impregnation and cross-linking copolymerization of AAm in the pores of Daisogel silica, followed by post-hydrolysis of amide with generation of COO⁻ functional groups (Dragan and Bucatariu 2016). The schematic representation of the formation of PAAm hydrogel inside the Daisogel microspheres is presented in Fig. 1.

The silica supported anionic hydrogels were tested in the loading/release of the LYS as macromolecular drug, *iep* is situated at pH around 11. As shown in Fig. 2, *H* type sorption isotherms of LYS onto the novel composites have been found, which support a very high affinity of the anionically charged composite for the positively charged protein. It was found that the textural characteristics of the composite sorbent had an influence on the amount of LYS sorbed at equilibrium, this being higher in the case of the composite based on silica particles having a higher initial surface area (CSP300PAAm10.h) (Dragan and Bucatariu 2016).

The LYS adsorption data were fitted, by the non-linear regression method, to four isotherm models: Langmuir, Freundlich, Dubinin-Radushkevich and Sips. A high degree of fitness of the Sips isotherm model on the experimental data was found for the anionic composites, this fact being attributed to a homogeneous distribution of the active sites inside the

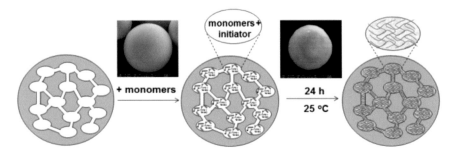

Fig. 1. Schematic representation of the composites formed by the impregnation of the Daisogel silica pores with anionic hydrogel (adapted from Dragan and Bucatariu 2016).

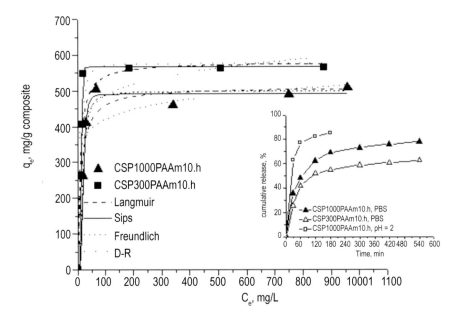

Fig. 2. Sorption isotherms of LYS onto Daisogel/PAAm10.h composites; the inset represents the profiles of cumulative release of LYS from Daisogel/PAAm. 10.h composites (adapted from Dragan and Bucatariu 2016).

composite. It was observed that both the morphology of Daisogel and the release medium of LYS had a strong influence on the profile of the release kinetics (the inset of Fig. 2). Thus, the release of LYS in PBS was faster in the case of the composite constructed with silica microspheres having a lower initial surface area and larger pores (CSP1000PAAm10.h) than in the case of the composite constructed with silica microspheres having a higher initial surface area and smaller pores (CSP300PAAm10.h). The influence of the textural properties of the sorbent on the release of LYS supports the distribution of protein molecules into the whole composite microsphere and not only on the surface. The faster release of LYS in pH 2 is attributed to the competition between protons and LYS for the COO⁻ groups in the composite at low pH. Decreasing the density of COO⁻ functional groups, the electrostatic interaction between the gel and LYS decreased and the release of LYS was promoted. Release mechanism of LYS as a function of the environment was a Fickian diffusion irrespective of the release medium and the morphology of Daisogel, supporting the feasibility of the anionically modified PAAm hydrogel confined in the silica pores as a promising sustained release system.

2.3 Films as macromolecular drugs carrier

Hydrogel films as drug carrier have been prepared either by synthesis of hybrid films such as kappa carrageenan (KC) and acrylic acid (AA) cross-linked with vinyltriethoxysilane (VTESi) (Rasool et al. 2010), or by the layer-by-layer (LbL) strategy (Dragan and Bucatariu 2010, Knipe and Peppas 2014, Zhao et al. 2011). The *in vitro* release profile of insulin from the hybrid films based on KC, AA and VTESi showed a negligible release of protein after the first 2 h in simulated gastric fluid (SGF), because the hydrogels have shrunk in the acidic media, while the insulin release has been consisted in SIF (pH 6.8), a sustained release being observed within 6 h (Rasool et al. 2010).

LbL deposition of oppositely charged species is a simple and versatile route to generate thin films with thickness and properties controlled at a molecular level (Bertrand et al. 2000, Dragan et al. 2010a). This technique is one of the most widely used to tailor surfaces with controlled loading and release of charged species, not only on hard (Bucatariu et al. 2013a, 2013b, Dragan and Bucatariu 2010, Macdonald et al. 2008, Macdonald et al. 2011) but also on soft substrates (Serizawa et al. 2002). The main characteristics of the films, such as thickness, roughness, morphology, stability and functional properties depend on the nature of the oppositely charged components, on the adsorption conditions, mainly on the charge density, pH and ionic strength, or post-fabrication treatments (Dragan et al. 2010a, Ghiorghita et al. 2016). Various LbL thin films based on microgels or micelles responsive to the external stimuli including light (Borges et al. 2014), pH (Kureha et al. 2016, Yusan et al. 2014, Zhao et al. 2011), and temperature (Clarke and Lyon 2013, Higashi et al. 2014, Hu and Lyon 2015, Kureha et al. 2016, Zhou et al. 2014) have been recently reported. A very interesting approach consists of the use of elastin-like peptides (ELP) as graft chains on poly(acrylic acid) (PAA) or PAAm as components of the thermo-responsive LbL films, whose lower critical solution temperature (LCST) could be precisely tuned by changing the amino acid in the penta-peptide sequence (Higashi et al. 2014). The layer thickness of these hybrid LbL films has been significantly affected by the deposition temperature, due to the presence of ELP, and the structural colour changes have been completely thermo-reversible. Zhou et al. have investigated the influence of film construction parameters such as number of layers, ionic strength, temperature and the outermost layer, on the drug release from the solid hexamethasone nanoparticles encapsulated in a model LbL assembly of tunable thickness consisting of poly(diallyldimethyl ammonium) chloride and poly(styrene sulfonate) (Zhou et al. 2014). The fine-tuning of the deswelling temperatures of the thermoresponsive microgel films based on N-isopropyl acrylamide (NIPAAm) and N-isopropyl methacrylamide within the range of 30–40°C has been demonstrated by Clarke and Lyon (Clarke and Lyon 2013). The films composed of more than one microgel building block have displayed multiple temperature responses, and response of the composite films consisting of microgels and polycation layers could be tuned not only by the microgel composition but also by the ratio between components.

Release of bioactive compounds such as proteins (Macdonald at al. 2008) and growth factors (Macdonald et al. 2011) from LbL thin films, in a controlled manner, has been achieved using hydrolytically degradable and biocompatible synthetic polycations and polysaccharide polyanions (heparin sulfate and chondroitin sulfate). LYS used as a model protein could be released with a linear trend over a period of approximately 14 days, this being very desirable for the drug delivery applications because it allows as constant and low levels of protein to be released from the surface (Macdonald et al. 2008). LbL encapsulation of proteins is also a candidate for the preservation of activity of encapsulated proteins due to the mild conditions used during the films' construction. The authors have found that 80%–100% of LYS activity has been preserved within the films. Thus, by combining hydrolytic degradability of a polycation directly with the protein of choice in LbL assembly (with heparin sulfate), it was possible to retain LYS for long periods of time.

Zhao et al. have fabricated composite microcapsules by the LbL deposition of insulin and alginate onto hydrocortisone (HC) crystals to prolong the release of HC under physiological conditions (Zhao et al. 2011). The core-shell structure has decomposed in PBS solution and the release rate of HC and insulin could be controlled by adjusting the number of insulin/alginate bilayers. The secondary structure of insulin has changed during the LbL construction and release process. Furthermore, the insulin release lagged behind the HC, decreasing hyperglycemia, which is the side effect of HC. This synergy effect might enable a novel way in using one carrier to deliver two kinds of drugs, simultaneously reducing their side effects (Zhao et al. 2011).

The interaction of proteins with LbL coated surfaces is a complex phenomenon, which has been widely investigated in the last decades to minimize or to enhance the protein adsorption onto the films. Thus, *in situ* cross-linked LbL films of poly(vinyl amine) (PVAm) as single component have been constructed onto silica microparticles and silicon wafers by selective cross-linking of PVAm chains in the films of PVAm/PAA, followed by the removal of PAA (Dragan and Bucatariu 2010, Dragan et al. 2010b). The highest amount of human serum albumin (HSA) has been adsorbed on the films constructed with low PVAm and high PAA. The decrease of the film roughness after the adsorption of HSA showed that the protein has been adsorbed into the (PVAm)$_n$ films making these films potential reservoirs for proteins. Single polycation cross-linked multilayer thin films have been also prepared by the 3,3′,4,4′-benzophenonetetracarboxylic dianhydride (BTCDA)–mediated electrostatic and hydrogen bonds LbL assembly with either poly(ethylene imine) (PEI) (Bucatariu et al. 2013a) or CS (Bucatariu et al. 2013b). In the fabrication of these films, BTCDA has played both the role of cross-linker and the supplier of carboxylic groups. The immobilization of pepsin (PEP) and LYS on the LbL films deposited onto silica microparticles showed that the amount of the attached enzyme significantly depended on the *iep* of the enzyme. Thus, PEP, an enzyme with *iep* in acidic region of pH, has been successfully immobilized onto the cross-linked LbL films of PEI (up to 90 mg PEP/g composite), where *iep* has been situated at around 8.0 (Bucatariu et al. 2013a), while LYS, an enzyme with *iep* in basic region of pH, has been preferentially immobilized onto the LbL films of CS, where *iep* has been located at around 4.5 (Bucatariu et al. 2013b).

3. Synthesis and Characterization of Porous Hydrogels

Macroporous hydrogels have been synthesized as a better alternative to the conventional hydrogels, of which main weak points are the slow kinetics of swelling and low mechanical strength. There are several main techniques used to create pores in hydrogels, including: (i) cross-linking polymerization in the presence of pore forming agents, when a phase separation occurs (Okay 2000); (ii) cross-linking in the presence of substances releasing gases (Caykara et al. 2007, Gürdag and Gökalp 2011, Kabiri and Zohurian Mehr 2004, Mahdavinia et al. 2009, Sun et al. 2015); (iii) porogen leaching (Dinu et al. 2013, Přádný et al. 2010, Přádný et al. 2014, Sokic et al. 2014, Zhang et al. 2012); (iv) freeze-drying (lyophilization) of the equilibrium swollen hydrogels (Baek et al. 2015, Buranachai et al. 2010, Dragan et al. 2009, Dragan et al. 2012a, Huang et al. 2011, Wang et al. 2008a, Wang et al. 2008b, Wang et al. 2013, Wu and Wang 2010, Zhang et al. 2011); (v) freezing/thawing (Jaiswal et al. 2013, Lee et al. 2011, Qi et al. 2015); (vi) cryogelation (ice templating) (Ak et al. 2013, Dinu et al. 2007, Dinu et al. 2013, Dragan

2014a, Dragan et al. 2016, Dragan and Cocarta 2016, Hu et al. 2014, Lozinsky 2014, Tylingo et al. 2016, Zhao et al. 2011). Some of the above mentioned techniques are presented in more detail in the next subsections.

3.1 Gas foaming and porogen leaching

Foaming technique consists of using a foaming agent such as $NaHCO_3$ (Gürdag and Gökalp 2011, Kabiri and Zohurian Mehr 2004), $CaCO_3$ (Mahdavinia et al. 2009, Sun et al. 2015), or supercritical CO_2 ($scCO_2$) (Rinki et al. 2009), able to generate CO_2 in mildly acidic solutions. The foaming/blowing agent is mixed into the prepolymer and generates gas bubbles *via* chemical reactions or by expelling from a pre-saturated gas/polymer mixture prepared at high pressure. Ammonium bicarbonate is another gas blowing agent that was used to produce macroporous hydrogels with interconnected pores *via* its decomposition into CO_2 and NH_3. A porous morphology with pores' sizes ranging from 100 to 500 µm can be formed by this technique (Bajaj et al. 2014). The blowing agents used for pore formation are generally friendly, this technique not involving the use of any organic solvents, which makes it appropriate for biomedical applications. The release kinetic of KNO_3 from a porous hydrogel prepared in the presence of $CaCO_3$ as foaming agent showed a faster release of the active compound from the porous gel compared with nonporous hydrogel, the release kinetic being closely related with the fast sorption of water (Mahdavinia et al. 2009).

The use of $scCO_2$ as 'green' medium to induce porosity inside of CS scaffolds (Rinki et al. 2009) was also reported. The $scCO_2$ method allows the preparation of porous scaffolds suitable for cell cultures directly upon depressurization. However, CO_2 generally has a low solubility in hydrophilic polymers. To improve the ability of this dense gas to diffuse into a hydrophilic polymer and produce porosity, various techniques, such as CO_2—water emulsion templating or the use of co-solvent systems, have been developed (Bajaj et al. 2014). One of the biggest advantages of this technique is the use of relatively inert foaming agents without the involvement of organic solvents. However, it has been reported that only 10–30% of the pores are interconnected, which highlights the diffusion limitations for hydrogels used as biomaterials (Bajaj et al. 2014).

According to the porogen leaching technique, the cross-linking polymerization takes place in the presence of soluble substances, usually as solid particles, including sucrose (Gurdag and Gokalp 2011), NaCl (Park et al. 2007, Přádný et al. 2010, Přádný et al. 2014), polymers (Kuo and Wang 2013, Phull et al. 2013, Sato et al. 2015, Sokic et al. 2014), SiO_2 (Serizawa et al. 2002, Yang et al. 2015, Zeng and Ruckenstein 1998), which are leached out from the hydrogel after polymerization. Interconnected (Přádný et al. 2010, Zhang et al. 2012) and non-interconnected micro-, macropores

(Kuo and Wang 2013, Phull et al. 2013, Sato et al. 2015, Sokic et al. 2014) could be generated by this method. The major advantage of porogen leaching technique consists of the facile control of pore size and overall porosity only by selecting the nature, size, geometry and concentration of the particles loaded into the prepolymer. The reduced control over the orientation and degree of pore interconnectivity, as well as the difficulties concerning the removal of soluble particles from the interior of 3D matrices are the major limitations associated with porogen leaching strategy. Moreover, it should be mentioned that, in most of the particle leaching methods, different organic solvents are involved (Park et al. 2007), which are highly toxic and require long drying times to assure their complete removal. However, macroporous 3D silk fibroin (SF) hydrogels have been recently prepared in the presence of NaCl by a salt-leaching procedure in organic solvent-free conditions (Zhang et al. 2012). The driving force in the generation of porosity in this case consists of the transformation of SF structure from a random coil to a β-sheet, the salt also having the role to promote the water loss from the hydrophobic domains, leading to enhanced chain-chain interactions and thus to β-sheet formation. The hydrogel morphology could be modulated by the concentration of SF and the ratio between NaCl and SF.

3.2 *Freeze-drying (lyophilization) and freezing-thawing*

Freeze-drying, also known as lyophilization, is a simple and efficient process to create porous hydrogels and consists in rapid freezing of hydrogel swollen at equilibrium in water followed by the sublimation of water under reduced pressure, and this leaves behind a highly porous polymeric structure with interconnected pores. The hydrogel morphology (pore size and shape, thickness of pore walls) is a function of the freezing regime, the concentration of the polymer (Pradny et al. 2010), the size of the ice crystals, and the solution pH (Bajaj et al. 2014). It was also demonstrated that the porosity could be modulated by the freeze-drying pressure. Thus, porous hydrogels based on the cross-linked pullulan/dextran containing pores with a mean diameter of 55 ± 4 µm and a porosity of 33 ± 12% have been prepared at high freeze-drying pressure (6.5 mbar), while hydrogels consisting of much larger pores with a mean diameter of 243 ± 14 µm and a porosity of 68 ± 3% have been obtained at low freeze-drying pressure (0.1 mbar) (Autissier et al. 2010). Porosity has been developed by lyophilization in various stimuli-responsive hydrogels, having potential in applications as intelligent drug carriers, either synthetic (Huang et al. 2011, Wang et al. 2008a, Wang et al. 2008b, Zhang et al. 2011) or composite hydrogels (Baek et al. 2015, Bocourt et al. 2011, Buranachai et al. 2010, Dragan et al. 2009, Dragan et al. 2012a, Dragan 2014a, Wang et al. 2013). Architectures with interconnected pores of various sizes have been reported for these hydrogels. The internal morphology and the pore size have been mainly influenced by the hydrogel cross-linking, the increase of the cross-linker ratio conducting to hydrogels with a more compact structure and smaller pore sizes (Dragan et al. 2012a, Wei et al. 2015a, Wei et al. 2015b). Another benefit of this technique is that it allows the incorporation of protein-based growth factors during the scaffold processing. However, there are some disadvantages of this technique including difficulties in the precise tuning of the hydrogel morphology, the low structural stability and weak mechanical properties.

Freezing-thawing is another technique used to modulate the morphology of the preformed hydrogels and consists in using some alternate freeze/thaw cycles, whose duration could be established according to the application requirements (Lee et al. 2011, Qi et al. 2015). The porous structure is formed during the first freeze/thaw cycle and involves not only the formation of ice crystals, but also the phase separation into a polymer-rich and a polymer-poor phase. However, the phase separation taking place during the initial freezing step is not complete, resulting in the formation of a polymer-poor phase that still contains important amounts of polymer. Therefore, to circumvent this drawback, the repetition of freezing–thawing cycles was used, an example being the preparation of composite hydrogels by the incorporation of salecan, a novel water-soluble microbial polysaccharide, into poly(vinyl alcohol) (PVA), three consecutive cycles of freezing at –20°C for 18 h and thawing at 25°C for 6 h being applied (Qi et al. 2015).

3.3 Cryogelation (ice templating)

Since Lozinsky et al. have coined cryogelation as a versatile and friendly technique to prepare porous hydrogels by covalent cross-linking under the freezing temperature of water (Lozinsky et al. 1982), this strategy has attracted numerous research groups (Ak et al. 2013, Dinu et al. 2007, Dinu et al. 2011, Dinu et al. 2013, Dragan 2014b, Dragan and Apopei Loghin 2013, Dragan et al. 2016, Dragan and Cocarta 2016, Hu et al. 2014, Lozinski et al. 2003, Tylingo et al. 2016, Zhao et al. 2011). Cryogelation is related to the technique of porogen leaching, the porogen in this case being constituted by the ice crystals, which leave the pores simply and fast by thawing after the cryogel synthesis (Henderson et al. 2013, Lozinsky 2014), unlike the porogen leaching which needs long time and sometimes toxic solvents to completely remove the porogen particles, the pores thus formed being often closed. In cryogelation, the microstructure of the gel is the negative replica of the ice crystals. Thus, cryogelation is a low cost and very friendly technique for the fabrication of supermacroporous gels. Cryogels can withstand high levels of deformations, being also characterized by superfast responsiveness to water absorption. A large variety of monomers and polymers, either synthetic or natural, have been used to prepare superporous hydrogels (cryogels), either as single networks or as composite cryogels including semi-interpenetrating polymer networks (semi-IPN) or IPN cryogels (Dinu et al. 2011, Dragan and Apopei 2013, Dragan et al. 2012b, Dragan 2014a, Dragan et al. 2016, Dragan and Cocarta 2016, Hu et al. 2014, Tylingo et al. 2016, Zhao et al. 2011). Cryogels, by their inter-connected pores, allow the unhindered diffusion of solutes or even colloidal particles. Therefore, from the beginning, cryogels have been very attractive in biomedicine and biotechnology including chromatographic materials, carriers for the immobilization of molecules and cells, matrices for cell separations, and cell culture. The most representative destinations of cryogels are biotechnological, including bioseparations and bioreactors (Kumar and Srivastava 2010, Lozinsky et al. 2001, Lozinsky et al. 2003), and biomedical applications, such as drug delivery, actuators, tissue engineering (cartilage, artificial organs), and so on (Dragan et al. 2016, Dragan and Cocarta 2016, Henderson et al. 2013, Jain et al. 2011, Jain et al. 2015, Kathuria et al. 2009), but their use as sorbents for the removal of various pollutants should also be mentioned (Dragan et al. 2012b, Dragan and Apopei Loghin 2013).

A combination of porogen leaching and cryogelation has been recently developed by Dinu et al. in order to generate 3D networks with permeable walls (having pores inside), which could allow the unrestricted diffusion of nutrients when macropores are filled with cells (Dinu et al. 2013). According to this strategy, the fractionated poly(methylmethacrylate) particles of different sizes have been enclosed within the pore walls of a CS network during the cross-linking with glutaraldehyde (GA) at −18°C, and were washed out from the cryogel by extraction, after the gel formation. CS cryogels have been thus prepared, having interconnected pores and less compact walls. A better control on the morphology of cryogels has been achieved by the unidirectional freezing of various systems including aqueous polymer solutions or composite systems consisting of water, organic polymer and inorganic particles, using various freezing agents such as liquid nitrogen, and frozen ethanol, when the ice crystals formed and grew unidirectionally. Micro-channeled structures aligned along the freezing direction have been thus obtained, characterized by well-defined morphologies (e.g., micro-honeycomb or lamellar) (Dinu et al. 2013, Zhang et al. 2015). The size of pores and the pore wall thickness have been adjusted by varying the initial monomer or polymer concentration, the molecular weight of polymer as well as the crystallization speed (Bai et al. 2013, Dinu et al. 2013, Zhang et al. 2015).

4. Porous Hydrogels as Carrier of Macromolecular Drugs

4.1 Overview of the preparation and characterization methods of porous hydrogels for delivery of macromolecular drugs

Macroporous temperature-sensitive poly(N-isopropylacrylamide) (PNIPAAm) hydrogels have been synthesized in the presence of PEG with molar mass of 2000–6000 g/mol, as pore-forming agent (Zhuo and Li 2003). The macroporous hydrogels have been characterized by swelling ratio, deswelling-reswelling kinetics, Fourier transform infrared spectroscopy (FTIR), differential scanning calorimetry (DSC), and scanning electron microscopy (SEM). It was found that the average pore size of the hydrogels increased with the increase of PEG molar mass, being in the range of 60–80 μm when PEG with 6000 g/mol has been used. The swelling, deswelling and reswelling kinetics have been influenced by the PEG content, irrespective of PEG molar mass, swelling ratio increasing with the increase of PEG content. The loading of BSA into macroporous hydrogels increased with the increase of the pore size and number, and the release profile of protein from the PNIPAAm macroporous hydrogels has showed a sustained release up to 120 h, the release rate increasing with the increase of the PEG molar mass.

CS affinity membranes are largely suggested for the immobilization of proteins and enzymes and therefore, there is a continuous interest in finding membranes whose properties could be tailored for desired applications. Porous CS-based membranes for protein separation have been prepared by leaching silica used as porogen in alkali solutions, taking the advantage of the insolubility of CS in basic pH (Chen et al. 2005, Zeng and Ruckenstein 1998). Porogen leaching technique has been also recently used by Yang et al. for the preparation of macroporous CS membranes, silica with sizes in the range 70–230 μm being used as porogen in silica/CS weight ratios of 1:15, 1:20 and 1:25 (Yang et al. 2015). Three different cross-linkers (1,4-butanediol diglycidyl ether, GA and epichlorohydrin (ECH) have been used for the chemical cross-linking of CS membranes, the membranes being used for the immobilization of BSA and *laccase*. Increasing the particle size of silica led to the increase of the pore size, the extent of enzyme immobilization increasing, and the relative enzyme activity being enhanced several folds of its original activity. Increasing the pH, the relative activity gradually decreased, and thus the enzymatic activity is stable at low pH only, while in the case of free enzymes, the relative activity sharply decreased on increasing the pH values. The higher stability against thermal and pH denaturation compared to that of free enzymes has been explained by the fact that the cross-linking prevented the unfolding of the enzymes under thermal and pH stress conditions (Yang et al. 2015). The results obtained from enzyme activity studies clearly indicated that increased pore size and thickness of the membrane facilitated the effective immobilization of enzyme as well as the enhanced relative enzyme activity. Both BSA and *laccase* showed similar trend of behaviour and hence both are equally capable of enhancing their activity upon immobilization.

As it has been already mentioned in Introduction, the low bioavailability of proteins at their oral administration demands their encapsulation in novel and advanced systems able to achieve sustained release, extended shelf-life, and reduction of adverse reactions. The repeated freezing-thawing cycles technique has been adopted to prepare poly(vinyl alcohol) (PVA)-poly(lactic)-*co*-glycolic acid (PLGA) core-shell particles for BSA encapsulation (Lee et al. 2011). It was reported that by increasing the number of cycles, the crystallinity of PVA increased, the hardening of the surface layer being the main cause for the sustained release kinetics of protein.

Chang et al. have reported the preparation of superabsorbent composite hydrogels consisting of carboxymethylcellulose sodium (CMC) and cellulose cross-linked together with ECH, which exhibited smart swelling and shrinkage in NaCl and $CaCl_2$ aqueous solutions (Chang et al. 2010). The size of pores increased with the increase of CMC content, suggesting that the electrostatic repulsion between the $-COO^-$ groups in CMC induced a more loose morphology while cellulose acted as strengthening for the composite hydrogel. The release behaviour of BSA could be tuned by changing the CMC content in the composite hydrogel, a faster release of protein being observed for the highest content in CMC, which shows that larger pores induced a faster release of BSA.

Yin et al. have synthesized superporous hydrogels (SPH) containing poly(AA-*co*-acrylamide)/O-CMC interpenetrating polymer networks (SPH-IPNs), the second network being formed by cross-linking O-CMC with GA. The hydrogels have been synthesized using $NaHCO_3$ as blowing agent to enhance the mechanical strength, *in vitro* muco-adhesive force and protein loading capacity (Yin et al. 2007, Yin et al. 2010). It was found an optimum ratio between O-CMC and acrylic monomers, homogeneous hydrogels with a high number of interconnected pores being obtained when the ratio was lower than 0.192, in the presence of Pluronic PF127 for foam stabilization. Insulin was used as a model protein to study the drug-loading capacities of the SPH-IPNs and drug release in SIF. Loading capacities with protein of the SPH-IPNs have been significantly higher than those of non-porous hydrogels. Furthermore, the IPN structure of the composite hydrogels prevented the protein-loaded hydrogel from collapsing during desiccation (Yin et al. 2007). The effect of polymer integrity on the efficacy of SPH-IPN as an oral protein delivery system has been evaluated by comparing integral-SPH-IPN with powdered-SPH-IPN, both *in vitro* and *in vivo*. Although I-SPH-IPN and P-SPH-IPN had comparable *in vitro* enzymatic inhibition capacities, I-SPH-IPN possessed notable superiority to P-SPH-IPN in *in vivo* enzymatic inhibition, permeation enhancing effect, and intestinal retention as a result of its preferable physical integrity that exerted stronger mechanical pressures to the intestinal epithelia. Thus, a significant increase in the undegraded insulin has been observed in the presence of integral-SPH-IPN, indicating that the physical integrity of SPH-IPN has been important for the *in vivo* enzymatic inhibition capacity and insulin stability (Yin et al. 2010).

Various macroporous IPN hydrogels, having pores generated by lyophilization, have been promoted, in the last decade, as vehicles for oral delivery of macromolecular drugs (Bocourt et al. 2011, Dutta et al. 2016, Hu et al. 2016, Kundu et al. 2012, Liu and Cui 2011, Wu and Wang 2010). Bocourt et al. have prepared CS/poly(AA-*co*-AAm) IPNs hydrogels, the effect of monomer feed composition and alkaline hydrolysis being investigated not only on the composite morphology and water uptake but also in terms of the hydrogels' abilities for loading/release of BSA as model protein (Bocourt et al. 2011). Hydrogels' swelling was controlled by the interaction between the amide groups of AAm and the carboxylic groups of AA. Higher loadings have been achieved for samples with lower AA content, while samples richer in AA exhibited lower swelling due to the higher density of carboxylate on their surface, which could hamper BSA adsorption by anionic electrostatic repulsion. BSA loading capacity was higher in the hydrolyzed hydrogels due to their high water content and greater porosity. BSA release from the composite hydrogels has been evaluated at pH 1.2 (SGF), pH 6.8 (SIF), and pH 7.4 (PBS). BSA release experiments showed that these composite hydrogels have been capable of sustained release at pH 6.8 and 7.4 for more than 10 h. BSA released from all hydrogels maintained its structural integrity at 6.7 and 7.4, which is a desirable requirement for preserving protein activity. The fact that hydrolyzed hydrogels exhibited limited BSA release in SGF and sustained release in SIF showed that they are good candidates as matrices for colon-specific sustained protein release formulations.

Last decade, the natural polymers including CS, cellulose, alginate, gelatin, guar gum, SF have attracted an increasing interest in the development of new biomaterials and devices for the biomedical and pharmaceutical applications owing to their intrinsic advantages of renewability, biodegradability, and low toxicity. In this context, macroporous and biocompatible IPN hydrogels composed of a protein and a synthetic hydrophilic polymer including SF/PVA (Kundu et al. 2012), soy protein/PNIPAm (Liu and Cui 2011) and silk sericin/PMAA (Wu and Wang 2010) attracted the interest as vehicles for macromolecular drugs such as proteins. The thermosensitive soy protein/PNIPAm IPN hydrogels have been prepared by free radical polymerization of NIPAm in the presence of GA and N,N'-methylenebisacrylamide (BAAm) as the cross-linking agents and ammonium persulfate as the initiator. It was found that increasing the content of soy protein led to stronger intermolecular hydrogen bonds. The IPN hydrogels had good miscibility and high porosity and interconnectivity (honey like morphology), the volume phase transition temperatures (VPTT) of all composite hydrogels being located at around 32°C. The release of BSA from the hydrogels has been strongly temperature dependent, and could be modulated by controlling the content of soy protein or BAAm. The analysis of the release mechanism revealed that the Fickian diffusion controlled release was dominant under the experimental conditions (Liu and Cui 2011).

Macroporous pH-responsive silk sericin/PMAA IPN hydrogels were prepared by the simultaneous strategy (Wu and Wang 2010). The swelling of the IPNs revealed that the hydrogels displayed definite pH sensitivity under physiological conditions, as well as sharp changes in the mesh size of their network as a function of composition and medium pH. In all cases, it was found that the release rate of BSA was lower in acidic media and higher in basic media. These composite hydrogels showed potential as protein delivery system because they undergo a significant volume transition from pH 2.6 to 7.4 and have been partially degraded *in vivo*.

Fabrication of a newer type of drug releasing photo-crosslinked hydrogel based on a semi-IPN consisting of PVA-methacrylate and SF, possessing tailorable structural and release properties has been reported by Kundu et al. Fluorescein isothiocyanate (FITC)–dextrans of different molar masses have been chosen as model drugs to evaluate the release behaviour of macromolecular drugs from these composite hydrogels (Kundu et al. 2012). SEM images revealed that all the samples had 3-D morphologies with uniform porous structures within the PVA/SF semi-IPN hydrogels. Decreasing the PVA content resulted in the decrease of the pore density. However, the hydrogels containing higher SF contents (about 30 wt.%) have larger pores and an irregular shape with a long axis dimension in the range 40–60 μm. The release of FITC–dextrans from the composite hydrogels was dependent on the SF content and on the molar mass of the encapsulated molecules. The morphology of the hydrogels dramatically affects the drug release behaviour of the composite hydrogel. It is known that the release rate of the solute could be retarded either increasing the molecular weight of the solute or increasing the cross-linking density of the network. The effects of hydrogel composition on the *in vitro* drug release behaviour of the composite hydrogels have been investigated at 37°C, in PBS for more than 7 days. All hydrogels in this study exhibited an initial burst release, due to the instantaneous release of drug from the surface of the hydrogel. It was found that FITC–dextrans have been released at a faster rate from gels with higher SF contents.

Novel pH, temperature and redox responsive semi-IPN hydrogels having CMC entrapped in PNIPAAm matrix cross-linked with BAAm or N,N'-bis(acryloyl)cystamine (CBA) have been recently reported (Dutta et al. 2016). Temperature dependent swelling studies revealed that semi-IPN hydrogels exhibited a VPTT around 32°C. CBA cross-linked hydrogels showed higher swelling in comparison to those cross-linked with BAAm. With the increase of CMC content in the hydrogels, pore size increased, because the increase of CMC content caused a higher hindrance in the formation of PNIPAAm network resulting in the increase of the porosity. The encapsulation efficiency of LYS after 48 h at pH ~7.4 at 25°C increased with the increase in CMC content in the composite hydrogels. Such behaviour has been attributed to the strong interactions between LYS, positively charged at pH ~7.4, and CMC which is negatively charged at this pH. *In vitro* release of LYS has been studied in SIF (pH = 7.4) and SGF (pH = 1.2) at 25°C and 37°C, in the presence and absence of glutathione (GSH). The maximum cumulative release was found to be 80%, the release profile being fast in the first 10 h, followed by a slow release over the next 72 h. The release rate of LYS at pH = 7.4 was slower than that at pH = 1.2 (about 21% LYS compared with 42.8%, after 10 h). The LYS release reached maximum values of about 67.5% and 27% at pH = 1.2 and pH = 7.4 respectively, after 72 h, hence the degree of ionization of CMC in water decreases significantly on decreasing pH from 7.4 to 1.2. The interaction between LYS and CMC at pH 1.2 becomes weaker compared to pH 7.4 because the pK_a of the -CH_2-COO^- groups in CMC is around 4.3 and, therefore, the release of LYS has become faster. Similarly, at a temperature below the VPTT (i.e., at 25°C) of the hydrogels, the protein release rate was higher than at 37°C. GSH is the most abundant low-molecular-weight intracellular reducing molecule. It was also observed that the presence of 20 mM GSH as a reducing agent led to a faster release of LYS when CBA has been used as cross-linker but had no influence in the case of BAAm. About 58.2% LYS has been released in 10 h at 25°C and pH = 1.2, whereas in the absence of GSH ~42.8% LYS was released in the same period of time. After 72 h, the LYS release amount was found to be 67.48% and 78.2% in pure buffer solution and buffer solution containing GSH respectively. Similar observation was also found at 37°C. The results show that in the presence of GSH as a reducing agent, a higher release of LYS was mainly attributed to the degradation of the di-sulphide bonds of the cross-linker.

Composite alginate/CMCS beads for oral delivery of proteins have been prepared by dual ionic cross-linking consisting of cross-linking of alginate with Ca^{2+} ions and of CCMCS with β-GP (Hu et al. 2016). The absence of new peaks in the FTIR spectra of the sodium alginate/CMCS composite beads indicated that the gels have been formed exclusively by physical cross-linking. The composite beads have slightly swollen in SGF but at high extent in SIF, due to the electrostatic repulsion between COO⁻ groups and the relaxation of chains. The chemical degradation in SIF at 37°C showed that the SA/CMCS composite beads have lost a large dry weight within 12 h, the degradation rate increasing with the increase of beads swelling ratio (Hu et al. 2016). The SA-CMCS composite beads cross-linked with increasing amounts of β-GP have been loaded with BSA as a model macromolecular drug during the cross-linking (before the beads formation in $CaCl_2$ solution). Dried test samples were set to swell in SGF and subsequently in SIF, at 37°C. The release of BSA from the composite beads indicated a pH-dependent behaviour. Thus, at pH 1.2, the amount of released drug was lower than 10%, while at pH 7.4, the content of released BSA have strongly increased for all beads. The high content of released drug at pH 7.4 can be assigned to the higher swelling of the gel beads in the neutral solution, the drug release time being prolonged for more than 11 h. The largest cumulative release ratio was 97%, i.e., in the case of the beads with the highest swelling ratio in SIF. However, for the pure SA/Ca^{2+} beads taken as reference, BSA has been completely released within 6 h due to the rapid disintegration of SA network. Thus, the authors have demonstrated that the SA/CMCS composite beads allowed a better controlled and sustained protein release (Hu et al. 2016).

Electron beam (EB) has been used as a clean route to prepare stimuli-responsive hydrogels having potential as oral delivery systems for proteins, in this way eliminating any potential toxic effects associated with chemical cross-linkers (Ahmad et al. 2014, LoPresti et al. 2011). Thus, bacterial cellulose-*g*-PAA (BC-*g*-PAA) hydrogels have been prepared, the degree of cross-linking, swelling, pore size, mechanical strength, and drug release profiles being tuned by varying the EB irradiation dose (Ahmad et al. 2014). The loading efficiency of BSA into the BC-*g*-PAA hydrogels has been 40–55%, increasing with the increase of the swelling ratio. Limited BSA release (<10%) was observed in SGF (for 2 h) from all hydrogels. However, when the hydrogels have been moved to SIF (pH 6.8), a rapid increase in BSA release was observed due to higher swelling of the hydrogels at higher pH. In addition, incorporation of mucoadhesive polymers into the hydrogel structure has been shown to prolong the duration of hydrogel residence in the intestine, thereby enhancing the absorbance of protein by maintaining intimate contact with mucus (Ahmad et al. 2014).

Very recently, Zhao et al. have developed a one-pot synthetic methodology for fabricating magnetic field-responsive hemicellulose hydrogels (MFRHHs) consisting of the *in situ* formation of magnetic iron oxide (Fe_3O_4) nanoparticles during the covalent cross-linking of O-acetyl-galactoglucomannan (Zhao et al. 2015b). The MFRHHs exhibited a much larger BSA adsorption capacity than the pure hemicellulose hydrogels. Thus, the MFRHHs containing 15% (w/w) Fe_3O_4 nanoparticles exhibited a BSA adsorption capacity of 146.5 mg/g. Upon the release of BSA, a burst release during the initial stage has been observed because the BSA loaded near the hydrogel surface could be immediately released in PBS (pH = 7.2–7.4). Based on the release curves, BSA was released more rapidly from the hydrogels during the first 12 h. More than 80% of BSA has been released from the gel without Fe_3O_4 nanoparticles, and less than 74% of BSA has been released from the composite hydrogel having 15% (w/w) Fe_3O_4 nanoparticles after 5 days. Thus, MFRHHs with tunable and controllable adsorption and release properties having potential applications in controlled release of proteins have been prepared (Zhao et al. 2015b).

A novel physically stabilized composite hydrogel has been prepared by the electrostatic interaction (polyelectrolyte complexation) between N-[(2-hydroxy-3-trimethylammonium) propyl] chitosan chloride (HTCC) and GP (Shi et al. 2011). Surface morphology analysis demonstrated that HTCC/GP hydrogels had 3D porous structures with pores in the range of 5 of 40 μm. The insulin has been entrapped during the formation of hydrogel. *In vitro* release of insulin was controlled by modifying the composition, drug loading, and pH conditions (Shi et al. 2011). It was found that the hydrogels dissolved and released insulin quickly under acidic condition, whereas it released drug slowly under neutral or basic conditions, the polyelectrolyte complex being stable under these conditions.

The delivery of insulin by noninvasive methods including transdermal, nasal, oral, ocular, and rectal routes is limited by its short half-life, low permeation rates, and digestion by various proteolytic enzymes (Khafagy et al. 2007). The transdermal drug delivery (TDD) of insulin can avoid its metabolism and the first-pass effect with a long and sustained release feature and may thus be the optimum route of administration. To enhance the permeation rate of insulin through the skin, Zu et al. have used the micronization of drug particles by the supercritical antisolvent (SAS) process (Zu et al. 2012). The nano-insulin-loaded CS–PVA blend hydrogels were prepared with GA as the cross-linking agent. The morphologies of the freeze-dried hydrogel films prepared using different cross-linking ratios showed a porous honeycomb-like structure for the hydrogel films having 3.6% and 4.8% cross-linking ratios, the pore diameter being about 20 μm and 5 μm, respectively. SEM images of the freeze-dried nano-insulin-loaded hydrogel showed a highly porous hydrogel film structure, i.e., the morphology of hydrogel remained unchanged after the loading of insulin nanoparticles, and this supports the miscibility between the hydrogel and the nano-insulin and that the loose pore structure facilitates the penetration of the nano-insulin into the hydrogel film. A linear relationship between the cumulative release profile and time has been observed, and the release coefficient of insulin was 4.421 μg/(cm^2 h). Thus, the *in vitro* insulin release supports the possibility to design a suitable TDD system for insulin administration in the diabetes chemotherapy (Zu et al. 2012).

Cryostructuration technique has been recently used to fabricate macroporous carriers for macromolecular drugs, either by freezing-thawing repeated cycles (physical cryogels) (Lazaridou et al. 2015), or by covalent cross-linking under the freezing temperature of the solvent (chemical cryogels) (Dragan et al. 2016, Huo et al. 2010, Kudaibergenov et al. 2016). Macroporous amphoteric cryogels based on DMAEM and MAA have been recently reported by Kudaibergenov et al., their particular advantage being the capability to adsorb both positively and negatively charged species by playing with the pH of the environment (Kudaibergenov et al. 2016). Thus, at pH 5.3, which has been lower than the *iep* of the cross-linked amphoteric macroporous cryogels (the value of *iep* depended on the molar ratio between the two comonomers, being 7.1 for the cryogel having DMAEM in excess) the negatively charged species such as methyl orange (MO) and an anionic surfactant have been adsorbed, while the adsorption of LYS and methylene blue (MB) was carried out in buffer solution at pH 9.5. The reason is the P(DMAEM-*co*-MAA) is positively charged at pH 5.3 due to ionization of tertiary amine groups and negatively charged at pH 9.5 due to ionization of carboxylic groups, being electroneutral at the *iep* (pH 7.1). The release of all ionic species reached up to 98% at the *iep* of amphoteric cryogel (pH$_{iep}$ = 7.1), because at the *iep* of the amphoteric cryogel, the cooperativity of intrachain interactions between the acidic and basic groups (formation of inner salt) exceed the interchain interactions between cryogel and ionic species (LYS, surfactant and dyes), resulting in the release of all species irrespective of their charge. Therefore, a negligible amount of molecules have been retained within the pores of cryogel at its *iep*.

The potential of PMAA/CS composite hydrogels in controlled DDSs has been recently supported by the preparation of novel IPNs hydrogels consisting of either P(MAA-*co*-AAm) or P[(MAA)-*co*-2-hydroxyethylmethacrylate (HEMA)] as the 1st network and covalently cross-linked CS as the 2nd network (Dragan et al. 2016). The 1st network has been synthesized by cryogelation at –18°C, and the 2nd network was generated by an amine/epoxy addition reaction between the primary amine groups of CS and the epoxy groups in poly(ethyleneglycol) diglycidyl ether (PEGDGE), in basic medium (Scheme 1).

It is known that, the pore size and the pore walls can affect the sorption/release properties of the hydrogels to a great extent. The SEM images presented in Fig. 3 show the differences between the interior morphology of the gels as a function of the synthesis conditions, for single network cryogels (SNCs) (up), and for the corresponding IPN gels (down).

A sponge-like morphology has been found in all SNCs, the average diameter of pores being 63 μm, 42 μm, 63 μm, and 95 μm for A55.20.5, A55.20.10, A73.20.5, and H73.20.10, respectively. The average pore diameter has been influenced by the MAA content at a lesser level but significantly

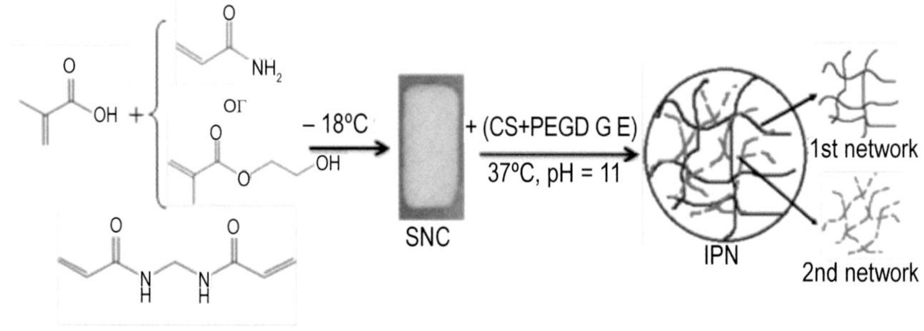

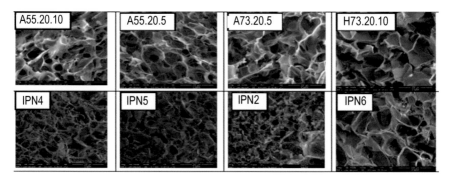

Scheme 1. Schematic representation of the synthesis of single network cryogels (SNC) and of the IPN gels by the sequential strategy (adapted from Dragan et al. 2016).

| A55.20.10 | A55.20.5 | A73.20.5 | H73.20.10 |
| IPN4 | IPN5 | IPN2 | IPN6 |

Fig. 3. SEM images of SNCs (up) and IPNs (down); mag 500x and scaling bare 200 µm (adapted from Dragan et al. 2016).

decreased with the increase of the monomer concentration. Using HEMA instead of AAm, led to much larger pores (Dragan and Bucatariu 2016). It is evident in Fig. 3 (down) that the average diameter of pores decreased in all composite hydrogels compared to the SNCs, because part of the pore volume has been occupied by the 2nd network. A strong difference can be observed between the morphology of IPN4, derived from A55.20.10, and IPN6 derived from H73.20.10, the pores in IPN4 being filled with fibers like polymer forming a tissue, while the interior of IPN6 kept its macroporous morphology. It seems that in the case of the composite gels having HEMA as comonomer ion the SNC, the 2nd network was mainly formed in/on the walls of the 1st network than in the pores. Figure 4 summarizes the swelling kinetics data of the SNCs and IPN gels.

The equilibrium of swelling has been attained in few seconds in the case of SNCs, while the macroporous IPN hydrogels needed a longer time to reach the equilibrium of swelling, the SR_{eq} values being much lower than those of the corresponding SNCs (Fig. 4). The decreasing of swelling has been attributed to the presence of the 2nd network, which limits the

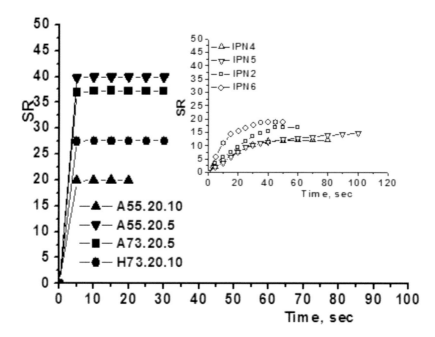

Fig. 4. Swelling kinetics of the SNCs and of the corresponding IPNs gels (the inset) (adapted from Dragan et al. 2016).

mobility of the 1st network by the entanglements of the chains, the size of pores decreasing after the formation of the second network.

LYS was selected for the investigations of the protein sustained release from SNCs and IPNs because its *iep* is located at pH around 11, and therefore, LYS is positively charged before this pH and can electrostatically interact with the gels containing COO^- groups. The highest amount of LYS has been loaded on SNCs obtained with the lowest concentration of monomers (637 mg LYS/g A55.20.5 compared with 385 mg LYS/g A55.20.10). Much lower amounts of LYS have been sorbed onto the IPNs gels, ranging between (84.6 mg LYS/g IPN5 and 157 mg LYS/g IPN4), because the pores have been partially occupied by the 2nd network, which, furthermore, reject the positively charged protein.

When the ratio between MAA and AAm or HEMA was 70:30, no protein release from SNCs was found at pH 2, because the higher density of COO^- groups required a higher concentration of H^+ ions to compete with LYS. However, the cumulative release of LYS from A73.20.5, at pH 1, was 55.56% in 48 h, and 65.4% in 30 h, respectively, while from H73.20.10 has been only 33.32% in 30 h (Fig. 5A). The initial concentration of monomers had a strong influence on the protein release from the IPNs gels (Fig. 5B). Thus, the decrease of the monomer concentration from 10 wt/v% to

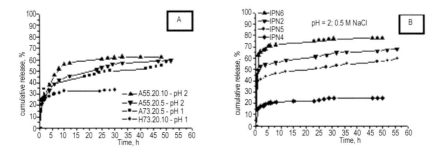

Fig. 5. Cumulative release of LYS from SNCs (A) and from IPN gels (B) (adapted from Dragan et al. 2016).

5 wt/v%, for the same MAA/AAm mole ratio (IPN4 compared to IPN5, Fig. 5B) led to the faster release of protein. This behaviour has been attributed to the fact that the relaxation and movement of polymer chains was more restrictive at a higher concentration of polymer in the 1st network, the whole composite being tighter. This tight structure makes the diffusion of water molecules into the hydrogels slower, resulting in the slower release and lower cumulative release of LYS. Increasing the ionic strength of the release environment could increase the release rate of the active principle by the screening of the electrostatic interactions between the opposite charges (Fig. 5B). For example, the cumulative release of LYS from IPN6 in pH 2 containing 0.5 M NaCl has been 77.8%, in 48 h. The differences in the protein release have been also correlated with the gels morphology. The sponge-type morphology of IPN2 and IPN6 could be responsible for the faster release of LYS, while the slower release from IPN4 might be attributed to the more compact morphology (SEM images in Fig. 3, down). The steady protein release observed in the case of IPN2 and IPN6 recommend them as promising systems for sustained release of LYS.

The data regarding the release of protein from the SNCs and IPNS hydrogel composites have been kinetically analyzed by the semi-empirical equation proposed by Korsmeyer and Peppas (K-P) for the initial stages of release (~ 60% of fractional release). The values of the exponent n_r in the K-P equation, which gives information about the release mechanism, have been lower than 0.5, and this indicates a pseudo-Fickian diffusion of LYS from both SNCs and IPN gels (Dragan et al. 2016).

4.2 Current applications of porous hydrogels as carriers for macromolecular drugs

Table 2 summarizes the main porous hydrogels and composites lately fabricated and recommended as carriers for macromolecular drugs, mainly proteins.

Table 2. Porous hydrogels generated last decade as carrier for macromolecular drugs.

Macromolecular drug	Carrier system	Physical status	Optimum pH and place of release	References
Lysozyme	PNIPAAm/CMC semi-IPN	-	1.2; stomach	Dutta et al. 2016
Lysozyme	Macroporous IPN cryogel P(MAA-*co*-HEMA)/CS	cylinder	2–4; stomach	Dragan et al. 2016
Lysozyme	Macroporous amphoteric cryogel P(DMAEM-*co*-MAA)	cylinder	7.1	Kudaibergenov et al. 2016
BSA	CMCNa	cylinder	7.4	Chang et al. 2010
BSA	macroporous CS	membrane	3.0; stomach	Yang et al. 2015
BSA	Soy protein/PNIPAAm	cylinder	7.4; colon	Liu and Cui 2011
BSA	Silk sericin/PMAA IPN	membrane	7.4; colon	Wu and Wang 2010
BSA	CS/P(AA-*co*-AAm) IPN	cylinder	6.8 and 7.4; colon	Bocourt et al. 2011
BSA	Bacterial cellulose-*g*-PAA	disks	6.8; small intestine	Ahmad et al. 2014
BSA	MFRHHs	cylinder	7.4; colon	Zhao et al. 2015b
BSA	Alginate/P(CE-MAA-MEG)	not specified	6.8	Wang et al. 2010
BSA	Porous β-glucans	cylinder	water	Lazaridu et al. 2015
BSA	Porous P(NIPAM-*co*-AAm)	cylinder	7.4; colon	Huo et al. 2010
BSA	Alginate/CMCS	beads	7.4; colon	Hu et al. 2016
Horse myoglobin	P(N-2-hydroxyethyl-DL-aspartamide-*g*-maleic anhydride) (PHE-MA)	not specified	6.8; small intestine	LoPresti et al. 2011
FITC-dextrans	Silk fibroin/PVA	disks	-	Kundu et al. 2012
Insulin	HTCC/GP	beads	PBS	Shi et al. 2011
Insulin	CS-PVA blend cross-linked with GA	films	transdermal	Zu et al. 2012
Insulin	CS/β-GP	thermogel	parenteral	Kashyap et al. 2007

As can be seen in Table 2, the most porous carriers for macromolecular drugs have potential for oral delivery, and less for transdermal and parenteral routes. Therefore, the bioavailability of the encapsulated proteins is essential and needs intensive investigations.

4.3 Concluding remarks

The low bioavailability of proteins at their oral administration demands their encapsulation in novel and advanced systems to be able to achieve sustained release, extended shelf-life, and reduction of adverse reactions. Among the lately reported systems, superporous composites as monoliths, disks, microspheres, core-shell have to be mentioned, many of them being based on the natural polymers including CS, cellulose, alginate, gelatin, silk fibroin, etc. The morphology of the hydrogels dramatically affects the drug release behaviour of the composite hydrogel. It was found that the release rate of the solute decreased by either increasing the molecular weight of the solute or by increasing the cross-linking density of the network. There is an increased interest, nowadays, in the field of chronopharmacology, which is focused on coordinating the biological rhythm with the medical treatment. Pulsatile drug delivery systems, defined as rapid and transient release of a certain amount of drug within a short period of time immediately after a predetermined off-release period, are recommended in such situations. There are various internal and external stimuli which have been used as triggers in the site-specific drug therapy or pulsatile drug release, among them temperature being the best and the most investigated. The thermal signals could be the increase of body temperature in a disease state or due to modulated external temperature (in the form of heat-triggered subdermal implants when gelation occurs due to the increase of temperature from ambient to physiological, with no other chemical or environmental treatments). It was found that the drug properties such as solubility, size and the interactions between the drug and the hydrogel chains should be taken under consideration when a thermo-responsive hydrogel is chosen as a drug carrier.

Acknowledgement

This work was supported by Romanian National Authority for Scientific Research, CNCSIS-UEFISCDI, Grant number PN-II-ID-PCE-2011-3-0300.

Abbreviations

AA   :   acrylic acid
AAm   :   acrylamide

BAAm	:	N,N′-methylenebisacrylamide
BC-*g*-PAA	:	bacterial cellulose-*g*-poly-(acrylic acid)
BSA	:	bovine serum albumin
BTCDA	:	3,3′,4,4′-benzophenonetetracarboxylic dianhydride
CBA	:	N,N′-bis(acryloyl)cystamine
CMCS	:	carboxymethyl chitosan
CMC	:	carboxymethylcellulose sodium
CS	:	chitosan
DDS	:	drug delivery systems
DMAEM	:	N,N-dimethylaminoethyl methacrylate
DMAEMC	:	N-dimethylaminoethyl methacrylate hydrochloride
DSC	:	differential scanning calorimetry (DSC)
EB	:	electron beam
ELP	:	elastin-like peptides
ECH	:	epichlorohydrin
EPR	:	enhanced permeability and retention
GA	:	glutaraldehyde
GDGE	:	glycerol-1,3-diglycidyl ether
GOD	:	glucose oxidase
GP	:	α, β-glycerol phosphate
GSH	:	glutathione
HC	:	hydrocortisone
HEMA	:	2-hydroxyethyl methacrylate
HSA	:	human serum albumin
HTCC	:	N-[(2-hydroxy-3-trimethylammonium) propyl] chitosan chloride
iep	:	isoelectric point
IPN	:	interpenetrating polymer network
KC	:	kappa carrageenan
LbL	:	layer-by-layer
LCST	:	lower critical solution temperature
LYS	:	lysozyme
MAA	:	methacrylic acid
MFRHHs	:	magnetic field-responsive hemicellulose hydrogels
MIP	:	molecular imprinting
O-HTCC	:	O-(2-hydroxy)propyl-3-trimethylammonium chitosan chloride
OS	:	oxidized starch
PAA	:	poly(acrylic acid)
PAAm	:	poly(acrylamide)
PBS	:	phosphate buffered saline
P(CE-MAA -MEG)	:	poly(ε-caprolactone-methacrylic acid-methoxy-PEG)

PDEAEM   :   poly(diethylaminoethyl methacrylate)
PEC   :   polyelectrolyte complexation
PEG   :   poly(ethylene glycol)
PEP   :   pepsin
PHE-MA   :   poly(N-2-hydroxyethyl-DL-aspartamide-g-maleic anhydride)
PEI   :   poly(ethylene imine)
PNIPAAm   :   poly(N-isopropylacrylamide)
PLGA   :   poly(lactic-*co*-glycolic acid)
PVA   :   poly(vinyl alcohol)
PVAm   :   poly(vinyl amine)
SEM   :   scanning electron microscopy
SF   :   silk fibroin
SGF   :   simulated gastric fluid
SIF   :   simulated intestinal fluid
SMA   :   poly(styrene-*co*-maleic acid anhydride)
SNC   :   single network cryogel
STMP   :   sodium trimetaphosphate
SPH   :   superporous hydrogel
TEMED   :   N,N,N',N'-tetramethylethylenediamine
TMAEMC   :   N-trimethylaminoethylmethacrylate chloride
TPP   :   tripolyphosphate
VPTT   :   volume phase transition temperature
VTESi   :   vinyltriethoxysilane

References

Ahmad, N., M.C.I.M. Amin, S.M. Mohali, I. Ismail and V.T.G. Chuang. 2014. Biocompatible and mucoadhesive bacterial cellulose-*g*-poly(acrylic acid) hydrogels for oral protein delivery. Mol. Pharm. 11: 4130–4142.

Ak, F., Z.I. Karakutuk and O. Okay. 2013. Macroporous silk fibroin cryogels. Biomacromolecules. 14: 719–727.

Autissier, A., C.L. Visage, C. Pouzet, F. Chaubet and D. Letourneur. 2010. Fabrication of porous polysaccharide-based scaffolds using a combined freeze-drying/cross-linking process. Acta Biomater. 6: 3640–3648.

Bae, K.H., F. Lee, K. Xu, C.T. Keng, S.Y. Tan, Y.J. Tan et al. 2015. Microstructured dextran hydrogels for burst-free sustained release of PEGylated protein drugs. Biomaterials. 63: 146–157.

Baek, K., N.E. Clay, E.C. Qin, K.M. Sullivan, D.H. Kim and H. Kong. 2015. *In situ* assembly of the collagen-polyacrylamide interpenetrating network hydrogel: Enabling decoupled control of stiffness and degree of swelling. Eur. Polym. J. 72: 413–422.

Bai, H., A. Polini, B. Delattre and A.P. Tomsia. 2013. Thermoresponsive composite hydrogels with aligned macroporous structure by ice-templated assembly. Chem. Mater. 25: 4551–4556.

Bajaj, P., R.M. Schweller, A. Khademhosseini, J.L. West and R. Bashir. 2014. 3D Biofabrication strategies for TE and regenerative medicine. Annu. Rev. Biomed. Eng. 16: 247–76.

Bayer, C.L., E.P. Herrero and N.A. Peppas. 2011. Alginate films as macromolecular imprinted matrices. J. Biomater. Sci. Polym. Ed. 22: 1523–1534.

Bawa, P., V. Pillay, Y.E. Choonara and L.C. du Toit. 2009. Stimuli-responsive polymers and their applications in drug delivery. Biomed. Mater. 4: 1–15.

Bayat, A., B. Larijani, S. Ahmadian, H.E. Junginger and M. Rafice-Tehrani. 2008. Preparation and characterization of insulin nanoparticles using chitosan and quaternized derivatives. Nanomedicine: Nanotechnology, Biology and Medicine. 4: 115–120.

Bergmann, N.M. and N.A. Peppas. 2008. Molecularly imprinted polymers with specific recognition of macromolecules and proteins. Prog. Polym. Sci. 33: 271–288.

Bertrand, P., A. Jonas, A. Laschewsky and R. Legras. 2000. Ultrathin polymer coatings by complexation of polyelectrolytes at interfaces: suitable materials, structure and properties, Macromol. Rapid Commun. 21: 319–348.

Bhattarai, N., H.R. Ramay, J. Gunn, F.A. Matsen and M. Zhang. 2005. PEG-grafted chitosan as an injectable thermosensitive hydrogel for sustained protein release. J. Control. Release. 103: 609–624.

Bhattarai, N., J. Gunn and M. Zhang. 2010. Chitosan-based hydrogels for controlled, localized drug delivery. Adv. Drug Deliv. Rev. 62: 83–99.

Bocourt, M., W. Argüelles, J.V. Cauich-Rodriguez, A. May, N. Bada and C. Peniche. 2011. Interpenetrated chitosan-poly(acrylic acid-co-acrylamide) hydrogels. Synthesis, characterization and sustained protein release studies. Mater. Sci. Appl. 2: 509–520.

Borges, J., L.C. Rodrigues, R.L. Reis and J.M. Mano. 2014. Layer-by-layer assembly of light-responsive polymeric multilayer systems. Adv. Funct. Mater. 24: 5624–5648.

Bucatariu, F., C.A. Ghiorghita, F. Simon, C. Bellmann and E.S. Dragan. 2013a. Poly(ethyleneimine) cross-linked multilayers deposited onto solid surfaces and enzyme immobilization as a function of the film properties. Appl. Surf. Sci. 280: 812–819.

Bucatariu, F., C.A. Ghiorghita, M. Mihai, F. Simon and E.S. Dragan. 2013b. Pepsin and Lysozyme immobilization onto Daisogel particles functionalized with chitosan cross-linked multilayers. Rev. Chim. 64: 334–337.

Buranachai, T., N. Praphairaksit and N. Muangsin. 2010. Chitosan/polyethyleneglycol beads crosslinked with tripolyphosphate and glutaraldehyde for gastrointestinal drug delivery. AAPS Pharm. Sci. Tech. 11: 1128–1137.

Byrne, M.E. and V. Salian. 2008. Molecular imprinted within hydrogels II: Progress and analysis of the field. Int. J. Pharm. 364: 188–212.

Caykara, T.S., S. Kücüktepe and E. Turan. 2007. Swelling characteristics of thermosensitive poly[(2-diethylaminoethyl methacrylate)-co-(N,N-dimethylacrylamide)] porous hydrogels. Polym. Int. 56: 532–537.

Censi, R., T. Vermonden, P.D. Martino and W.E. Hennink. 2012. Hydrogels for protein delivery in tissue engineering. J. Control. Release. 161: 680–692.

Chang, C., B. Duan, J. Cai and L. Zhang. 2010. Superabsorbent hydrogels based on cellulose for smart swelling and controllable delivery. Eur. Polym. J. 46. 92–100.

Chen, L., Z. Tian and Y. Du. 2004. Synthesis and pH sensitivity of carboxymethyl chitosan-based polyampholyte hydrogels for protein carrier matrices. Biomaterials. 25: 3725–3732.

Chen, X., J. Liu, Z. Feng and Z. Shao. 2005. Macroporous chitosan/carboxymethylcellulose blend membranes and their application for Lysozyme adsorption. J. Appl. Polym. Sci. 96: 1267–1274.

Clarke, K.C. and L.A. Lyon. 2013. Modulation of the deswelling temperature of thermoresponsive microgel films. Langmuir. 29: 12852–12857.

Cleland, J.L. and R. Langer. 1994. Design and development strategies. pp. 1–19. In: Cleland, J.L. and R. Langer [eds.]. Formulation and Delivery of Proteins and Peptides. ACS Symposium Series, vol. 567, MIT Cambridge, MA.

Dinu, M.V., M.M. Ozmen, E.S. Dragan and O. Okay. 2007. Freezing as a path to build macroporous structures: Superfast responsive polyacrylamide hydrogels. Polymer. 48: 195–204.

Dinu, M.V., M.M. Perju and E.S. Dragan. 2011. Composite IPN ionic hydrogels based on polyacrylamide and dextran sulfate. React. Funct. Polym. 71: 881–890.

Dinu, M.V., M. Pradny, J. Michalek and E.S. Dragan. 2013. Ice-templated hydrogels based on chitosan with tailored porous morphology. Carbohydr. Polym. 94: 170–178.

Dragan, E.S. and S. Schwarz. 2004. Polyelectrolyte complexes. VI. Polycation structure, polyanion molar mass and polyion concentration effects on complex nanoparticles based on NaPAMPS. J. Polym. Sci. Part A: Polym. Chem. 42: 2495–2505.

Dragan, E.S., A. Nistor and M. Cazacu. 2009. Ionic organic/inorganic materials. III. Stimuli responsive hybrid hydrogels based on oligo(N,Ndimethylaminoethylmethacrylate) and chloroalkyl-functionalized siloxanes. J. Polym. Sci. Part A: Polym. Chem. 47: 6801–6813.

Dragan, E.S. and F. Bucatariu. 2010. Cross-linked multilayers of poly(vinyl amine) as a single component and their interaction with proteins. Macromol. Rapid Commun. 31: 317–322.

Dragan, E.S., S. Schwarz and K.J. Eichhorn. 2010a. Specific effects of the counterion type and concentration on the construction and morphology of polycation/azo dye multilayers. Colloids Surf. A. 372: 210–216.

Dragan, E.S., F. Bucatariu and G. Hitruc. 2010b. Sorption of proteins onto porous single-component poly(vinyl amine) multilayer thin films. Biomacromolecules. 11: 787–796.

Dragan, E.S., M.M. Lazar and M.V. Dinu. 2012a. Preparation and characterization of IPN composite hydrogels based on polyacrylamide and chitosan and their interaction with ionic dyes. Carbohydr. Polym. 88: 270–281.

Dragan, E.S., M.M. Lazar, M.V. Dinu and F. Doroftei. 2012b. Macroporous composite IPN hydrogels based on poly(acrylamide) and chitosan with tuned swelling and sorption of cationic dyes. Chem. Eng. J. 204–206: 198–209.

Dragan, E.S. and D.F. Apopei Loghin. 2013. Enhanced sorption of methylene blue from aqueous solutions by semi-IPN composite cryogels with anionically modified potato starch entrapped in PAAm matrix. Chem. Eng. J. 234: 211–222.

Dragan, E.S. 2014a. Design and applications of interpenetrating polymer network hydrogels. A review. Cem. Eng. J. 243: 572–590.

Dragan, E.S. 2014b. Advances in interpenetrating polymer network hydrogels and their applications. Pure Appl. Chem. 86: 1707–1721.

Dragan, E.S. and F. Bucatariu. 2016. Design and characterization of anionic hydrogels confined in Daisogel silica composites microspheres and their application in sustained release of proteins Colloids Surf. A 489: 46–56.

Dragan, E.S. and A.I. Cocarta. 2016. Smart macroporous IPN hydrogels responsive to pH, temperature and ionic strength: Synthesis, characterization, and evaluation of controlled release of drugs. ACS Appl. Mater. Interfaces. 8: 12018–12030.

Dragan, E.S., A.I. Cocarta and M. Gierszewska. 2016. Designing novel macroporous composite hydrogels based on methacrylic acid copolymers and chitosan and *in vitro* assessment of lysozyme controlled delivery. Colloids Surf. B: Biointerfaces. 139: 33–41.

Dutta, S., P. Samanta and D. Dhara. 2016. Temperature, pH and redox responsive cellulose based hydrogels for protein delivery. Int. J. Biol. Macromol. 87: 92–100.

Fundueanu, G., M. Constantin and P. Ascenzi. 2008. Preparation and characterization of pH- and temperature-sensitive pullulan microspheres for controlled release of drugs. Biomaterials. 29: 2767–2775.

George, M. and T.E. Abraham. 2006. Polyionic hydrocholoids for the intestinal delivery of protein drugs: Alginate and chitosan—a review. J. Control. Release. 114: 1–14.

Ghanem, A. and D. Skonberg. 2002. Effect of preparation method on the capture and release of biologically active molecules in chitosan gel beads. J. Appl. Polym. Sci. 84: 405–413.

Ghiorghita, C.A., F. Bucatariu and E.S. Dragan. 2016. Sorption/release of diclofenac sodium in/from free-standing poly(acrylic acid)/poly(ethyleneimine) multilayer films. J. Appl. Polym. Sci. 133: Art. 43752.

Gil, E.S. and S.M. Hudson. 2004. Stimuli responsive polymers and their bioconjugates. Prog. Polym. Sci. 26: 1173–1222.

Gilmore, K.A., M.W. Lamply, C. Boyer and E. Harth. 2016. Matrices for combined delivery of proteins and synthetic molecules. Adv. Drug Deliv. Rev. 98: 77–85.

Guo, B., J. Yuan, L. Yao and Q. Gao. 2007. Preparation and release profiles of pH/temperature-responsive carboxymethyl chitosan/P(2-(dimethylamino)ethyl methacrylate) semi-IPN amphoteric hydrogel. Colloid Polym. Sci. 285: 665–671.

Gürdag, G. and A. Gökalp. 2011. Effects of pore-forming agents and polymer composition on the properties of novel poly(N,N-dimethylaminoethyl methacrylate) sulfate-*co*-N,N-dimethylacrylamide) hydrogels. Ind. Eng. Chem. Res. 50: 8295–8303.

Henderson, T.M., K. Ladewig, D.N. Haylock, K.M. McLean and A.J. O'Connor. 2013. Cryogels for biomedical applications. J. Mater. Chem. B. 1: 2682–2695.

Higashi, N., K. Yasufuku, Y. Matsuo, T. Matsumoto and T. Koga. 2014. Thermo-responsive multilayer films from ionic polymers with elastin-like peptide as graft chains. Colloid Interface Sci. Commun. 1: 50–53.

Hu, X., L. Feng, A. Xie, W. Wei, S. Wang, J. Zhang et al. 2014. Synthesis and characterization of a novel hydrogel: salecan/polyacrylamide semi-IPN hydrogel with a desirable pore structure. J. Mater. Chem. B 2: 3646–3658.

Hu, X. and L.A. Lyon. 2015. Thin films constructed by centrifugal deposition of highly deformable, charged microgels. ACS Macro Lett. 4: 302–307.

Hu, Y., J. Peng, L. Ke, D. Zhao, H. Zhao and X. Xiao. 2016. Alginate/carboxymethyl chitosan composite gel beads for oral delivery. J. Polym. Res. 23: 129.

Huang, Y., M. Liu, L. Wang, C. Gao and S. Xi. 2011. A Novel triple-responsive poly(3-acrylamidephenylboronic acid-*co*-2-(dimethylamino)ethyl methacrylate)/(β-cyclodextrin-epichlorohydrin) hydrogels: Synthesis and controlled drug delivery. React. Funct. Polym. 71: 666–673.

Huo, D., J. Yang, C. Hou and M. Yang. 2010. Macroporous poly(N-isopropylamide-co-acrylamide) hydrogels prepared by two-step polymerization for drug delivery applications. Chem. Eng. Technol. 33: 1943–1949.

Imren, D., M. Gümüsderelioğlu and A. Güner. 2010. *In vitro* release kinetics of bovine serum albumin from highly swellable dextran hydrogels. J. Appl. Polym. Sci. 115: 740–747.

Jain, E., A.A. Karande and A. Kumar. 2011. Supermacroporous polymer-based cryogel bioreactor for monoclonal antibody production in continuous culture using hybridoma cells. Biotechnol. Prog. 27: 170–180.

Jain, E., A. Damania, A.K. Shakia, A. Kumar, S.K. Sarin and A. Kumar. 2015. Fabrication of macroporous cryogels as potential hepatocyte carriers for bioartificial liver support. Colloid Surf. B: Biointerfaces. 136: 761–771.

Jaiswal, M., S. Lale, N.G. Ramesh and V. Koul. 2013. Synthesis and characterization of positively charged interpenetrating double-network hydrogel matrices for biomedical applications. React. Funct. Polym. 73: 1493–1499.

Kabiri, K. and M.J. Zohurian-Mehr. 2004. Porous superabsorbent hydrogel composites: Synthesis, morphology and swelling rate. Macromol. Mater. Eng. 289: 653–661.

Kashyap, N., B. Viswanad, G. Sharma, V. Bhardwaj, P. Ramarao and M.N.V. Ravi Kumar. 2007. Design and evaluation of biodegradable, biosensitive *in situ* gelling system for pulsatile delivery of insulin. Biomaterials. 28: 2051–2060.

Kathuria, N., A. Tripathi, K.K. Kar and A. Kumar. 2009. Synthesis and characterization of elastic and macroporous chitosan-gelatin cryogels for tissue engineering. Acta Biomater. 5: 406–418.

Kaygusuz, H. and F.B. Erim. 2013. Alginate/BSA/montmorillonite composites with enhanced protein entrapment and controlled release efficiency. React. Funct. Polym. 73: 1420–1425.

Khafagy, E.S., M. Morishita, Y. Onuki and K. Takayama. 2007. Current challenges in non-invasive insulin delivery systems: A comparative review. Adv. Drug Deliv. Rev. 59: 1521–1544.

Kikuki, A. and T. Okano. 2002. Pulsatile drug release control using hydrogels. Adv. Drug Deliv. Rev. 54: 53–77.

Knipe, J.M. and N.A. Peppas. 2014. Multi-responsive hydrogels for drug delivery and tissue engineering applications. Regenerative Biomater. 57–65.

Knipe, J.M., F. Chen and N.A. Peppas. 2015. Enzymatic biodegradation of hydrogels for protein delivery targeted to the small intestine. Biomacromolecules. 16: 962–972.

Kono, H., I. Oeda and T. Nakamura. 2013. The preparation, swelling characteristics, and albumin adsorption and release behaviors of a novel chitosan-based polyampholyte hydrogel. React. Funct. Polym. 73: 97–107.

Kryscio, D.R. and N.A. Peppas. 2012. Surface imprinted thin polymer film systems with selective recognition for bovine serum albumin. Anal. Chim. Acta. 718: 109–115.

Kudaibergenov, S.E., G.S. Tatykhanova and A.N. Klivenko. 2016. Complexation of macroporous amphoteric cryogels based on N,N-dimethylaminoethyl methacrylate and methacrylic acid with dyes, surfactant, and protein. J. Appl. Polym. Sci. 133: Art. 43784.

Kumar, A. and A. Srivastava. 2010. Cell separation using cryogel-based affinity chromatography. Nat. Protoc. 5: 1737–1747.

Kundu, J., L.A. Poole-Warren, P. Martens and S.C. Kundu. 2012. Silk fibroin/poly(vinyl alcohol) photocrosslinked hydrogels for delivery of macromolecular drugs. Acta Biomaterialia. 8: 1720–1729.

Kuo, Y.C. and C.C. Wang. 2013. Guided differentiation of induced pluripotent stem cells into neuronal lineage in alginate–chitosan–gelatin hydrogels with surface neuron growth factor. Colloids Surf. B: Biointerfaces. 104: 194–199.

Kureha, T., T. Shibamoto, S. Matsui, T. Sato and D. Suzuki. 2016. Investigation of changes in the microscopic structure of anionic poly(N-isopropylacrylamide-*co*-acrylic acid) microgels in the presence of cationic organic dyes toward precisely controlled uptake/release of low-molecular-weight chemical compound. Langmuir. 32: 4575–4585.

Lazaridou, A., K. Kritikopoulou and C.G. Biliaderis. 2015. Barley β-glucan cryogels as encapsulation c arriers of proteins: Impact of molecular size on thermo-mechanical and release properties. Bioact. Carbohydr. Dietary Fibre. 6: 99–108.

Lee, M.K., H. Bae, S. Lee, N. Chung, H. Lee, S. Choi et al. 2011. Freezing/thawing processing of PVA in the preparation of structured microspheres for protein drug delivery. Macromol. Res. 19: 130–136.

Li, Y., R. de Vries, T. Slaghek, J. Timmermans, M.A. Cohen Stuart and W. Norde. 2009. Preparation and characterization of oxidized starch polymer microgels for encapsulation and controlled release of functional ingredients. Biomacromolecules. 10: 1931–1938.

Li, Y., R. de Vries, M. Kleijn, T. Slaghek, J. Timmermans, M.A. Cohen Stuart et al. 2010. Lysozyme uptake by oxidized starch polymer microgels. Biomacromolecules. 11: 1754–1762.

Lin, Y.-H., H.F. Liang, C.K. Chung, M.C. Chen and H.W. Sung. 2005. Physically crosslinked alginate/N,O-carboxylethyl chitosan hydrogels with calcium for oral delivery of protein drugs. Biomaterials. 26: 2105–2113.

Lin, Y.-H., F.-L. Mi, C.-T. Chen, W.-C. Chang, S.-F. Peng, H.F. Liang et al. 2007. Preparation and characterization of nanoparticles shelled with chitosan for oral insulin delivery. Biomacromolecules. 8: 146–152.

Lin, Y.-H., K. Sonaje, K.M. Lin, J.H. Juang, F.L. Mi, H.W. Yang et al. 2008. Multi-ion-crosslinked nanoparticles with pH-responsive characteristics for oral delivery of protein drugs. J. Control. Release. 132: 141–149.

Liu, J., X. Ying, H. Wang, X. Li and W. Zhang. 2016. BSA imprinted polyethylene glycol grafted calcium alginate hydrogel microspheres. J. Appl. Polym. Sci. 133/APP.43617.

Liu, Y. and Y. Cui. 2011. Thermosensitive soy protein/poly(N-isopropylacrylamide) interpenetrating polymer network hydrogels for drug controlled release. J. Appl. Polym. Sci. 120: 3613–3620.

Liu, Z., Y. Jiao and Z. Zhang. 2007. Calcium-carboxymethyl chitosan hydrogel beads for protein drug delivery system. J. Appl. Polym. Sci. 103: 3164–3168.

Lohani, A., G. Singh, S.S. Bhattacharya and A. Verma. 2014. Interpenetrating polymer networks as innovative drug delivery systems. J. Drug Deliv. Art. 583612.

LoPresti, C., V. Vetri, M. Ricca, V. Fodera, G. Tripodod, G. Spadaro et al. 2011. Pulsatile protein release and protection using radiation-crosslinked polypeptide hydrogel delivery devices. React. Funct. Polym. 71: 155–167.

Lozinsky, V.I., E.S. Vainerman and S.V. Rogozhin. 1982. Study of cryostructurization of polymer systems. II. The influence of freezing of reacting mass on the properties of products in the preparation of covalently cross-linked gels. Colloid Polym. Sci. 260: 776–780.

Lozinsky, V.I., F.M. Plieva, I.Yu. Galaev and B. Mattiasson. 2001. The potential of polymeric cryogels in bioseparation. Bioseparation. 10: 163–188.

Lozinsky, V.I., I.Y. Galaev, F.M. Plieva, I.N. Savina, H. Jungvid and B. Mattiasson. 2003. Polymeric cryogels as promising materials of biotechnological interest. Trends Biotechnol. 21: 445–451.

Lozinsky, V.I. 2014. A brief history of polymeric cryogels. Adv. Polym. Sci. 263: 1–48.

Ma, L. and C. Liu. 2010. Preparation of microspheres by ionotropic gelation under a high voltage electrostatic field for protein delivery. Colloids Surf. B: Biointerfaces. 75: 448–453.

Macdonald, M., N.M. Rodriguez, R. Smith and P.T. Hammond. 2008. Release of a model protein from biodegradable self assembled films for surface delivery applications. J. Control. Release. 131: 228–234.

Macdonald, M.L., R.E. Samuel, N.J. Shah, R.F. Padera, Y.M. Beben and P.T. Hammond. 2011. Tissue integration of growth factor-eluting layer-by-layer polyelectrolyte multilayer coated implants. Biomaterials. 32: 1446–1453.

Magnin, D., J. Lefebvre, E. Chornet and S. Dumitriu. 2004. Physicochemical and structural characterization of a polyionic matrix of interest in biotechnology, in the pharamaceutical and biomedical fields. Carbohydr. Polym. 55: 437–453.

Mahdavinia, G.R., S.B. Mousavi, F. Karimi, G.B. Marandi, H. Garabaghi and S. Shahabvand. 2009. Synthesis of porous poly(acrylamide) hydrogels using calcium carbonate and its application for slow release of potassium nitrate. eXPRESS Polym. Lett. 3: 279–285.

Marek, S.R. and N.A. Peppas. 2013. Insulin release dynamics from poly(diethylaminoethyl methacrylate) hydrogel systems. AIChE Journal. 59: 3578–3585.

Matricardi, P., C.D. Meo, T. Coviello, W.E. Hennink and F. Alhaique. 2013. Interpenetrating polymer networks polysaccharide hydrogels for drug delivery and tissue engineering. Adv. Drug Deliv. Rev. 65: 1172–1187.

Mocanu, G, D. Mihai, D. LeCerf, L. Picton and M. Moscovici. 2009. Cyclodextrin-Anionic polysaccharide hydrogels: Synthesis, characterization, and interaction with some organic molecules (water pollutants, drugs, proteins). J. Appl. Polym. Sci. 112: 1175–1183.

Moroz, E., S. Matoori and J.-C. Leroux. 2016. Oral delivery of macromolecular drugs: Where we are after almost 100 years of attempts. Adv. Drug Deliv. Rev. 101: 108–121.

Nam, Y.S., M.S. Bae, S. Kim, I. Noh, J.K.F. Suh, K.B. Lee et al. 2011. Mechanism of albumin release from alginate and chitosan beads fabricated in dual layers. Macromol. Res. 19: 476–482.

Nguyen, M.N. and E. Alsberg. 2014. Bioactive factor delivery strategies from engineered polymer hydrogels for therapeutic medicine. Prog. Polym. Sci. 39: 1235–1265.

Okay, O. 2000. Macroporous copolymer networks. Prog. Polym. Sci. 25: 711–779.

Park, J.S., D.G. Woo, B.K. Sun, H.M. Chung, S.J. Im, Y.M. Choi et al. 2007. *In vitro* and *in vivo* test of PEG/PCL-based hydrogel scaffold for cell delivery application. J. Control. Release. 124: 51–59.

Park, K., I.C. Kwon and K. Park. 2011. Oral protein delivery: Current status and future prospect. React. Funct. Polym. 71: 280–287.

Peppas, N.A., J.Z. Hilt, A. Khademhosseini and R. Langer. 2006. Hydrogels in biology and medicine: From molecular principles to bionanotechnology. Adv. Mater. 18: 1345–1360.

Peppas, N.A. and J.R. Clegg. 2016. The challenge to improve the response of biomaterials to the physiological environment. Regenerative Biomater. 1–5.

Phull, M.K., T. Eydmann, J. Roxburgh, J.R. Sharpe, D.J. Lawrence-Watt, G. Phillips et al. 2013. Novel macro-microporous gelatin scaffold fabricated by particulate leaching for soft tissue reconstruction with adipose-derived stem cells. J. Mater. Sci.: Mater. Med. 24: 461–467.

Přádný, M., M. Šlouf, L. Martinová and J. Michálek. 2010. Macroporous hydrogels based on 2-hydroxyethyl methacrylate. Part 7: Methods of preparation and comparison of resulting physical properties. e-Polymers. 043: 1–12.

Přádný, M., M. Dušková-Smrčková, K. Dušek, O. Janoušková, Z. Sadakbayeva, M. Šlouf et al. 2014. Macroporous 2-hydroxyethyl methacrylate hydrogels of dual porosity for cell cultivation: morphology, swelling, permeability, and mechanical behavior. J. Polym. Res. 21: 567–579.

Rasool, N., T. Yasin, J.Y.Y. Heng and Z. Akhter. 2010. Synthesis and characterization of novel pH-, ionic strength and temperature-sensitive hydrogel for insulin delivery. Polymer. 51: 1687–1693.

Rinki, K., S. Tripathi, P.K. Dutta, J. Dutta, A.J. Hunt, D.J. Macquarrie et al. 2009. Direct chitosan scaffold formation *via* chitin whiskers by a supercritical carbon dioxide method: a green approach. J. Mater. Chem. 19: 8651–8655.

Qi, X., X. Hu, W. Wei, H. Yu, J. Li, J. Zhang et al. 2015. Investigation of Salecan/poly(vinyl alcohol) hydrogels prepared by freeze/thaw method. Carbohydr. Polym. 118: 60–69.

Qian, F., F. Cui, J. Ding, C. Tang and C. Yin. 2006. Chitosan graft copolymer nanoparticles for oral protein drug delivery: preparation and characterization. Biomacromolecules. 7: 2722–2727.

Sajeesh, S. and C.P. Sharma. 2006. Interpolymer complex microparticles based on polymethacrylic acid-chitosan for oral insulin delivery. J. Appl. Polym. Sci. 99: 506–512.

Sarmento, B., A. Ribeiro, F. Veiga, D. Ferreira and R. Neufeld. 2007. Oral bioavailability of insulin contained in polysaccharide nanoparticles. Biomacromolecules. 8: 3054–3060.

Sato, R., R. Noma and H. Tokuyama. 2015. Preparation of macroporous poly(N-isopropylacrylamide) hydrogels using a suspension–gelation method. Eur. Polym. J. 66: 91–97.

Sokic, S., M. Christenson, J. Larson and G. Papavasiliou. 2014. *In situ* generation of cell-laden porous MMP-sensitive PEGDA hydrogels by gelatin leaching. Macromol. Biosci. 14: 731–739.

Serizawa, T., K. Wakita, T. Kaneko and M. Akashi. 2002. Thermoresponsive properties of porous poly(Nisopropylacrylamide) hydrogels prepared in the presence of nanosized silica particles and subsequent acid treatment. J. Polym. Sci. Part A Polym. Chem. 40: 4228–4235.

Shi, L., S. Khondee, T.H. Linz and C. Berkland. 2008. Poly(N-vinylformamide) nanogels capable of pH-sensitive protein. Macromolecules. 41: 6546–6554.

Shi, W., Y. Ji, X. Zhang, S. Shu and Z. Wu. 2011. Characterization of pH- and thermosensitive hydrogel as a vehicle for controlled protein delivery. J. Pharm. Sci. 100: 886–895.

Shi, X., Y. Du, L. Sun, B. Zhang and A. Dou. 2006. Polyelectrolyte complex beads composed of water soluble chitosan/alginate: Characterization and their protein release behavior. J. Appl. Polym. Sci. 100: 4614–4622.

Sun, X.F., Z. Gan, Z. Jing, H. Wang, D. Wang and Y. Jin. 2015. Adsorption of methylene blue on hemicellulose-based stimuli-responsive porous hydrogel. J. Appl. Polym. Sci. 132: Art. 41606.

Tessmar, J.K. and A.M. Göpferich. 2007. Matrices and scaffolds for protein delivery in tissue engineering. Adv. Drug Deliv. Rev. 59: 274–291.

Torchilin, V. 2011. Tumor delivery of macromolecular drugs based on the EPR effect. Adv. Drug Deliv. Rev. 63: 131–135.

Tylingo, R., G. Gorczyca, S. Mania, P. Szweda and S. Milewski. 2016. Preparation and characterization of porous scaffolds from chitosan-collagen-gelatin composite. React. Funct. Polym. 103: 131–140.

Ungaro, F., M. Biondi, I. d'Angelo, L. Indolfi, F. Quaglia, P.A. Netti et al. 2006. Microsphere-integrated collagen scaffolds for tissue engineering: effect of microsphere formulation and scaffold properties on protein release kinetics. J. Control. Release. 113: 128–136.

Vermonden, T., R. Censi and W.E. Hennink. 2012. Hydrogels for protein delivery. Chem. Rev. 112: 2853–2888.

Wan, A., Y. Sun and H. Li. 2009. Characterization of novel quaternary chitosan derivative nanoparticles loaded with protein. J. Appl. Polym. Sci. 114: 2639–2647.

Wang, B., X.D. Xu, Z.C. Wang, S.X. Cheng, X.Z. Zhang and R.X. Zhuo. 2008a. Synthesis and properties of pH and temperature sensitive P(NIPAAm-*co*-DMAEM) hydrogels. Colloids Surf. B: Biointerfaces. 64: 34–41.

Wang, Z.C., X.D. Xu, C.S. Chen, G.R. Wang, B. Wang, X.Z. Zhang et al. 2008b. Study of novel hydrogels based on thermoresponsive PNIPAAm with pH sensitive PDMAEM grafts. Colloids Surf. B: Biointerfaces. 67: 245–252.

Wang, K., X. Xu, Y.J. Wang, G. Guo, M.J. Huang, F. Luo et al. 2010. *In vitro* release behavior of bovine serum albumin from alginate/P(CE-MAA-MEG) composite hydrogel. Soft Mater. 8: 307–319.

Wang, J., X. Zhou and H. Xiao. 2013. Structure and properties of cellulose/poly(N-isopropylacrylamide) hydrogels prepared by SIPN strategy. Carbohydr. Polym. 94: 749–754.

Wei, W., X. Hu, X. Qi, H. Yu, Y. Liu, J. Li et al. 2015a. A novel thermo-responsive hydrogel based on salecan and poly(N-isopropylacrylamide): Synthesis and characterization. Colloids Surf. B: Biointerfaces. 125: 1–11.

Wei, W., X. Qi, Y. Liu, J. Li, X. Hu, G. Zuo et al. 2015b. Synthesis and characterization of a novel pH-thermo dual responsive hydrogel based on salecan and poly(N,N-diethylacrylamide-co-methacrylic acid). Colloids Surf. B: Biointerfaces. 136: 1182–1192.

Wu, W. and D. Wang. 2010. A fast pH-responsive IPN hydrogel: Synthesis and controlled drug delivery. React. Funct. Polym. 70: 684–691.

Yang, J., J. Chen, D. Pan, Y. Wan and Z. Wang. 2013. pH-sensitive interpenetrating network hydrogels based on chitosan derivative and alginate for oral drug delivery. Carbohydr. Polym. 92: 719–725.

Yang, W.Y., M. Thirumavalavan and J.F. Lee. 2015. Effects of porogen and cross-linking agents on improved properties of silica-supported macroporous chitosan membranes for enzyme immobilization. J. Membr. Biol. 248: 231–240.

Yin, L., L. Fei, Y. Hu, F. Cui, C. Tang and C. Yin. 2007. Superporous hydrogels containing poly(acrylic acid-co-acrylamide)/O-carboxymethyl chitosan interpenetrating polymer networks. J. Appl. Polym. Sci. 108: 1238–1248.

Yin, L., J. Ding, J. Zhang, C. He, C. Tang and C. Yin. 2010. Polymer integrity related absorption mechanism of superporous hydrogel containing interpenetrating polymer networks for oral delivery of insulin. Biomaterials. 31: 3347–3356.

Yuan, Y., B.M. Chesnutt, G. Utturkar, W.O. Haggard, Y. Yang, J.L. Ong et al. 2007. The effect of cross-linking of chitosan microspheres with genipin on protein release. Carbohydr. Polym. 68: 561–567.

Yusan, P., I. Tuncel, V. Butun, A. Levent Demirel and I. Erel-Goktepe. 2014. pH-responsive layer-by-layer films of zwitterionic block copolymer micelles. Polym. Chem. 5: 3777–3787.

Zeng, Z. and E. Ruckenstein. 1998. Cross-linked macroporous chitosan anion-exchange membranes for protein separations. J. Membr. Sci. 148: 195–205.

Zhao, L., Y. Chen, W. Li, M. Lu, S. Wang, X. Chen et al. 2015a. Controlled uptake and release of lysozyme from glycerol diglycidyl ether cross-linked oxidized starch microgel. Carbohydr. Polym. 121: 276–283.

Zhao, Q., J. Sun, X. Wu and Y. Lin. 2011. Macroporous Double-Network Cryogels: Formation Mechanism, Enhanced Mechanical Strength and Temperature/pH Dual Sensitivity. Soft Matter. 7: 4284–4293.

Zhao, W., K. Odelius, U. Edlund, C. Zhao and A.C. Albertsson. 2015b. *In situ* synthesis of magnetic field-responsive hemicellulose hydrogels for drug delivery. Biomacromolecules. 16: 2522–2528.

Zhang, L., J. Guo, X. Peng and Y. Jin. 2004. Preparation and release behavior of carboxymethylated chitosan/alginate microspheres encapsulating bovine serum albumin. J. Appl. Polym. Sci. 92: 878–882.

Zhang, N., M. Liu, Y. Shen, J. Chen, L. Dai and C. Gao. 2011. Preparation, properties, and drug release of thermo- and pH-sensitive poly((2-dimethylamino)ethyl methacrylate)/poly(N,N-diethylacrylamide) semi-IPN hydrogels. J. Mater. Sci. 46: 1523–1534.

Zhang, X., C. Cao, X. Ma and Y. Li. 2012. Optimization of macroporous 3-D silk fibroin scaffolds by salt-leaching procedure in organic solvent-free conditions. J. Mater. Sci.: Mater. Med. 23: 315–324.

Zhang, Y., W. Yan, Z. Sun, C. Pan, X. Mi, G. Zhao et al. 2015. Fabrication of porous zeolite/chitosan monoliths and their applications for drug release and metal ions adsorption. Carbohydr. Polym. 112: 657–665.

Zhou, J., M.V. Pishko and J.L. Lutkenhaus. 2014. Thermoresponsive layer-by-layer assemblies for nanoparticle-based drug delivery. Langmuir. 30: 5903–5910.

Zhuo, R.X. and W. Li. 2003. Preparation and characterization of macroporous poly(N-isopropylacrylamide) hydrogels for the controlled release of proteins. J. Polym. Sci. Part A: Polym. Chem. 41: 152–159.

Zu, Y., Y. Zhang, Y. Zhao, C. Shan, S. Zu and K. Wang. 2012. Preparation and characterization of chitosan-polyvinyl alcohol blend hydrogels for controlled release of nano-insulin. Int. J. Biol. Macromol. 50: 82–87.

Biopolymer-based Interpenetrating Network Hydrogels for Oral Drug Delivery

*Sabyasachi Maiti** and *Sougata Jana*

ABSTRACT

Interpenetrating network is composed of two hydrophilic polymers, which are cross-linked in the presence of other to give a three-dimensional hydrogel network producing free volume for easy encapsulation of drugs. The hydrogels swell but do not dissolve in simulated biological fluids due to chemical or physical crosslinks. The swelling ability of hydrogel network enables them to regulate the release of encapsulated drugs over an extended period by controlling the degree of crosslinking. Now-a-days, naturally occurring polymers are preferred to synthetic materials due to their non-toxicity and biodegradability. Further, the biopolymers are easily amenable to chemical crosslinking/modification due to the presence of a variety of functional groups in the monomer units. Homopolymers alone cannot meet the demand in terms of both properties and drug delivery performance. Therefore, biopolymer-based interpenetrating network (IPN) hydrogels appears to be a better approach. This chapter discusses the design of biopolymer-based IPN hydrogels and their oral controlled drug delivery applications reported in the literature in the last decade.

Keywords: interpenetrating network, polysaccharides, sodium alginate, gellan gum, chitosan, graft copolymers, glutaraldehyde, hydrogels, locust bean gum, drug delivery

Department of Pharmaceutics, Gupta College of Technological Sciences, Ashram More, G.T. Road, Asansol-713301, West Bengal, India.
* Corresponding author: sabya245@rediffmail.com

1. Introduction

The oral route is the most convenient and comfortable way of administering drugs due to various advantages like better patient compliance, ease of self-medication, pharmacoeconomic suitability, and painless delivery, which all combines to make this route suitable for chronic therapy (Das and Chaudhury 2011). As oral route is the most popular route of administration, emphasis is given to the development of oral controlled drug delivery systems.

The use of novel types of polymers provides newer approaches for the development of controlled release formulations with an ultimate goal to achieve desired therapeutic results with minimum side effects (Garcia et al. 2000). Among the synthetic and natural polymers, the polysaccharides represent a class of macromolecules that can be used to optimize drug release rate. The polysaccharides are available in a large variety of compositions, and are enriched with a number of different functional groups that may allow desirable chemical modifications to generate a special class of biomaterials called hydrogels. Hydrogels are three-dimensional hydrophilic networks that are capable of absorbing a large amount of water without dissolving because of the presence of crosslinks (Chen and Metters 2006). The characteristic features of hydrogels are their ability to alter their volumes and properties in response to the external stimuli such as pH, temperature, ionic strength and electric field. The low interfacial tension with the surrounding biological fluids and tissues makes hydrogels biocompatible that minimizes the driving force for protein absorption and cell adhesion (Ganji and Vasheghani-Farahani 2009). The high water content makes them biocompatible. However, their inherent drawbacks such as poor mechanical strength, uncontrolled degradation, and extensive water uptake properties results in uncontrolled and unpredictable release rates of the active ingredients (Kumbar et al. 2003). However, their swelling propensity and the ability to release encapsulated drug can be regulated by monitoring the crosslinking that makes them attractive as materials for controlled drug delivery (Henriksen et al. 1996). The hydrogels composed of cross-linked polysaccharides and their derivatives have been studied for the design of novel drug carriers (Coviello et al. 2007, Vermonden et al. 2012).

Furthermore, smart hydrogels have been investigated to release the entrapped drug in response to specific physiological triggers such as pH, temperature, etc. (Qiu and Park 2001). Since the homopolymers alone cannot meet divergent demand in terms of mechanical, thermal and other smart properties and drug delivery performances, the development of interpenetrating network (IPN) appears to be a better approach and one of the easiest ways for modification of the properties of polysaccharides. IPN hydrogel structures are primarily created for the purpose of combining the properties of each network, to obtain better mechanical strength (Lee and Chen 2001), and to enhance the drug release performance of hydrogels. In some cases, entirely new properties that are not observed in either of the two single networks alone are exhibited by the IPNs (Myung et al. 2008). Interpenetration of the two networks may result in a higher mechanical strength than in the homopolymer network (Zhang and Peppas 2000). Furthermore, IPNs provide free volume space for the easy encapsulation of drugs in their network structure (Kulkarni et al. 2001).

IPN is a composite of two polymers, which is obtained when at least one polymer network is synthesized or cross-linked independently in the immediate presence of the other (Agnihotri and Aminabhavi 2005). There are two reactive phases in an IPN. If both phases are cross-linked, it is called a full IPN, while if one is cross-linked and the other is linear, it is called semi IPN. A semi-IPN, instead, is composed of one cross-linked polymer system in which free polymer chains are dissolved.

In recent years, polysaccharide-based IPN hydrogels have emerged as a rapidly developing branch of polymer technology for drug delivery. The reasons that polysaccharides are utilized for the development of IPN structures with specific characteristics are their abundance, low cost of production and peculiar and complex properties. Moreover, the chemical derivatization of polysaccharide functional groups can impart new material characteristics such as stimuli responsiveness, gelling property, thermal stability, viscosity, etc. to the polymer systems, such as networks obtained by crosslinking of chains (Matricardi et al. 2013). In particular, alginate, chitosan, gellan gum, locust bean gum and, to a lesser extent, other polysaccharides, received attention for the development of IPNs in order to control the release of drugs (Prabaharan and Mano 2006, Bajpai et al. 2008, Hoare and Kohane 2008). These natural polymer-based materials are very much susceptible to environmental condition than synthetic polymers. These materials are usually biodegradable and biocompatible (Bhardwaj et al. 2000). The controlled swelling property of IPN materials due to chemical or physical cross-links can help in achieving extended drug release profiles in simulated biological fluids (Ray et al. 2010a). In the swollen state, they become soft and rubbery, resemble living tissues, and exhibit excellent biocompatibility (Athawale et al. 2003). It must be remembered that a judicious selection of polymer combination such as natural-natural and natural-synthetic is crucial in designing delivery systems to control the release of short half-lived drugs under physiological conditions (Lohani et al. 2014).

Recently, the concept of interpenetrating network (IPN) opens up the doors to develop novel multi-particulate drug delivery systems. The multiple unit controlled drug delivery systems have been found to be superior to single unit systems as they can be mixed with gastrointestinal

(GI) tract fluids and are distributed over a large area (Setty et al. 2005). Recently, the use of natural polymers to prepare multi-unit controlled release dosage forms has been the focus of research because of their capability to meet the needs of spatial and temporal delivery of drug molecules with minimum fluctuation of plasma drug concentration (Dashevsky and Mohamad 2006). To make a multi-particulate delivery system, which will be able to deliver the active ingredients for a prolonged period, the delivery device should have sufficient integrity during its GI residence. A sufficient integrity during GI residence can be provided to the particulate delivery device after crosslinking. Moreover, any damage to multi-particulate devices only affects the release behaviour of the subunit involved, which represents a small part of the total dose, reducing the likelihood of safety problems that may arise due to dose dumping of single-unit dosage form (Dey et al. 2008). They are distributed throughout gastrointestinal (GI) tract, prevent exposure to a high drug concentration, and thereby minimize local irritation to the absorbing mucosa and ensure uniform drug absorption (Tang et al. 2005). The polysaccharides are hydrophilic and hence, the particulate systems can be developed in a completely aqueous environment by ionotropic gelation method. This, in turn, will avoid the use of organic solvents during their development and minimize the exposure of toxic organic solvents to the working personnel. However, the IPN polymers can also be used as matrix forming material for tablet dosage forms.

In recent years, the chemical and physical combination of natural or synthetic polymers for the fabrication of IPNs has been of great research interest. Different combinations have been tested for controlled release of a variety of drugs. This chapter highlights the recent progress in the design and drug delivery performance of IPNs of polysaccharides such as alginate, gellan, chitosan and locust bean gum. The IPN combination of natural polysaccharides either in native or modified form and IPNs of polysaccharide-synthetic copolymer are discussed under each head. The delivery attributes of some other least studied polysaccharides are also summarized.

2. Drug Delivery Application of IPN Networks

This section covers the controlled drug delivery potential of some natural polysaccharide-based IPN structures. Only four polysaccharides—sodium alginate, gellan gum, chitosan and locust bean gum are described in detail in subsequent section. Each biopolymer has been described under two heads, i.e., IPNs of polysaccharide blends and IPNs of polysaccharide and synthetic polymer combination.

2.1 ALG-based IPN networks

Sodium alginate (ALG) is a linear polymer, obtained from brown seaweed and marine algae. It is composed of 1, 4-linked β-D-mannuronic acid and α-L-guluronic acid residues (Lee et al. 2003). The structure of sodium alginate is given in Fig. 1.

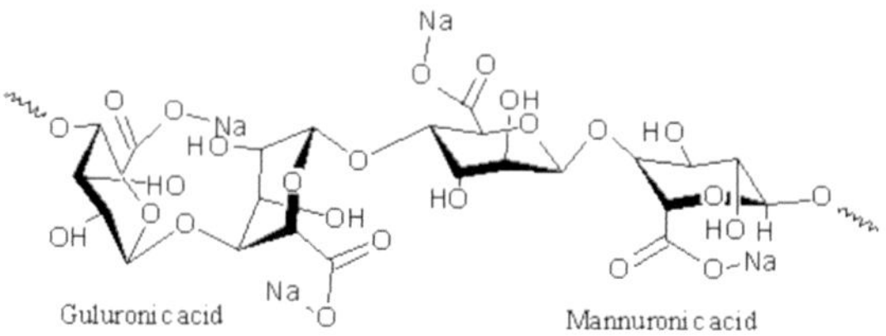

Fig. 1. Chemical structure of sodium alginate.

The gelling ability of this polysaccharide in presence of divalent counter ions leads to formation of hydrogels. ALG hydrogels have been widely studied in pharmaceutics as drug delivery vehicles. However, drug leaching during hydrogel preparation and rapid dissolution of alginate at higher pH are the major limitations, as it results in very low entrapment efficiency and burst release of entrapped protein drug, once it enters the intestine. To overcome the limitations, the mechanical properties of ALG have been tailored by designing IPNs with other natural or synthetic polymers to make it useful for controlled drug delivery applications.

2.1.1 ALG and other biopolymers

Kulkarni and colleagues (2001) described an IPN system of ALG with gelatin or egg albumin for the delivery of cefadroxil. They produced hydrogel beads after drop wise addition of polymer solution into methanol containing GA and HCl. The spherical beads ranged in size from 750–850 μm. SEM analysis did not reveal the existence of any pores on the smooth bead surface. They reported 83–88% DEE. Because IPN bead formation was carried out in methanol in which cefadroxil was insoluble, the possibility of drug leaching was less during encapsulation and resulted in higher DEE. They noticed a higher water uptake for egg albumin-based IPNs than gelatin-based IPNs. However, IPN formation with gelatin or egg albumin reduced the swelling and extent of drug release of non-IPN ALG beads. Gelatin IPNs released only about 63% drug in 400 min at phosphate buffer solution (pH 7.4). On the contrary, about 75% drug released from albumin IPN in the same period. Further, an anomalous transport mechanism was involved in drug release process.

ALG is a non-toxic polysaccharide with favourable pH sensitive properties for intestinal delivery of protein drugs. George and Abraham (2007) designed a pH-sensitive ALG: guar gum (3:1) hydrogel using 0.5% (w/v) GA as cross-linker that ensured 100% encapsulation efficiency and controlled delivery of a model protein, bovine serum albumin (BSA). Protein release from freeze-dried hydrogels was minimal at pH 1.2 (~20%), but was significantly higher (~90%) at pH 7.4. The presence of guar gum and GA crosslinking increased protein entrapment efficiency and prevented rapid dissolution of ALG in higher pH of the intestine, ensuring a controlled release of the entrapped protein drug. Mohamadnia et al. (2007) encapsulated betamethasone acetate into the IPN hydrogel network beads of ALG and carrageenan (sulfate esters of galactose and 3,6-anhydrogalactose copolymers). The variation in pH and temperature of gelling medium allowed ~71% drug loading efficiency at pH 4.8 and 55°C. The *in vitro* release profiles of IPNs was comparable with that of the non-IPN alginate-Ca^{2+} and carrageenan-K^+ hydrogels at pH 1.2 and pH 7.4. Matricardi and coworkers (2007) prepared borax-cross-linked ALG-scleroglucan (SCLG) semi-IPN hydrogel loaded with theophylline (TPH). The resulting hydrogels were frozen with liquid nitrogen, freeze-dried, and then used for the preparation of 230 ± 10 mg tablets with diameter and thickness of 13.00 ± 0.05 mm and 1.40 ± 0.10 mm, respectively. TPH was completely released after 2 hr from the ALG/borax system, while the release from SCLG/borax was complete only after 8 hr in simulated intestinal fluid (SIF, phosphate buffer pH 7.4). The delivery was complete after about 8 hr for SCLG/borax and roughly, 7 hr were needed for SCLG/ALG/borax. The burst effect was higher for the SCLG/borax system than that obtained with the SCLG/ALG/borax system. ALG influenced the release rate of TPH from semi-IPN to a lesser extent.

Ray et al. (2010b) adopted Al^{+3}-mediated ionotropic gelation method for IPN fabrication using ALG and carboxymethyl xanthan gum (CXM). They investigated the effect of polymer concentration, gelation time, $AlCl_3$ concentration and drug load on the release of a non-steroidal anti-inflammatory drug ibuprofen. The drug entrapment efficiency (DEE) increased from 93.46 to 99.50% with increase in the amount of polymer blend (1:1). Prolonged gelation lowered DEE irrespective of total polymer concentration. The use of higher amount of cross-linker (2–8%) and drug affected DEE marginally. X-ray diffraction studies suggested that no amorphization of the drug took place in the IPNs. Only 8.82–14.09% drug was released in pH 1.2 in 2 hr; however, in phosphate buffer (pH 6.8), complete drug release occurred in 210–300 min as a function of total polymer concentration. Increasing polymer blend from 2.0 to 4.0% and gelation period from 0.5 to 2.0 hr slowed down the drug release in both media. It may be due to the formation of a compact gel system with a greater crosslinking density in the matrix (Liu et al. 2005). As a result, free volume of matrix decreased (Agnihotri and Aminabhavi 2005) and hindered easy transport of drug. However, an unusual drug release behaviour was noticed as the concentration of $AlCl_3$ was raised from 2.0 to 8.0% in that the drug release rate was increased. They postulated that an outer thick gel layer, formed around the periphery, resisted influx of Al^{+3} ions and a less dense matrix core was formed. Once the gel layer eroded, the drug release occurred very fast. It is usual that a higher concentration gradient is established at higher drug load and results in faster drug diffusion. However, they noticed a decreased drug release tendency with increasing drug load (20–60% w/w of total polymer). In their opinion, low drug loading created larger pore fraction and allowed faster solvent penetration resulting in polymer swelling/ relaxation with consequent rapid release of release in both media. They hinted that IPNs could be used to minimize drug release in acidic medium and modulate drug release in phosphate buffer solution.

They further disclosed the effect of CMX: ALG IPN composition on ibuprofen release in another report (Ray et al. 2010c) and compared the drug release data with homopolymer beads. The average DEE was found to be $101.43 \pm 1.89\%$. The drug release was rapid from Al-CMX beads (42.5% in pH 1.2) and lowest for Al-ALG beads (25.4% in 2 hr) in acidic medium. Higher proportion of ALG in 3% total polymer blend slowed down drug release rate in acidic medium. The extent of interaction between carboxyl groups and aluminum ions determined the gel strength of the beads. Due to low degree of carboxymethyl substitution (0.8), a large number of –OH groups in AL-CMX remained free, making the gum more hydrophilic and very less ionic interaction ensued. Thus, the percentage of swelling of Al-CMX was high. On the contrary, the hydrophilicity of Al-alginate was less due to less number of OH groups and greater cationic interaction with guluronic acid residues of ALG. Therefore, as the amount of ALG was increased, the swelling and drug release of the beads decreased; and least swelling was noted for Al-ALG beads. Although the swelling of Al-ALG beads was the lowest in phosphate buffer, the drug release from IPN beads was found to be less than homopolymer beads. Their study clearly suggested that IPN hydrogel beads were more suitable than homopolymer beads in sustaining drug release.

2.1.2 *ALG and synthetic copolymers*

Poly(vinyl alcohol) (PVA) based IPN systems have been found encouraging due to its inherent non-toxicity, non-carcinogenicity, biocompatibility and desirable physical properties such as sufficient mechanical strength and high degree of swelling in aqueous solution (Hassan and Peppas 2000). A combination of PVA with natural polymer may provide the system with better stability and improved mechanical strength to meet the major objectives of controlled release of drug delivery. Hua and coworkers (2010) used Ca^{2+} crosslinking and freeze-thawing (FT) cycle techniques to prepare ALG alginate/poly(vinyl alcohol) (ALG/PVA) hydrogel beads. Ca^{2+} crosslinked ALG/PVA beads were subjected to freezing–thawing cycles for further crosslinking. The data indicated that the encapsulation efficiency of the beads was greatly improved when the ratio of PVA to ALG was 3:1 and FT process was included. The swelling and degradation of the beads was influenced by pH of the test medium and PVA content. FT cycling slowed the release of diclofenac sodium from the dual cross-linked beads compared with Ca^{2+}-ALG beads without PVA.

The grafting of synthetic polymers onto natural polymers is a vital approach to use natural polymers for controlled and targeted drug delivery application. The copolymers obtained through grafting will possess new/improved properties than their native characteristics. On grafting, the host polymer gains some of the desired properties of monomer used for grafting (Kurkuri et al. 2002). The structures of some of the synthetic polymers used in design of IPNs are shown in Fig. 2.

Babu and group (2006) synthesized ALG-g-acrylic acid (AA) copolymer for the encapsulation and pH-sensitive oral delivery of an anti-inflammatory drug ibuprofen. IPN microgels were developed by water-in-liquid paraffin emulsion-GA crosslinking method. They investigated the amount of AA, GA and drug loading on the size, DEE, and drug release kinetics of the IPN particles. DEE increased from 48.36% to 62.19%; however, mean size of the particles decreased from 113 to 58 µm with consequent increase in the amount of GA from 2.5 to 7.5 ml. DEE value and particle size increased with increasing drug load from 25% to 75% while keeping the amount of GA at intermediate value and ranged 51.85–83.82% and 81–167 µm, respectively. The variation in the amount of AA exhibited similar trend in these values. In general, a systematic increase in % release with increase in composition AA was observed. The use of 30% AA produced almost 100% drug release in 12 hr whereas the same was ~90% for 20% AA at pH 7.4 in same duration. Only about 40–50% drug released in pH 1.2 in 12 h; however, the trend of drug release as a function of AA amount remained the same. They swelled more with increasing amount of AA due to loosely cross-linked chains of AA in the microgels. The % drug release was quite faster at low GA. At higher GA, polymeric chains became rigid due to contraction of microvoids and therefore, there is decreased swelling and drug release through polymer matrices. The formulation with 75%

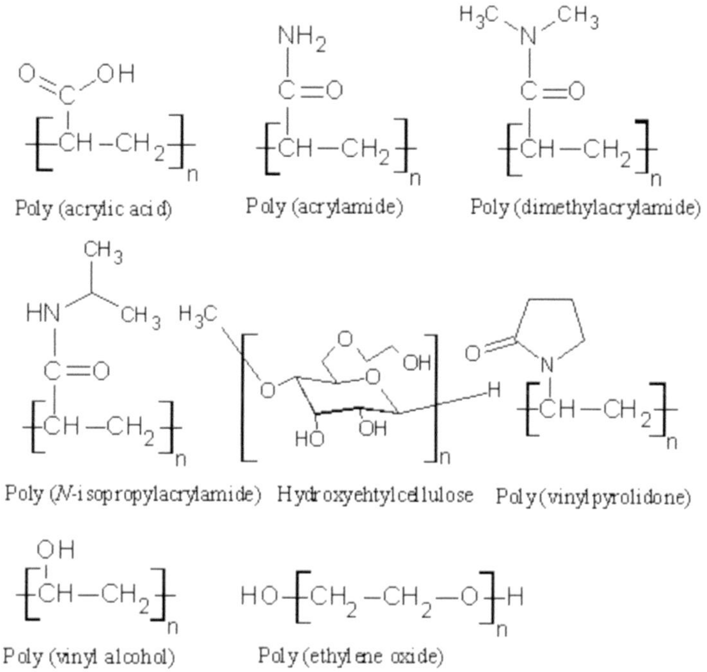

Fig. 2. Chemical structures of synthetic polymeric counterparts of biopolymer-based IPNs.

drug load displayed faster drug release rates. A prolonged release was observed for formulation containing 25% drug load. The release rate became slower at lower amount of drug in the matrix because of availability of more free void spaces through which lesser number of drug molecules was transported. By increasing the pH from 1.2 to 7.4, a considerable increase in % drug release was observed for all microgels. At higher pH, above pK_a of microgels, the –COOH groups ionized increasingly, an osmotic pressure was built up inside microgels and ultimately caused higher swelling and drug release. They highlighted that the microspheres had low densities and thus could be retained in gastric environment for >12 hr which might help to improve bioavailability of ibuprofen. The IPNs of graft copolymers and ALG may be advantageous because it comprises of two crosslinked polymer chains in complex structure resulting in three-dimensional pH-sensitive matrix with more free volume for increased entrapment efficiency and better mechanical strength. The grafting of polyacrylamide (PAAm) on polysaccharides may yield the new copolymer, combining the properties of both natural and synthetic polymers. This graft copolymer can also be converted into ionic form through the hydrolysis of amide groups resulting in pH-responsive copolymer (Kaur and Chatterji 1990) which can then be used for smart drug delivery.

Gum ghatti (GG) is an anionic polysaccharide, obtained from the exudation of Anogeis-suslatifolia tree pertaining to combretaceae family. The composition of GG includes 1→6 linked D-galactopyranose major units and alternating 4-*O*-subsituted and 2-*O*-subsituted-D-mannopyranose units along with a single L-arabinofuranose unit as side chain (Kaith et al. 2012). Boppana et al. (2015) developed pH-sensitive IPN microbeads using alkali hydrolyzed polyacrylamide-g-gum ghatti (PAAm-g-GG) and ALG for gastro-protective controlled delivery of ketoprofen. They prepared ketoprofen-loaded IPN microbeads by crosslinking the polymers with Ca^{2+} ions and GA. With an increase in the amounts of PAAm-g-GG and ketoprofen, ionically cross-linked microbeads demonstrated rough and dense surface; however, dual crosslinking provided smooth surface along with few surface foldings but the surface roughness had disappeared. The size of IPN microbeads persisted in the range of 820–931 µm. The size of microbeads increased due to formation of large drops following extrusion of highly viscous polymer dispersion. The DEE of IPN microbeads ranged between 78–91%. They noticed that the DEE of IPN microbeads prepared with lesser amount of Ca^{2+} ions was lower. They pointed out that the matrix might be saggy and leaky due to inadequate crosslinking, resulting in leakage of drug from IPN matrix during the production of microbeads. On the other hand, as PAAm-g-GG copolymer was increased, the DEE was slightly increased. IPN microbeads liberated a larger amount of drug in buffer solution (pH 7.4) than in solution of pH 1.2. Dual cross-linked microbeads showed slower drug release than the ionically crosslinked IPN beads. Only 17% drug was released in pH 1.2 solution and 83% of drug was released in pH 7.4 buffer solutions in a controlled fashion up to 12 hr. The IPN microbeads exhibited higher AUC values than pristine ketoprofen, suggesting the better bioavailability of ketoprofen from IPN microbeads due to controlled release of ketoprofen. The pH-sensitive controlled release of ketoprofen from IPN microbeads was also revealed *in vivo*. Because a small amount of drug was released in stomach from IPNs, the IPN microbeads showed lower plasma drug concentration up to 2 hr as compared to pristine ketoprofen. Once the beads moved from stomach into alkaline environment of intestine, they underwent ionization and maximum swelling and drug release occurred. They observed only 10.23% edema inhibition up to 2 h, which was slowly increased to 90.23% at the end of 7 hr, and then decreased to 84.40% at the end of 12 hr in anti-inflammatory pharmacodynamics. Pristine ketoprofen showed 88.6% inhibition of carrageenan-induced paw edema up to 2 h, and then the same decreased to 7.21% at the end of

12 hr. Moreover, the adverse effects like ulcers, hemorrhage and mucosal erosion associated with pristine ketoprofen were reduced when ketoprofen was formulated as pH-sensitive IPN microbeads. Kulkarni et al. (2012) used another copolymer poly(acrylamide)-g-carrageenan with ALG for the production of ketoprofen-loaded IPN hydrogel beads. To do that, an aqueous solution of polymer blends was dropped into mixtures of aqueous solutions of $CaCl_2$ and KCl. These ionically crosslinked hydrogel beads were incubated in a solution containing GA and 1.0 N HCl for 30 min at 50°C to introduce covalent crosslinks. The PAAm-g-CG beads were spherical into counter ion medium, but they lost their shape and looked like flat disks after drying. The IPN beads were spherical in shape having surface folding; this may be due to improved mechanical strength of particles after formation of IPN with ALG. In case of IPN, the PAAm-g-CG and ALG were closely knotted with the help of crosslinking agents to form stronger network. The hydrogel beads had size range of 903 to 1132 µm. At higher counter-ion concentration, smaller hydrogel beads were produced. The treatment of the beads with GA reduced the size further. The DEE of hydrogel beads ranged 76–90%. DEE of the hydrogel beads dropped with the use of low concentration of counter ions. DSC and XRD analyses suggested the amorphous dispersion of the drug after entrapment into IPN matrix. A reversible swelling–de-swelling behaviour was noted as pH of the medium was changed between 1.2 and 7.4, possibly due to the presence of carboxylate groups on the backbone of graft copolymer. ALG hydrogel beads discharged the entire drug within 4 hr in alkaline pH, and about 25% drug in acidic pH; while PAAm-g-CG hydrogel beads extended the drug release up to 7 hr as did the IPN beads. The release of drug in solution of pH 1.2 was slower as compared to that in pH 7.4 buffer solution due to a higher swelling of hydrogel beads in alkaline pH. IPN hydrogel beads treated with GA released the drug more slowly in a controlled manner as compared to ionically crosslinked IPNs. Overall, the dual cross-linked IPN beads showed a maximum of 10% of drug release in pH 1.2, and a major portion (about 90%) of drug was released in pH 7.4 solution in a controlled manner. In stomach histopathology, very mild congestion and mucosal erosions were noticed for animals treated with drug-loaded IPN hydrogel beads. However, the hemorrhage, perforation, edema, and necrosis were not observed. While plain ketoprofen induced ulcer and hemorrhage, and caused erosion of gastric mucosa, these side effects were reduced after entrapment of ketoprofen into pH-responsive IPN hydrogel beads.

The presence of thermosensitive synthetic polymer in ALG-based semi-interpenetrating structures has also been investigated for tailoring the release of drugs (Zhang et al. 2004). These polymers can undergo reversible transition from a hydrophilic (sol) to a more hydrophobic (gel) material triggered by small changes in environmental temperature. The transition from a hydrogel to sol occurred when the temperature is lowered below a certain temperature, called lower critical solution temperature (LCST). The most commonly used thermosensitive polymer poly(*N*-isopropylacrylamide) (pNIPAAm) has LCST of 32–37°C (Schmaljohann 2006). Choi et al. (2008) synthesized Ca^{2+} ions cross-linked hydrogel beads of ALG in combination with poly(*N*-isopropylacrylamide) (pNIPAM), *N*-isopropylacrylamide-methacrylic acid (p(NIPAM-co-MAA)) copolymer, and N-isopropylacrylamide-methacrylic acid-octadecyl acrylate (p(NIPAM-co-MAA-co-ODA)) copolymer. The release of entrapped blue dextran from freeze-dried beads was in the order of alginate bead < ALG/pNIPAM bead ≈ ALG/p(NIPAM-co-MAA) bead < ALG/p(NIPAM-co-MAA-co-ODA) bead in distilled water. The drug release correlated well with the degree of swelling. Only ALG/p(NIPAM-co-MAA-co-ODA) bead exhibited pH-dependent release. Due to weak inter- and intra-electrostatic repulsion at acidic condition, p(NIPAM-co-MAA-co-ODA) readily assembled into an aggregate, which reduced the pore of bead matrix, and consequently led to a suppressed release of the model drug. In a study, Reddy et al. (2008) produced ALG-*N*-isopropylacrylamide (NIPAAm) semi-IPNs by water-in-oil (w/o) emulsification method using glutaraldehyde as a crosslinker for ALG instead of Ca^{2+} ions. 5-fluorouracil was loaded into hydrogel microspheres and its extent of release was studied at temperatures below and above the LCST of pNIPAAm. A slower drug release rate was evident in phosphate buffer (pH 7.4) at 37°C, releasing only 60% drug in 12 hr. Monodisperse simultaneous IPN beads was also reported (Park and Choi 1998). The aqueous solution of ALG, NIPAAm and the chemical crosslinker *N,N'*-bis(acryloy1) cystamine was added drop wise into an aqueous $CaCl_2$ and radical polymerization initiator (ammonium persulfate) solution, thus causing immediate and simultaneous gelation of ALG, polymerization and chemical crosslinking of NIPAAm. The beads had Ca-ALG hydrogel enriched outer shell as compared to the core because the diffusion of Ca^{2+} ions into the droplets slowed down as the gelation proceeded. On the contrary, pNIPAAm was more abundant in the inner core of the beads during the formation of the beads. They found that homogeneous opaque IPN beads below the LCST turned into heterogeneous core-shell type beads above the LCST (32°C). The formation of the white core region generated above the LCST was due to the collapse and shrinkage of pNIPAAm network out of the IPN composite structure. Accordingly, the opaque shell layer in the beads is believed to be Ca-alginate rich network. The temperature-induced formation of pNIPAAm-rich core and alginate-rich shell layer was fully reversible with the variation of temperature. The thermally reversible formation of the core-shell double structure in the IPN hydrogel beads was applied for the temperature modulated drug release using indomethacin.

At 25°C, the release rate from the IPN beads was slower than that from the homo-pNIPAAm beads up to 7.5 hr due to the presence of the Ca-alginate chain network. At 37°C, the drug release rate from the IPN beads was much faster than that from the homo-pNIPAAm beads, because the former developed a core-shell type, double-walled structure within hydrogel microbeads at 37°C in 0.01 M Tris buffer (pH 7.4).

2.2 Gellan-based IPN structures

Gellan gum is an anionic, bacterial exopolysaccharide, which consists of repeating tetrasaccharide units of β-D-glucose, β-D-glucuronic acid, and α-L-rhamnose residues in molar ratio of 2:1:1 (Fig. 3) (Izumi et al. 1996) and produced by *Pseudomonas elodea*.

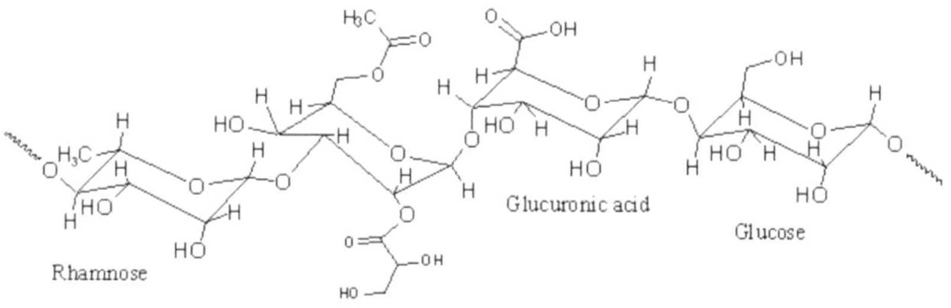

Fig. 3. Structural features of gellan polysaccharide.

It has been mainly investigated as ophthalmic drug delivery and oral controlled release preparations. However, we restrict our discussion to the use of gellan gum as a component of IPN structures for oral drug delivery.

2.2.1 Gellan and other biopolymers

There is little evidence on gellan and other biopolymer IPN system in literature towards their controlled drug delivery applications. Kulkarni et al. (2011) reported GG and albumin (ALB) IPNs for the controlled release of diltiazem hydrochloride (half-life of 3–4 hr) in the management of angina pectoris and hypertension. Because the drug is administered three to four times daily (Shivkumar et al. 2006), it would be beneficial to develop controlled release formulations to improve the patient compliance. In this study, a cation exchange resin Indion 254® was bound with diltiazem HCl to form reversible complex and the resulting drug–resin complex was entrapped within Ca^{2+}-GA treated gellan gum-egg ALB IPN microcapsules.

The microcapsules were spherical but rough and dense surface along with folding was evident. The DEE for the prepared IPN microcapsules (841–1118 µm) was found to be in the range of 68.02–89.06%. The size of ionically crosslinked microcapsules (987 µm) decreased after dual crosslinking (962 µm). With an increase in concentration of GA (5–15 ml), the size of the microcapsules also decreased from 962 to 876 µm. This may be due to the formation of more rigid polymer network at higher crosslink densities. By increasing the concentration of ALB, an increase in size of the microcapsules was observed, which could be attributed to the formation of bigger droplets due to increase in viscosity of the solution. On the other hand, as the amount of resinate increased, the size of microcapsules increased because resinate might have occupied the interstitial spaces between polymer segments. This was in accordance with the study published by Halder and Sa (2006).

Increase in concentration of $CaCl_2$ decreased the DEE, which may be due to the displacement of bound diltiazem HCl by Ca^{2+} ions; higher the concentration of $CaCl_2$ solution, larger the amount of Ca^{2+} ions diffused inwardly into the resinate loaded microcapsules and consequently the larger the amount of drug displaced from the resinate by Ca^{2+} ions. The free drug diffused out of the microcapsules resulted in decreased DEE. The results were quite similar to that reported by Halder et al. (2005) for polyethyleneimine-treated calcium alginate beads. On the other hand, DEE of the microcapsules prepared by ionic crosslinking was little higher than those prepared by dual crosslinking. In case of dual cross-linked microcapsules, DEE of the microcapsules prepared with lower concentration of GA was lowest as compared to those prepared with higher concentration of GA. At lower concentration of GA, the IPN matrix might have larger pores due to insufficient crosslinking, causing higher leakage of drug into crosslinking solution. On the contrary, the IPN matrix was stiff and leakage of drug from matrix was low at higher concentration of GA, resulting in high DEE. Rokhade et al. (2007) found similar results for chitosan and methylcellulose IPN microspheres. Swelling of the ionically cross-linked beads was greater than the dual cross-linked beads. The ionically cross-linked microcapsules could maintain the drug release up to 9 hr, while the dual cross-linked microcapsules released the drug up to 15 hr depending upon GG:ALB mass ratio, $CaCl_2$ and GA concentration. The ionically crosslinked microcapsules discharged their content quickly up to 9 hr whereas, dual crosslinked microcapsules extended the drug release up to 15 hr, depending upon GG:ALB mass ratio, $CaCl_2$ and GA concentration. The microcapsules prepared with higher concentration of GA released the drug more slowly. The GG–ALB IPN microcapsules could be used as versatile carriers for controlled release of water-soluble drugs. Wen et al.

(2014) developed a new IPN bio-hydrogel of gellan gum and gelatin using a combined enzymatic and ionic crosslinking approach. The resulting IPN hydrogel exhibited significantly increased and tunable mechanical strength, decreased swelling ratios and lower degradation rate compared with pure gelatin gel. The composite hydrogels supported the attachment and proliferation of L929 fibroblasts *in vitro*. However, they did not demonstrate controlled drug delivery potential of this bio-hydrogel system.

2.2.2 Gellan and synthetic copolymers

Some reports are available where copolymers have been used as a component of gellan gum-based IPN hydrogels. Agnihotri and Aminabhavi (2005) reported IPN microspheres of gellan and PVA for the controlled delivery of an antihypertensive drug carvedilol. They employed water-in-oil emulsion crosslinking method for drug encapsulation in the microspheres, improving mechanical strength and maintenance of swelling degree with consequent slow drug release pattern. The mass ratio of GG:PVA (1:4, 1:1.5 and 1:0.66) and GA concentration (0.001–0.003 ml/mg polymer) did not influence the DEE significantly. Despite the variation, the DEE values lied in narrow range of 83–87%. However, the size of the particles decreased with increasing GA concentration at each level of GG:PVA ratio, probably due to formation of more rigid network structures. Higher proportion of GG in the IPN caused the formation of bigger droplets during emulsification and therefore, the particle size increased from 276 to 346 µm at 0.001 ml/mg polymer concentration of GA. Both DSC and X-ray analyses suggested crystalline dispersion of drug into polymer matrix after entrapment. At higher GA concentration, free volume of the matrix would be less, thereby it might hinder the easy transport of drug molecules through the matrix into simulated gastric fluid (SGF) and simulated intestinal fluid (SIF). Although, the initial rate of drug release was slower up to 10 hr, thereafter, there was no appreciable difference in drug release rate and almost entire drug was released in 12 hr. The drug release rate became slower when higher amount of GG was used in IPN. Probably, stiffer polymer chain entanglements at higher GG reduced the rate of swelling and consequently the release of drug. There was no significant difference in swelling of microspheres in SGF and SIF. Interestingly, the drug release rate was faster at SGF. Because saturation solubility of carvedilol was almost double in SGF, the difference in drug release was attributed to the differences in solubility of drug. Oral dosage formulation of carvedilol in the form of GG: PVA IPNs could be developed for controlling the drug release. Mundargi et al. (2010) designed thermoresponsive semi-IPN microspheres of gellan gum-P(NIPAAm) by ionic crosslinking to study the controlled release of atenolol, an antihypertensive drug. Scanning electron microscopy (SEM) indicated spherical nature and smooth surfaces of the hydrogel matrix with some debris attached on their surfaces. The pulsatile trends in swelling and drug release at 25°C and 37°C in phosphate buffer (pH 7.4) exhibited thermoresponsive nature of the polymer particles (34–76 µm). It was observed that the drug release could be extended up to 12 hr at both the temperatures. A recent study highlighted the potential of crosslinked semi-IPN xerogel matrix tablet (Hoosain et al. 2014). Chemical crosslinking of poly(ethylene) oxide (PEO) and gellan gum by epichlorohydrin allowed sustained release of sulpiride from the hydrophilic semi-IPN xerogel matrix system. The matrix tablets displayed zero-order release kinetics, extending over 24 h. The drug release occurred primarily by swelling and surface erosion of the matrix. Surface morphology of the crosslinked system depicted a porous network, displaying water uptake of 450–500%. The physiochemical properties of the PEO and GG were sufficiently modified to allow for 100% drug release at 24 h in a controlled manner. They further investigated the ability of these semi-IPNs to sustain drug release and enhance bioavailability of sulpiride *in vivo* by evaluating the plasma drug concentration over 24 h in the large pig model (Hoosain et al. 2016). The optimized formulation exhibited greater intestinal absorption of sulpiride than the marketed product with a peak plasma concentration (C_{max}) of 830.58 ng/mL after 15 hr.

2.3 Chitosan IPN

Chitosan is a cationic polysaccharide, obtained by alkaline deacetylation of chitin (Muzzerelli 1993). It is composed of α-1,4-linked 2-amino-2-deoxy-α-D-glucose (Fig. 4) (Jana et al. 2014).

It is a very promising biomaterial as carrier material for controlled drug delivery due to its non-toxic, biocompatible and biodegradable nature (Ravikumar 2000, Alves and Mano 2008). However, it has a limited capacity for controlling the release of drug from oral dosage forms due to its fast dissolution in the stomach. To overcome this disadvantage, modification of chitosan is required for the development of drug delivery systems.

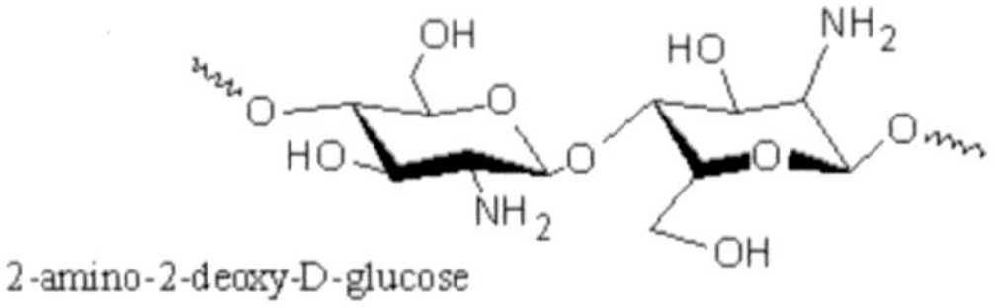

2-amino-2-deoxy-D-glucose

Fig. 4. Chemical structure of chitosan.

2.3.1 Chitosan-based Bio-IPNs

Kumari and Kundu (2008) reported *in vitro* release of chlorpheniramine maleate from semi-IPNs of chitosan and glutamic acid. They extruded a homogeneous mixture of CS and glutamic acid (GLA) in acetic acid drop wise into NaOH-methanol (1:20) solution for the formation of beads. The beads were cross-linked with GA to form CS-GA-GLA IPNs. The swelling rate of CS-GA-GLA IPNs having equal mass ratio of CS:GLA decreased with increasing GA concentration from 3.1% to 25.0% in pH 2.0. The extent of swelling was higher in pH 7.4 solution than in acidic solution. Perhaps, the free carboxylic ends of CS-GLA semi IPN were ionized and caused swelling due to generation of electrostatic repulsive forces. The swelling tendency decreased with increasing concentration of CS at the same GA concentration. The slowest drug release rate was observed in case of higher concentration of CS. As the amount of GLA spacers decreased, the pore size of the beads narrowed and penetration of solution into beads became difficult resulting in lesser degree of swelling. The IPNs showed burst release of chlorpheniramine maleate in the first hour, followed by a moderate release for next 5 hr and then at constant rate over 48 hr in both acidic and alkaline media. The drug release rate was slower for IPNs cross-linked with higher % GA in both media. At pH 2.0, IPNs swelled less and thus the drug entrapped did not easily escape from IPNs. However, at pH 7.4, the beads swelled to higher extent leading to faster release of drug. Overall, they suggested that the desired drug release rate could be maintained by varying mass ratio of CS:GLA and concentration of GA.

Tamarind seed polysaccharide (TSP) is a natural polysaccharide, obtained from the endosperm of *Tamarindus indica* L. seeds, and belongs to the family Leguminosae. It is composed of $(1\rightarrow4)$-β-D-glucan backbone substituted with side chains of α-D-xylopyranose and β-D-galactopyranosyl $(1\rightarrow2)$-α-D-xylopyranose linked $(1\rightarrow6)$ to glucose residues. TSP is non-carcinogenic, biocompatible and extraordinarily stable even in the acid pH range (Pal and Nayak 2012). Jana et al. (2013) evaluated GA cross-linked chitosan-tamarind seed polysaccharide (TSP) IPN microparticles for prolonged release of aceclofenac. The drug entrapment efficiency of the microparticles was found between 85.84 to 91.97% and their average particle sizes ranged from 490 to 621 μm. Chitosan:TSP (1:2) IPN microparticles released aceclofenac over 8 hr in phosphate buffer (pH 6.8). Chitosan-TSP IPN microparticles slowly inhibited edema and exhibited sustained anti-inflammatory activity in carrageenan-induced rat-paw edema model after oral administration. They further compressed IPN microparticles with excipients to make tablets (Jana et al. 2014). The matrix tablets showed sustained release of aceclofenac over 8 hr. This could be beneficial in reducing dosing frequency and side effects associated with long-term treatment. Sirajudheen et al. (2015) tested a novel pH-independent IPN system of chitosan and guar gum for the treatment of angina pectoris, hypertension and cardiac arrhythmia. They used calcium chloride as crosslinking agent for the encapsulation of propranolol HCl. A higher chitosan: guar gum combination exhibited sustained drug release up to 12 hr under simulated bio-fluids.

2.3.2 Chitosan-synthetic copolymers

The crosslinked chitosan swells in acidic solutions due to protonation of free amino groups and the hydrogels are widely used in controlled release of drugs in stomach *via* oral route (Thacharodi and Rao 1993).

Risbud et al. (2000) developed a pH-sensitive chitosan/polyvinyl pyrrolidone (PVP) based controlled drug release system for antibiotic delivery. Chitosan and PVP blend were cross-linked with GA to form semi-IPN. Amoxicillin containing hydrogels were either freeze-dried or air-dried. Porous freeze-dried hydrogels (pore diameter, 39.20 µm) exhibited superior pH-dependent swelling properties over non-porous air-dried hydrogels. Increased swelling of hydrogels under acidic conditions was due to the protonation of a primary amino group on chitosan. Freeze-dried membranes released ~73% of the amoxicillin (33% by air-dried) in 3 hr at pH 1.0 and thus, had superior drug-release properties to air-dried hydrogels. Freeze-dried hydrogels could serve as potent candidates for stomach-targeted delivery of antibiotic for treating *H. pylori* infections.

Rao et al. (2006) introduced microgels based on chitosan and hydrolyzed or non-hydrolyzed acrylamide-*g*-PVA for the controlled delivery of an antibiotic, cefadroxil. The drug was loaded into IPN microspheres by water-in-liquid paraffin emulsion method using GA as crosslinking agent. The use of non-hydrolyzed copolymer ensured 88–92% drug entrapment efficiency of the 124–160 µm-sized IPNs. However, the hydrolyzed copolymer improved the drug entrapment efficiency of the IPNs (141–182 µm) from 89% to 95%. Higher drug loadings (25% to 100%) caused an improvement in DEE and large particle size. X-ray diffraction studies indicated amorphous state of the encapsulated drug. The equilibrium swelling increased from 249 to 252% in pH 1.2 and 290–292% in pH 7.4 as the drug loading was increased for the IPNs of non-hydrolyzed copolymer. The incorporation of hydrophilic PVA segments along with polyacrylamide chains into IPN matrix perhaps caused higher swelling of the blends. In case of IPN of CS with hydrolyzed copolymer, the equilibrium swelling became constant to 242% due to complexation between CS amine and acidic group of copolymer in pH 1.2. Hydrolyzed amide groups in IPNs were responsible for higher swelling (360–367%) of IPNs in pH 7.4 media with increased drug loading. In pH 7.4, the swelling decreased from 393% to 337% with increasing amount of GA from 2.5 to 7.5 ml. Nevertheless, the swelling degree was <243% in pH 1.2. This may be due to higher crosslinking density and decreased pore volume of IPNs with increasing amount of GA in the matrix. Increasing amount of GA in the matrix caused lowering of encapsulation efficiency from 93% to 85%, due to lesser free volume space available in the matrix at higher crosslinking density. Only 40% drug was released at 10 hr for 25% drug-loaded CS-hydrolyzed PVA-g-AAm IPNs in pH 1.2 media compared to 62% drug release in pH 7.4 media in the same duration. The data supported that the use of CS microgels with hydrolyzed copolymer were promising materials for controlled drug release application.

Babu et al. (2008) prepared pH-sensitive novel semi-interpenetrating networks (semi-IPN) of *N,N´*-dimethylacrylamide (NNDMA) and chitosan (CS) in the form of microspheres by water-in-oil (w/o) emulsion and GA crosslinking technique. The size of CS-NNDMA particles ranged from 80 to 190 μm and was higher than the plain chitosan. The DEE (57.5%), as was observed for plain chitosan microspheres, was higher (61.5–84.6%) for the IPN formulations. The DEE increased with increasing amount of NNDMA in the microspheres. The DEE of microspheres crosslinked with 2.5, 5 and 7.5 mL of GA, was 74%, 61.5% and 51.9%, respectively. Such a decreasing trend might be due to an increased crosslink density and rigidity that reduced the free volume spaces within the polymer matrix and hence, lower encapsulation efficiency was obtained. By increasing the pH from 1.2 to 7.4, a considerable increase in the cumulative release was observed for the microspheres. The drug release was faster with the use of lower amount of GA during the preparation of microspheres. The slow drug release at higher amount of GA was extended up to 12 hr. The IPNs containing highest amount of drug (30%, w/w) displayed faster and higher release rates than those containing a relatively lower amount of chlorthiazide. The prolonged drug release was observed for formulation containing lower amount of drug. This could be due to availability of more free void spaces in the matrix through which lesser number of drug molecules could transport.

Angadi et al. (2010) prepared GA crosslinked IPN blend microspheres of chitosan (CS) and hydroxyethyl cellulose (HEC) in the form of microspheres (66–82 μm dia) and investigated the potential for controlled release of isoniazid (INH), an antituberculosis drug. The microspheres encapsulated 50 to 66% of fed drug. X-ray data indicated the absence of INH crystals in the drug-loaded matrices. As the amount of GA in the matrices was increased from 5 ml to 10 ml, equilibrium swelling in water decreased significantly from 88 to 58% due to the formation of a more rigid IPN blend matrix. Higher amount of HEC exhibited higher swelling due to presence of higher amount of more hydrophilic HEC than CS. The sequential drug release pattern in SGF (pH 1.2 for 2 hr) and SIF (pH 7.4 for 14 hr) was influenced by the strength of crosslinker, IPN composition and drug loading. The devices released up to 75% drug in 16 hr and thus the IPN matrix could control the drug release following oral ingestion. In a study by Sekhar et al. (2011), guar gum-g-acrylamide (GG-g-AAm) copolymer was incorporated as a part of semi IPN chitosan microspheres. They followed water-in-liquid paraffin oil emulsion and GA crosslinking method for the loading of 5-fluorouracil (5-FU), an anticancer drug in these semi-IPNs. The crystalline nature of drug persisted after encapsulation into semi IPNs. The spherical IPNs of 112–185 µm size provided a maximum drug encapsulation efficiency of 57%. As graft polymer was increased from 20 to 40%, the average size of microspheres and DEE increased from 158–185 µm and 49–54%, respectively. Increasing GA content during the formation of microspheres decreased the trend in drug encapsulation efficiency. As the amount of crosslinker (GA) in the polymer matrices was increased from 2.5 to 7.5 ml, equilibrium water uptake decreased significantly due to the formation of a rigid network structure. The formulations containing higher amount of GG-g-AAm showed higher swelling rates than those formulation without GG-g-AAm due to the extremely hydrophilic nature of GG-g-AAm/CS polymer matrix. Higher amount of GG-g-AAm and GA provided prolonged drug release characteristics to the IPNs for more than 12 hr in buffer medium (pH 7.4). Kajjari et al. (2011) blended acrylamide-*g*-guar gum (pAAm-*g*-GG) with chitosan (CS) to form IPN hydrogel microspheres by the same method. The microspheres encapsulated up to 74% of an antibiotic ciprofloxacin (CFX) and extended CFX release up to 12 hr. Fourier transform infrared spectroscopy (FTIR) confirmed the grafting reaction as well as chemical stability of CFX in the blend IPN hydrogel microspheres. *In vitro* release of CFX in pH 1.2 and 7.4 media was dependent on composition of the IPN, extent of crosslinking as well as initial drug loading. Non-Fickian transport of CFX was assumed through the blend IPN hydrogel microspheres.

Li et al. (2012) synthesized thermo- and pH-sensitive semi-IPN p(NIPAM-co-NVP)/CS hydrogels for the loading and release of an anionic non-steroidal anti-inflammatory (NSAID) drug, naproxen (NAP). They employed free radical polymerization technique using *N,N*-methylenebisacrylamide (MBA) as cross-linker and potassium persulfate/ N,N,N′,N′-tetramethylethylenediamine (TEMED) as redox-initiator pair at 40°C. The hydrogels were swollen in NAP solutions for 48 hr for drug loading purpose.

The amount of NAP loaded by semi-IPN hydrogels increased with the increase of CS contents in hydrogels with DEE values ranging from 42.6 to 51.5%. This was attributed to the good binding affinity of semi-IPN hydrogels to NAP. On one hand, the addition of CS improved the swelling ratio of hydrogels, which favoured the permeating of NAP into hydrogels. On the other hand, interactions of CS with NAP encapsulated more drugs resulting in high entrapment efficiency. Chitosan is a basic polysaccharide (pK$_a$ 6.5) and NAP is a weak acidic drug (pK$_a$ ~4.2). As the hydrogels swelled in water, both CS and NAP were ionized, and resulted in the formation of electrostatic interactions (COO– on NAP and NH^{3+} on CS) as well as the hydrogen bonds between OCH$_3$, COOH on NAP and partly unionized amino groups or hydroxyl groups on CS. The release of NAP from the hydrogels was studied in buffer solution at different pH and temperatures. At temperatures above LCST (32°C), PNIPAM chains assumed a contracted formation and thereby significantly reduced the tendency of water uptake, which then slowed down the diffusion of drug. Only a small portion of NAP was released from p(NIPAM-co-NVP)/CS semi-IPN hydrogels at the initial stage; thereafter, there was no or very slow release up to 36 hr in pH 5.0. Strong electrostatic interactions between CS and NAP at pH 5.0 prevented NAP release from hydrogels. In contrast, NAP released from p(NIPAM-co-NVP) hydrogel was rapid at the initial time being due to lack of the interactions between NAP with CS. However, the amount of NAP release at pH 2.2 was slightly higher than that observed at pH 5.0. The protonation of NAP at pH 2.2 might lead to the partial dissociation of electrostatic interactions between CS and NAP. Nevertheless, due to the collapse of pNIPAM chains at 37°C, the hydrophobic interactions or hydrogen bonds between NAP and hydrogels were still capable of retaining much of loaded drugs. Increasing pH to 7.4, CS was deprotonated leading to the dissociation of interactions between CS and NAP. On the other hand, carboxylic groups of NAP were gradually ionized at pH 7.4, which favoured NAP diffusion from hydrogels into outer surrounding. The release of NAP from hydrogels showed a pronounced burst behaviour at the first 8 hr, during which 85–90% of NAP was released at 25°C. The release rate of NAP at 37°C was slower than that observed at 25°C. Only ~50% of NAP was released in the initial 8 hr; thereafter, a continuous release still occurred over 36 hr exhibiting a sustained release feature. This was most likely because the phase transition of pNIPAM occurred at 37°C and the hydrophobic interactions hindered the diffusion of drugs. The presence of CS in semi-IPN networks provided a high affinity for anionic drugs, which favoured the stabilization and migration of encapsulated drugs in hydrogels. At pH 7.4 and 37°C, deprotonation of CS and collapsed pNIPAM resulted in the controlled release of drugs without burst diffusion compared to that occurred at pH 2.2 and pH 5.0. This type of smart material could be very useful in designing novel controlled drug delivery system.

2.3.3 *Modified chitosan-synthetic polymers*

To combine the advantages of synthetic and natural polymers and at the same time maintain the favourable properties of natural polymers such as biodegradation and bioactivity, Guo and Gao (2007) synthesized pH- and temperature-sensitive hydrogels with CMCS and poly(N-isopropylacrylamide) using MBA as the crosslinking agent. They used coenzyme A (CoA) as the model drug that modulates the metabolism of sugar, fat, and protein.

The swelling of the hydrogels decreased as a function of temperature both at pH 2.1 and 7.4. Since the semi-IPN hydrogel swells differently at different solution temperatures, they investigated temperature-dependent swelling properties of semi-IPNs. The IPN hydrogel swelled reversibly at 25°C and 37°C in pH 7.4. The semi-IPN hydrogels swelled much more at 25°C in pH 7.4 solution than that in pH 2.1 solution. This was explained by the fact that –COOH could form an H-bond between the –OH groups in the CMCS and the –NHCO in pNIPAm in acidic solution. Although –NH$_2$ is positively charged in pH 2.1 solution, there is electrostatic repulsion in the polymer network. However, the degree of substitution of CMCS is very high (1.08), and the amount of residual –NH$_2$ is rather limited, so the H-bond was dominant in the polymer network system and the hydrogel shrank. At pH 7.4, –COOH was negatively charged and H-bonds between –COOH and –OH, –NHCO groups were dissociated due to electrostatic repulsion between the –COO- groups and the hydrogel swelled dramatically. The swelling of pNIPAm was always larger than that of the semi-IPN hydrogels in acid solution, and the swelling ratio of pNIPAm was always smaller than that of the semi-IPN hydrogels in basic solution. The swelling of the semi-IPN hydrogel increased with the CMCS content in pH 7.4 solutions at various temperature. Increasing CMCS content from 5–30% accelerated CoA release at 25°C in pH 7.4, while maintaining drug release over 24 hr.

Though the swelling was higher at 25°C, the drug release rate was slower up to 24 hr in pH 7.4. They reasoned that as pNIPAm chains became more hydrophobic near or above the LCST, the effective crosslinking density of the CMCS/pNIPAm network might be reduced by the precipitation of pNIPAm. Hence, the porous size of the hydrogel was enlarged after collapsing of PNIPAm chains inside the semi-IPN hydrogel, which accelerated the CoA release (Muniz and Geuskens 2001, Soppimath et al. 2002).

Another possible reason was that there was an electrostatic repulsion between phosphates in CoA and –COO- in the hydrogel, and it accelerated CoA release at pH 7.4. At 25°C, the substitute of phosphate in CoA could form an H-bond with the –OH, –NHCO, and –NH$_2$ groups in the hydrogel. With increasing temperature of the release medium, the H-bond became weaker, and accelerated the release of CoA from the hydrogel. As a result, the release rate in pH 7.4 buffer solution at 37°C was faster than that at 25°C. Semi-IPN could swell and shrink with changing pH between pH 2.1 and 7.4, which was similar to the temperature-sensitivity. The CoA release profile of semi-IPN in solutions of pH 2.1 was slower than that in pH 7.4 at

37°C over a period of 24 hr. The CoA released from the hydrogel was 16.5% within 3 hr in SGF (pH 2.1), and the release rate in SIF (pH 7.4) reached nearly 81.4% of the initial drug content 6 hr after changing the medium. This implied that this polymer had the desired protective effect for oral delivery of the drug, as a significant fraction of the drug remained in the polymer as the hydrogels passed through the low-pH environment of the stomach. The results suggested that the hydrogel had great potential as oral drug delivery systems. After 24 hr, ~88.6% CoA was released. This was because some CoA molecules might be entrapped within the hydrogel network, and were not released unless the polymer matrixes degraded.

Superporous hydrogels containing poly(acrylic acid-co-acrylamide)/ carboxymethyl chitosan (CMCS) IPNs (SPH-IPNs) were prepared by crosslinking CMCS with GA after superporous hydrogel (SPH) was synthesized. Due to the cross-linked *O*-CMCS network, *in vitro* mucoadhesive force and mechanical properties, including compression and tensile modulus of the SPH-IPN were greatly improved when compared with the SPH without CMCS. The loading capacities of the SPH-IPNs were significantly improved and could be modulated by varying the CMCS content. More than 90% of the insulin was released within 1 hr and the remaining drug was almost released in another hour in PBS (pH 7.4). SPH-IPN exhibited immense potential to be used as mucoadhesive system for peroral delivery of peptide and protein drugs. Ajish et al. (2016) irradiated an aqueous solution of 5% (w/v) D-glucose based monoacrylamide (Glc-acryl) and 0.1% (w/v) bisacrylamide (Glc-bis) up to 29.5 kGy in Co-60 γ-source to synthesize glycopolymeric hydrogel (Glc-gel). Ca^{2+} cross-linked *N*-succinyl chitosans (NSCs) beads were coated with *in situ* forming IPN of Glc-acryl and Glc-bis gel following a total irradiation dose of 1.68 kGy. Doxorubicin (DOX) was loaded into beads and the best DOX encapsulation was observed after 12 hr of incubation. The DOX encapsulation efficiency of the beads was dependent on the degree of succinylation in the NSCs (75% and 88%). The encapsulation efficiency of the NSC88/Glc-gel and NSC75/Glc-gel beads was 92.7% and 75%, respectively. This suggested that the mechanism of loading was governed mainly by the electrostatic interaction between the COO– groups in the polymer and the NH_2 group of DOX (Das et al. 2013, Hu et al. 2015). After an initial release of pysisorbed DOX molecules from the hydrogel matrix, a slow and sustained DOX delivery profile was observed for both types of beads, with greater release rate at pH 5.0. The DOX release from the NSC75/Glc-gel beads at pHs 5.0 and 7.4 were 76% and 36% in 18 d, respectively. The respective values with the NSC88/Glc-gel beads were 88% and 79%. Hence, NSC75/Glc-gel beads were considered ideal matrices for localized cancer therapy.

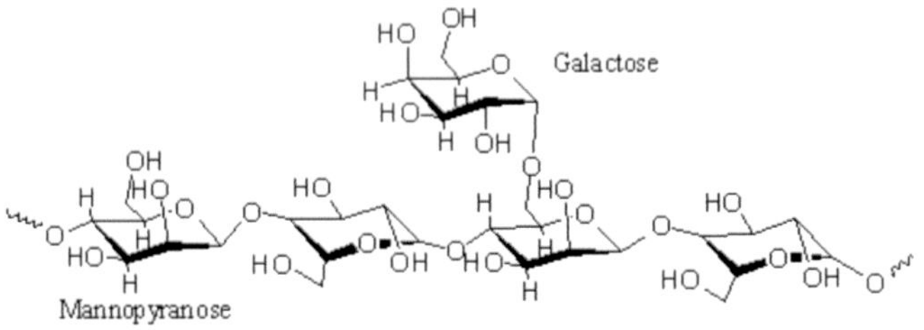

Fig. 5. Possible structure of LBG with monosaccharide units.

2.4 Locust bean gum IPNs

Locust bean gum (LBG) is another high molecular weight branch polysaccharide, extracted from the seeds of carob tree *Ceratonia siliqua*. Figure 5 depicts the structural information about this biopolymer.

It consists of (1,4)-linked β-D-mannopyranose backbone with branch points from their 6-positions linked to α-D-galactose (1,6-linked α-D-galactopyranose) (Parvathy et al. 2005). Locust bean gum finds wide application in drug formulation due to its non-toxic potential.

2.4.1 LBG-other polysaccharides

Dey et al. (2013a) compared the drug delivery performance of Al^{3+} ions crosslinked IPNs of ALG and carmoxymethyl LBG (CMLBG) with homopolymer hydrogel networks. IPNs allowed about 94% entrapment of glipizide and exhibited slower drug release profiles up to 8 hr. Al^{3+}-ALG network almost completed the release of embedded drug in 3.5 hr; however, the homopolymer Al^{3+}-CMLBG network discharged their content at a slow, uniform rate up to 8 hr like the IPNs in phosphate buffer (pH 7.4). Moreover, IPNs gained appreciation for their better mechanical strength (63.79 ± 1.59 MPa) than Al^{3+}-CMLBG network. Hence, Al^{3+}-ELBG and IPNs could be useful in controlling diabetes for longer periods. They further evaluated *in vivo* hypoglycemic activity of the IPN in male Wistar rats (Dey et al. 2013b). IPN beads, composed of CMLBG:ALG (3:1) ensured about 96.91% DEE and provided the slowest drug-release profile. A maximum reduction of 58.96% in the blood glucose level was observed at the 8th hr after oral administration of the IPN beads. The hypoglycemic activity was significant between the 2nd and 10th hr. They concluded that the IPNs of ALG with CMLBG could replace Ca^{2+}–ALG beads in terms of prolonged control of diabetes. Dey and groups (2015) also investigated the effect of gelation time during synthesis of glipizide-loaded carboxymethyl LBG and ALG IPN beads by ionic crosslinking in aqueous aluminium chloride salt solution. The longer exposure of the IPN beads caused a considerable loss of drug, and affected their drug release performance. IPNs cured for 0.5 hr exhibited slower drug release kinetics in HCl (pH 1.2) and phosphate buffer (pH 7.4) solution than those incubated for 1–2 hr. The higher swelling of IPN was associated with faster release rate in phosphate buffer solution (pH 7.4) and continued for at least 8 hr. Thus, the delivery of BCS class II anti-diabetic can be controlled by modulating gelation period. Jana et al. (2015) prepared ALG–LBG IPN microspheres which were prepared by calcium ion (Ca^{+2}) induced ionotropic gelation technique for prolonged release of aceclofenac. The drug entrapment efficiency of 406–684 µm size microspheres lied in between 59–93%. Increasing concentration of LBG in IPN progressively increased DEE due to the formation of dense matrix and uniform encapsulation of insoluble aceclofenac within ALG-LBG IPN. The microspheres prepared using ALG:LBG of 1:1 showed low entrapment of aceclofenac (59–63%). The microspheres provided sustained release of aceclofenac in phosphate buffer solution (pH 6.8) over a period of 8 hr. The initial burst release of ALG beads was reduced by increasing the concentration of LBG. The standard aceclofenac exhibited comparatively rapid inhibition of rat paw oedema than that of the IPN microspheres indicating rapid anti-inflammatory activity up to 3 hr and then declined. IPN microspheres showed slower oedema inhibition and gradually % inhibition increased up to 5 hr after oral administration indicating sustained action of aceclofenac.

2.4.2 *LBG and synthetic polymers*

Kaity and associated research workers (2013) developed IPN microspheres of LBG and PVA for oral controlled release of buflomedil hydrochloride (BH) by emulsion crosslinking method using GA as crosslinker. The DEE was highly dependent on gum:PVA ratio and the amount of crosslinker and ranged 29.73–68.59%. The arithmetic mean diameter varied from 734 to 293 µm. As the amount of LBG was increased, the swelling capacity of the hydrogel network was increased in parallel due to hydrophilic nature of native gum. The amount of PVA did not affect the water uptake because of its low water uptake capacity compared to LBG. The amount of crosslinker significantly influenced the water uptake capacity of the microspheres. A lowering of LBG:PVA ratio (3:1 to 1:3) reduced the drug release rate, which indicated the role of LBG in the swelling of microspheres in dissolution medium. In formulations with fixed gum:PVA ratio (3:1), the amount of GA added (2.5–7.5 mL) resulted in reduction of drug release from 85.23% to 81.64% to 75.36%. They argued that higher crosslinker concentration increased the rigidity of the network, prevented the imbibition of buffer into the polymer matrix leading to reduction of drug release in pH 6.8. The drug release also increased from 65.24% to 74.66% as the amount of drug loading was increased from 50 to 75%. The same decreased to 63.42% when drug loading was decreased to 25%. In acidic medium, less than 20% drug release was approximated. Regardless of the variation, the drug release could be prolonged up to 12 hr.

The drug entrapment efficiency (DEE) of carboxymethyl LBG-PVA IPN did not significantly improve to that of LBG-PVA IPN (Kaity and Ghosh 2013). The drug release rate was faster due to porous nature of IPN particles. However, acrylamide grafted LBG-PVA (Am-g-LBG-PVA) IPN microspheres showed improvement in both DEE and drug release.

In another study, they developed a biodegradable, biocompatible and stable IPN system of acrylamide-grafted-LBG (Am-g-LBG) and PVA by emulsion crosslinking method for controlled oral delivery of BH (Kaity and Ghosh 2016). They used microwave-assisted technique for grafting acrylamide onto LBG using ceric ammonium nitrate as free radical generator. DSC study with placebo microspheres did not reveal peaks of individual components, rather a broad endothermic peak was observed at about 288°C. This was indicative of the formation of a polymer composite, which degraded at a temperature other than the degradation points of individual components. The drug entrapment capacity was found to depend on the gum:PVA, cross-linker and drug loads. A higher amount of Am-g-LBG led to reduced DEE due to increased hydrophilicity of the system and inability of GA to crosslink the total system. Regardless of the variables, the mean drug entrapment efficiency of Am-g-LBG-PVA IPN microspheres was in the range of 51.32–73.51%. An increased amount of GA assisted in the entrapment of higher amount of drug due to the formation of rigid polymer matrix. Interestingly, an increased drug loading showed least effect on the DEE of the IPN microspheres. The presence of higher amount of grafted gum in microspheres resulted in higher swelling both in pH 1.2 and 6.8 buffer solutions. However, the swelling of particles in acidic media (pH 1.2) was less than that in phosphate buffer (pH 6.8). The arithmetic mean diameter of IPN particles varied from 371 µm to 766 µm. The sequential release of drug from the IPN microspheres were investigated in pH 1.2 for the initial 2 hr, followed by phosphate buffer of pH 6.8. When the blend ratio of IPN particles were changed from 1:2 to 1:1 at a fixed crosslinker and % drug loading, the drug release increased up to 87% in 12 hr. On the contrary, the particles composed of only PVA showed 74% drug release in 12 hr. As usual, higher crosslinking of the matrix at higher amount of GA (2.5 to 5.0 ml) prevented solvent imbibition and network erosion leading to slow drug release property.

Moreover, they focused on the comparative bio-safety and pharmacokinetics of BH-loaded LBG-PVA, carboxymethyl LBG-PVA and Am-g-LBG-PVA IPNs (Kaity and Ghosh 2015). During acute oral toxicity study on Swiss albino mice, no animals died during an observation period of 14 d following administration of a single dose of 2000 mg/kg body weight of IPNs. Because LD50 value was greater than 2000 mg/kg dose of IPNs, the test product fell under the *Category 5* and hence, toxicity rating was zero as per "Organization of Economic Co-operation and Development (OECD)" guidelines. Further, the histological sections of heart, kidney, liver and spleen appeared to be almost similar to that of control group on 15th d of toxicity study. Therefore, IPNs were considered safe for oral use. In biodegradability study, the test plates showed gradual evidence of fungal growth in all IPNs. The microscopic study showed apparent fungi growth on 0, 3, 7, 14 and 21 d in the entire test Petridishes. Since the media was not having a component, which can provide carbon for the growth of the *Aspergillus niger* fungi, it could be said that the evidence of fungal growth in IPN containing plates was a result of carbon utilization from the particles. Therefore, it was inferred that all three IPNs were biodegradable in nature. Among three optimized IPN microspheres, the Am-g-LBG showed highest growth of microbes in comparison to others. The CMLBG-PVA IPN microspheres showed evidence of less microbial growth than the other IPNs. LBG-PVA IPN microspheres showed normal growth of microbes due to biodegradable nature of LBG.

Pharmacokinetic study on rabbit model revealed that T_{max}, i.e., time to reach peak plasma drug concentration from LBG-PVA and Am-g-LBG-PVA IPNs was greater than that of both BH oral suspension and CMLBG-PVA IPN but there was no significant difference between BH oral suspension and CMLBG-PVA IPN. Therefore, the rate of absorption from LBG-PVA IPN and Am-g-LBG-PVA IPN was delayed though there was no significant difference of their C_{max} value suggesting that both dosage forms were capable of releasing the required amount of drug to attain minimum effective concentration, satisfying the loading dose concept of sustained release dosage form. The absorption rate was high but the extent of absorption was low for CMLBG-PVA IPN. The enzymatic degradation rate was lower for LBG-IPN and Am-g-LBG-PVA IPN suggesting low rate of absorption and high extent of absorption, satisfying the behaviour of ideal sustained release dosage form.

Some other polysaccharides have also been used as a component of IPNs for drug delivery applications. The IPN fabrication methods and the properties of the drug delivery devices are summarized in Table 1.

Table 1. Some other natural polymer-based IPN hydrogel systems for potential applications in controlled drug delivery

IPN polymers/ drug	Methods of hydrogel fabrication	Study outcomes	References
Gelatin & poly(acrylamido glycolic acid)/curcumin	Free radical emulsion polymerization	• Curcumin encapsulation efficiency of 100 nm size IPN nanogels (NGs) was 42–48%. The same decreased with increasing acrylamidoglycolic acid (AGA) content in the NGs due to the more rigid network formed during polymerization. • Curcumin release increases with increasing AGA content in the NGs because of the hydrophilicity of AGA (30–55% in PH 1.2 gastric fluid & 80–90% in pH 7.4 PBS 96 h). • High water dispersible CUR-loaded NGs exhibited enhanced anti cancer activity on the colorectal cancer cells than pristine CUR. • pH-sensitive NGs can be applied for colorectal cancer drug delivery applications.	Rao et al. 2015
κ-carrageenan and sodium carboxymethyl cellulose (SCMC)/Ibuprofen	Water-in-water emulsion gelation process using AlCl3	• The drug entrapment efficiency was found to be in the range between 78.68 ± 1.14% and 89.42 ± 1.44%. IPN beads prepared with a higher amount of SCMC exhibited lower drug entrapment efficiency. • Swelling ability and drug release of beads in alkaline medium was substantial as that of acidic medium. • About 65–90% drug released sequentially in release medium (2 hr in pH 1.2 & then 10 hr in pH 7.4). • pH-sensitive IPN beads retarded NSAID release in acidic medium and thus, could minimize the gastric side effects of the model ibuprofen.	Lohani et al. 2016
κ-carrageenan and poly(methacrylic acid)/ poly(N, N-diethylacrylamide)/ None	Free radical polymerization	• Increase of κ-carrageenan-g-poly(methacrylic acid) component improved thermo- and pH-sensitivity of into poly(diethylacrylamide) hydrogel. • Pore size of hydrogel became larger with the increase in κ-carrageenan-g-poly(methacrylic acid). • Expected to have potential application in controlled drug delivery systems.	Chen et al. 2009

Polymer/Drug	Method	Observations	Reference
Carboxymethyl cellulose and polyacrylamide-g-xanthan/ketoprofen	Ionotropic gelation using AlCl$_3$	• Drug entrapment efficiency of the beads was 81.8–92.9%. • Use of higher AlCl$_3$ strength (5–15%w/v) slowed the drug release (About 90% drug released in 10 hr). • Higher amount of graft copolymer caused faster drug release. • Swelling and drug release significantly increased with change in medium from acidic (pH 1.2) to alkaline (pH 7.4). • May be useful as pH-sensitive drug delivery systems.	Kulkarni and Sa 2008
Guar gum and poly(vinyl alcohol)/nifedipine	Emulsion cross linking with glutaraldehyde (GA)	• Drug entrapment efficiency of 300 µ size microspheres varies depending upon drug loading method. • Drug loading before crosslinking produced higher 20–62% DEE. • By loading higher percentage of drug before cross linking, the drug release can be prolonged.	Soppimath et al. 2000
Poly(acrylamide)-*grafted*-Guar Gum and chitosan/Ciprofloxacin	Emulsion crosslinking method using GA	• The microspheres encapsulated up to 74% of ciprofloxacin (CFX) antibiotic. • The release of CFX from microspheres was extended up to 12 hr. • CFX release in pH 1.2 and 7.4 media was dependent on IPN composition, extent of crosslinking as well as initial drug loading.	Kajjari et al. 2011
Guar gum (GG) and chitosan (CS)/Cefadroxil	water-in-oil (w/o) emulsion crosslinking with GA	• The drug is dispersed at the molecular level in the semi-IPN matrix. • Sustained and controlled release of cefadroxil from semi-IPN microspheres up to 10 hr in pH 7.4 buffer. • CS-GG composition of the blend and the amount of crosslinking agent affected the release of cefadroxil from the semi-IPN microspheres.	Reddy et al. 2006
Gelatin and polyethylene glycol diacrylate (PEG-DA575)/nystatin	Electrospun method	• Gelatin nanofiber scaffolds possessed improved structural stability. • Scaffold possessed greatest mucoadhesion properties at 4 times higher PEG-DA concentration @575 g mol^{-1}. • Semi-IPN scaffold slowly released an anti-fungal reagent nystatin. • Nanofiber scaffolds was suitable for oral mucosal drug delivery.	Aduba Jr et al. 2013

Table 1 contd. ...

...Table 1 contd.

IPN polymers/ drug	Methods of hydrogel fabrication	Study outcomes	References
carboxymethyl pullulan and poly(N-isopropylacrylamide) (PNIPAAm) / diphenhydramine (DPH)	Chemical crosslinking followed by additional reticulation of polysaccharide	• IPN hydrogels responded to both temperature and pH, reversibly. • DPH release rate was higher at pH 10 buffer solution than at pH 7.4 and 1.2. • In pseudo physiological conditions, DPH was quickly released from the hydrogel at 20°C, and showed a sustained release profile at 37°C.	Asmarandei et al. 2013
Delonix regia seed polysaccharide (DRG) and sodium alginate/Diclofenac sodium (DS)	Ionotropic gelation method using calcium chloride	• DEE of the beads was found in the range 32.79–56.54%. • Swelling of beads was higher in phosphate buffer (pH 6.8) than in 0.1 N HCl (pH 1.2). • DRG-alginate IPN beads exhibited sustained release of DS for 8 hr in phosphate buffer (pH 6.8).	Dias et al. 2015
Gum ghatti and poly(methacrylic acid-aniline)/ amoxicillin trihydrate	Free radical and simple oxidative polymerization	• Hydrogel network showed a pH-dependent swelling behaviour. • Less release in acidic and neutral media than in basic media. • Suitable as carriers for colon specific controlled release of drug.	Sharma et al. 2015
Gum ghatti and poly(vinyl alcohol)(PVA)/ ranitidine HCl	Emulsion crosslinking with GA	• Drug encapsulation of up to 87.80% was achieved. • The percentage mucoadhesivity was increased with increase in the ratio of gum:PVA. • The release of ranitidine HCl depends on the extent of crosslinking of the matrix as well as the ratio of Gum:PVA present in the matrix. • IPN mucoadhesive microspheres provided oral controlled release of ranitidine HCl in 0.1 N HCl solution (pH 1.2). • Uniform drug absorption could be achieved from oral controlled release IPNs.	Jain and Banik 2015

Xanthan gum and PVA / diclofenac sodium	Emulsion crosslinking with GA	• Depending on GA and XG concentration, DEE was 60–84%. • Mean particle size ranged between 310–477 μm. • Slow drug release for IPNs with higher amount of GA. • Increase in the xanthan gum caused higher swelling and faster drug release. • IPN microspheres provided oral controlled release of water-soluble DS over 12 hr in pH 6.8. • Oral absorption was significantly higher with IPN microparticles in rabbit model.	Ray et al. 2010
Gum ghatti, poly(acrylic acid) and polyaniline/amoxicillin trihydrate and paracetamol	Radical copolymerization & oxidative-radical copolymerization	• Release of amoxicillin trihydrate and paracetamol from hydrogels was found more at pH 9.2 as compared to that at pH 2.4 and pH 7.0. • Maximum conductivity was found to be 2.5×10^{-6} S cm^{-1} at 1.5 N HCl concentration. • Conducting hydrogel appeared to be a good drug delivery device for both drugs in alkaline pH. • Hydrogel showed lower release in acidic (pH 2.4) and neutral media than in basic media (pH 9.2), making those suitable carriers for colon-specific drug delivery.	Sharma et al. 2015
Dextran-*g*-acrylamide (Dex-*g*-AAm) and PVA/abacavir sulfate	emulsion cross-linking	• Size of semi-IPN microspheres ranged between 80 and 100 μm. • Controlled release (CR) of an anti-HIV agent.	Sullad et al. 2011
Guar gum-*g*-acrylic acid and PVA/isoniazid	water-in-oil (w/o) emulsification	• pH-sensitive microspheres of ~10 μm size were produced. • Release of the antituberculosis drug was increased to 8 hr from its nascent plasma half-life of 0.5–1.6 hr.	Sullad et al. 2010
Pectin and carboxymethyl xanthan Gum/Diltiazem HCl	Ionic (Al^{3+} ions) and covalent crosslinking with GA	• Increasing the GA content in the IPN beads decreased their degradation rate. • Higher swelling and drug release were observed in pH 6.8 buffer solutions than in pH 1.2. • Hydrogel beads minimized the drug release in pH 1.2 buffer and release < 80% drug in 8 hr.	Giri et al. 2013

3. Conclusion

The multi-component drug delivery systems have been developed for potential therapeutic applications. Semi-interpenetrating polymer networks (semi-IPNs) and IPNs have emerged as innovative biomaterials for drug delivery. The network properties could be tailored by the type and concentration of polymers, drug, crosslinker, type of crosslinking (ionic or covalent or both), and mass ratio of IPN polymers. In most of the cases, the polysaccharides were chemically and physically crosslinked, both for the formation of IPN hydrogel networks. Several biopolymers were critically reviewed and it was apparent that the polysaccharides were suitable building block materials for the design of stimuli-responsive hydrogel networks. The dual biopolymers and combination of natural-synthetic polymers have been tested to improve the mechanical strength, drug entrapment efficacy and controlled drug release properties. Despite the non-toxic and biodegradable nature of native biomaterials, the major concerns that must be addressed for effective applications of new systems are the biocompatibility and biodegradability of their interpenetrating networks. Moreover, some polysaccharides possess inherent bioactivity that may be exploited to improve the performances of the prepared hydrogels. However, the synergistic behaviour of the combined polysaccharide networks must also be evaluated. The presence of a large number of functional groups in the polysaccharide structures can be tailored to generate novel IPN systems for successful delivery of drugs.

References

Aduba, Jr, D.C., J.A. Hammer, Q. Yuan, W.A. Yeudall, G.L. Bowlin and H. Yang. 2013. Semi-interpenetrating network (sIPN) gelatin nanofiber scaffolds for oral mucosal drug delivery. Acta Biomater. 9: 6576–6584.

Agnihotri, S.A. and T.M. Aminabhavi. 2005. Development of novel interpenetrating network gellan gum-poly(vinyl alcohol) hydrogel microspheres for the controlled release of carvedilol. Drug Dev. Ind. Pharm. 31: 491–503.

Ajish, J.K., K.S.A. Ajish Kumar, S. Chattopadhyay and M. Kumar. 2016. Glycopolymeric gel stabilized N-succinyl chitosan beads for controlled doxorubicin delivery. Carbohydr. Polym. 144: 98–105.

Alves, N.M. and J.F. Mano. 2008. Chitosan derivatives obtained by chemical modifications for biomedical and environmental applications. Int. J. Biol. Macromol. 43: 401–414.

Angadi, S.C., L.S. Manjeshwar and T.M. Aminabhavi. 2010. Interpenetrating polymer network blend microspheres of chitosan and hydroxyethyl cellulose for controlled release of isoniazid. Int. J. Biol. Macromol. 47: 171–179.

Asmarandei, I., G. Fundueanu, M. Cristea, V. Harabagiu and M. Constantin. 2013. Thermo- and pH-sensitive interpenetrating poly(N-isopropylacrylamide)/carboxymethyl pullulan network for drug delivery. J. Polym. Res. 20: 293.

Athawale, V.D., S.L. Kolekar and S.S. Raut. 2003. Recent developments in polyurethanes and poly(acrylates) interpenetrating polymer networks. J. Macromol. Sci. Part. C. Polym. Rev. 43: 1–26.

Babu, V.R., K.S.V.K. Rao, M. Sairam, B.V.K. Naidu, K.M. Hosamani and T.M. Aminabhavi. 2006. pH sensitive interpenetrating network microgels of sodium alginate-acrylic acid for the controlled release of ibuprofen. J. Appl. Polym. Sci. 99: 2671–2678.

Babu, V.R., K.M. Hosamani and T.M. Aminabhavi. 2008. Preparation and *in vitro* release of chlorothiazide novel pH-sensitive chitosan-N,N´-dimethylacrylamide semi-interpenetrating network microspheres. Carbohydr. Polym. 71: 208–217.

Bajpai, A.K., S.K. Shukla, S. Bhanu and S. Kankane. 2008. Responsive polymers in controlled drug delivery. Prog. Polym. Sci. 33: 1088–1118.

Bhardwaj, T.R., M. Kanwar, R. Lal and A. Gupta. 2000. Natural gums and modified natural gums as sustained-release carriers. Drug Dev. Ind. Pharm. 26: 1025–1038.

Boppana, R., G.K. Mohan, U. Nayak, S. Mutalik, B. Sa and R.V. Kulkarni. 2015. Novel pH-sensitive IPNs of polyacrylamide-g-gum ghatti and sodium alginate for gastro-protective drug delivery. Int. J. Biol. Macromol. 75: 133–143.

Chen, C.C. and A.T. Metters. 2006. Hydrogels in controlled release formulations: network design and mathematical modeling. Adv. Drug Deliv. Rev. 58: 1379–1408.

Chen, J., M. Liu and S. Chen. 2009. Synthesis and characterization of thermo- and pH-sensitive kppa-carrageenan-g-poly(methacrylic acid)/poly(N,N-diethylacrylamide) semi-IPN hydrogel. Mater. Chem. Physic. 115: 339–346.

Choi, J.-H., H.Y. Lee and J.-C. Kim. 2008. Release behavior of freeze-dried alginate beads containing poly(N-isopropylacrylamide) copolymers. J. Appl. Polym. Sci. 110: 117–123.

Coviello, T., P. Matricardi, C. Marianecci and F. Alhaique. 2007. Polysaccharide hydrogels for modified release formulations. J. Control. Release. 119: 5–24.

Das, D., R. Das, P. Ghosh, S. Dhara, A.B. Panda and S. Pal. 2013. Dextrin crosslinked with poly(HEMA): A novel hydrogel for colon specific delivery of ornidazole. RSC Adv. 3: 25340–25350.

Das, S. and A. Chaudhury. 2011. Recent advances in lipid nanoparticle formulations with solid matrix for oral drug delivery. AAPS PharmSciTech. 12: 62–76.

Dashevsky, A. and A. Mohamad. 2006. Development of pulsatile multiparticulate drug delivery systemcoated with aqueous dispersion Aquacoat® ECD. Int. J. Pharm. 318: 124–131.

Dey, N.S., S. Majumdar and M.E.B. Rao. 2008. Multiparticulate drug delivery systems for controlled release. Trop. J. Pharm. Res. 7: 1067–75.

Dey, P., S. Maiti and B. Sa. 2013a. Novel etherified locust bean gum-alginate hydrogels for controlled release of glipizide. J. Biomater. Sci. Polym. Ed. 24: 663–683.

Dey, P., S. Maiti and B. Sa. 2013b. Gastrointestinal delivery of glipizide from carboxymethyl locust bean gum–Al^{3+}–alginate hydrogel network: *in vitro* and *in vivo* performance. J. Appl. Polym. Sci. 128: 2063–2072.

Dey, P., B. Sa and S. Maiti. 2015. Impact of gelation period on modified locust bean-alginate interpenetrating beads for oral glipizide delivery. Int. J. Biol. Macromol. 76: 176–180.

Dias, R.J., V.S. Ghorpade, V.D. Havaldar, K.K. Mali, N.H. Salunkhe and J.H. Shinde. 2015. Development and optimization of interpenetrating network beads of delonix regia gum and sodium alginate using response surface methodology. J. Appl. Pharm. Sci. 5: 56–64.

Ganji, F. and E. Vasheghani-Farahani. 2009. Hydrogels in controlled drug delivery systems. Iranian Polym. J. 18: 63–88.

Garcia, M.O., D. Blanco, J.A. Martin and J.M. Teijon. 2000. 5-Fluorouracil trapping in poly(2-hydroxyethyl methacrylate) hydrogels: *In vitro* drug delivery studies. Eur. Polym. J. 36: 111–122.

George, M. and T.E. Abraham. 2007. pH sensitive alginate-guar gum hydrogel for the controlled delivery of protein drugs. Int. J. Pharm. 335: 123–129.

Giri, T.K., C. Choudhary, A. Alexander, Ajazuddin, H. Badwaik, M. Tripathy et al. 2013. Sustained release of diltiazem hydrochloride from cross-linked biodegradable IPN hydrogel beads of pectin and modified xanthan gum. Indian J. Pharm. Sci. 75: 619–627.

Guo, B.-L. and Q.-Y. Gao. 2007. Preparation and properties of a pH/temperature-responsive carboxymethyl chitosan/poly(N-isopropylacrylamide) semi-IPN hydrogel for oral delivery of drugs. Carbohydr. Res. 342: 2416–2422.

Halder, A., S. Mukherjee and B. Sa. 2005. Development and evaluation of polyethyleneimine-treated calcium alginate beads for sustained release of diltiazem. J. Microencapsul. 22: 67–80.

Halder, A. and B. Sa. 2006. Preparation and *in vitro* evaluation of polystyrene-coated diltiazem–resin complex by oil-in-water emulsion solvent evaporation method. AAPS PharmSciTech. 7: E4-105–E112.

Hassan, M.C. and N.A. Peppas. 2000. Structure and applications of poly(vinyl alcohol) hydrogel produced by conventional crosslinking or by freezing/thawing methods. Adv. Polym. Sci. 153: 37–62.

Henriksen, I., K.L. Green, J.D. Smart, G. Smistad and J. Karlsen. 1996. Bioadhesion of hydrated chitosan: An *in vitro* and *in vivo* study. Int. J. Pharm. 145: 231–240.

Hoare, T.R. and D.S. Kohane. 2008. Hydrogels in drug delivery: progress and challenges. Polymer. 49: 1993–2007.

Hoosain, F.G., Y.E. Choonara, P. Kumar, L.K. Toma, C. Tyagi and L.C. du Toit. 2014. An epichlorohydrin-crosslinked semi-interpenetrating GG-PEO network as a xerogel matrix for sustained release of sulpiride. AAPS PharmSciTech. 15: 1292–1306.

Hoosain, F.G., Y.E. Choonara, P. Kumar, L.K. Toma, C. Tyagi and L.C. du Toit. 2016. *In vivo* evaluation of a PEO-gellan gum semi-interpenetrating polymer network for the oral delivery of sulpiride. AAPS PharmSciTech. (in press).

Hu, X., W. Wei, X. Qi, H. Yu, L. Feng, J. Li et al. 2015. Preparation and characterization of a novel pH-sensitive Salecan-g-poly(acrylic acid) hydrogel for controlled release of doxorubicin. J. Mater. Chem. B. 3: 2685–2697.

Hua, S., H. Ma, X. Li, H. Yang and A. Wang. 2010. pH-sensitive sodium alginate/poly(vinyl alcohol) hydrogel beads prepared by combined Ca^{2+} crosslinking and freeze thawing cycles for controlled release of diclofenac sodium. Int. J. Biol. Macromol. 46: 517–523.

Izumi, Y., N. Kikuta, K. Sakai and H. Takezawa. 1996. Phase diagrams and molecular structures of sodium-salt-type gellan gum. Carbohydr. Polym. 30: 121–127.

Jain, N. and A. Banik. 2013. Novel interpenetrating polymer network mucoadhesive microspheres of gum ghatti and poly(vinyl alcohol) for the delivery of ranitidine HCl. Asian J. Pharm. Clin. Res. 6: 119–123.

Jana, S., A. Saha, A.K. Nayak, K.K. Sen and S.K. Basu. 2013. Aceclofenac-loaded chitosan-tamarind seed polysaccharide interpenetrating polymeric network microparticles. Colloids Surf. B. Biointerfaces. 105: 303–309.

Jana, S., K.K. Sen and S.K. Basu. 2014. *In vitro* aceclofenac release from IPN matrix tablets composed of chitosan-tamarind seed polysaccharide. Int. J. Biol. Macromol. 65: 241–245.

Jana, S., S. Manna, A.K. Nayak, K.K. Sen and S.K. Basu. 2014. Carbopol gel containing chitosan-egg albumin nanoparticles for transdermal aceclofenac delivery. Colloids Surf. B. Biointerfaces. 114: 36–44.

Jana, S., A. Gandhi, S. Sheet and K.K. Sen. 2015. Metal ion-induced alginate–locust bean gum IPN microspheres for sustained oral delivery of aceclofenac. Int. J. Biol. Macromol. 72: 47–53.

Kaith, B.S., R. Jindal, H. Mittal and R. Kumar. 2012. Synthesis of crosslinked networks of gum ghatti with different vinyl monomer mixtures and effect of ionic strength of various cations on its swelling behavior. Int. J. Polym. Mater. 61: 99–115.

Kaity, S. and A. Ghosh. 2013. Carboxymethylation of locust bean gum: Application in interpenetrating polymer network microspheres for controlled drug delivery. Ind. Eng. Chem. Res. 52: 10033–10045.

Kaity, S., J. Isaac and A. Ghosh. 2013. Interpenetrating polymer network of locust bean gum-poly(vinyl alcohol) for controlled release drug delivery. Carbohydr. Polym. 94: 456–467.

Kaity, S. and A. Ghosh. 2015. Comparative bio-safety and *in vivo* evaluation of native or modified locust bean gum-PVA IPN microspheres. Int. J. Biol. Macromol. 72: 883–893.

Kaity, S. and A. Ghosh. 2016. Facile preparation of acrylamide grafted locust bean gum-poly(vinyl alcohol) interpenetrating polymer network microspheres for controlled oral drug delivery. J. Drug Deliv. Sci. Technol. 33: 1–12.

Kajjari, P.B., L.S. Manjeshwar and T.M. Aminabhavi. 2011. Novel interpenetrating polymer network hydrogel microspheres of chitosan and poly(acrylamide)-*grafted*-guar gum for controlled release of ciprofloxacin. Ind. Eng. Chem. Res. 50: 13280–13287.

Kaur, H. and R.R. Chatterji. 1990. Interpenetrating hydrogel networks. 2. Swelling and mechanical properties of the gelatin-polyacrylamide interpenetrating networks. Macromolecules. 23: 4868–4871.

Kulkarni, A.R., K.S. Soppimath, T.M. Aminabhavi and W.E. Rudzinski. 2001. *In vitro* release kinetics of cefadroxil-loaded sodium alginate interpenetrating network beads. Eur. J. Pharm. Biopharm. 51: 127–133.

Kulkarni, R.V. and B. Sa. 2008. Evaluation of pH-sensitivity and drug release characteristics of (polyacrylamide-grafted-xanthan)-carboxymehtyl cellulose-based pH-sensitive interpenetrating network hydrogel beads. Drug Dev. Ind. Pharm. 34: 1406–1414.

Kulkarni, R.V., B.S. Mangond, S. Mutalik and B. Sa. 2011. Interpenetrating polymer network microcapsules of gellan gum and egg albumin entrapped with diltiazem–resin complex for controlled release application. Carbohydr. Polym. 83: 1001–1007.

Kulkarni, R.V., R. Boppana, G.K. Mohan, S. Mutalik and N.V. Kalyane. 2012. pH-responsive interpenetrating network hydrogel beads of poly(acrylamide)-g-carrageenan and sodium alginate for intestinal targeted drug delivery: Synthesis, *in vitro* and *in vivo* evaluation. J. Colloid Interface Sci. 367: 509–517.

Kumari, K. and P.P. Kundu. 2008. Studies on *in vitro* release of CPM from semi-interpenetrating polymer network (IPN) composed of chitosan and glutamic acid. Bull. Mater. Sci. 31: 159–167.

Kumbar, S.G., A.M. Dave and T.M. Aminabhavi. 2003. Release kinetics and diffusion kinetics of solid and liquid pesticides through interpenetrating polymer network beads of plyacrylamide-g-guar gum with sodium alginate. J. Appl. Polym. Sci. 90: 451–457.

Kurkuri, M.D., S.G. Kumbar and T.M. Aminabhavi. 2002. Synthesis and characterization of polyacrylamide-grafted sodium alginate copolymeric membranes and their use in pervaporation separation of water and tetrahydrofuran mixtures. J. Appl. Polym. Sci. 86: 272–281.

Lee, D.W., S.J. Hwang, J.B. Park and H.J. Park. 2003. Preparation and release characteristics of polymer-coated and blended alginate microspheres. J. Microencapsul. 20: 179–192.

Lee, W.-F. and Y.-J. Chen. 2001. Studies on preparation and swelling properties of the *N*-isopropylacrylamide/chitosan semi-IPN and IPN hydrogels. J. Appl. Polym. Sci. 82: 2487–796.

Li, G., L. Guo, X. Chang and M. Yang. 2012. Thermo-sensitive chitosan based semi-IPN hydrogels for high loading and sustained release of anionic drugs. Int. J. Biol. Macromol. 50: 899–904.

Liu, Y.H., H.-F. Lian, C.-K. Chung, M.-C. Chen and H.-W. Sung. 2005. Physically cross-linked alginate/N,O-carboxymethyl chitosan hydrogels with calcium for oral delivery of protein drugs. Biomaterials. 26: 2105–2113.

Lohani, A., G. Singh, S.S. Bhattacharya and A. Verma. 2014. Interpenetrating polymer networks as innovative drug delivery systems. J. Drug Deliv. 1: 1–11.

Lohani, A., G. Singh, S.S. Bhattacharya, R.R. Hegde and A. Verma. 2016. Tailored-interpenetrating polymer network beads of k-carrageenan and sodium carboxymethyl cellulose for controlled drug delivery. J. Drug Deliv. Sci. Tec. 31: 53–64.

Matricardi, P., I. Onorati, G. Masci, T. Coviello and F. Alhaique. 2007. Semi-IPN hydrogel based on scleroglucan and alginate: drug delivery behavior and mechanical characterization. J. Drug Deliv. Sci. Technol. 17: 193–197.

Matricardi, P., C.D. Meo, T. Coviello, W.E. Hennink and F. Alhaique. 2013. Interpenetrating polymer networks polysaccharide hydrogels for drug delivery and tissue engineering. Adv. Drug Deliv. Rev. 65: 1172–1187.

Mohamadnia, Z., M.J. Zohuriaan-Mehr, K. Kabiri, A. Jamshidi and H. Mobedi. 2007. pH-Sensitive IPN hydrogel beads of carrageenan-alginate for controlled drug delivery. J. Bioact. Compatib. Polym. 22: 342–356.

Mundargi, R.C., N.B. Shelke, V.R. Babu, P. Patel, V. Rangaswamy and T.M. Aminabhavi. 2010. Novel thermoresponsive semi-interpenetrating network microspheres of gellan gum-poly(N-isopropylacrylamide) for controlled release of atenolol. J. Appl. Polym. Sci. 116: 1832–1841.

Muniz, E.C. and G. Geuskens. 2001. Compressive elastic modulus of polyacrylamide hydrogels and semi-IPNs with poly(*N*-isopropylacrylamide). Macromolecules. 34: 4480–4484.

Muzzarelli, R.A.A. 1993. Biochemical significance of exogenous chitins and chitosans in animals and patients. Carbohydr. Polym. 20: 7–16.

Myung, D., D. Waters, M. Wiseman, P.-E. Duhamel, J. Noolandi, C.N. Ta et al. 2008. Progress in the development of interpenetrating polymer network hydrogels. Polym. Adv. Technol. 19: 647–657.

Pal, D. and A.K. Nayak. 2012. Novel tamarind seed polysaccharide-alginate mucoadhesive microspheres for oral gliclazide delivery: *in vitro-in vivo* evaluation. Drug Deliv. 19: 123–131.

Park, T.G. and H.K. Choi. 1998. Thermally induced core–shell type hydrogel beads having interpenetrating polymer network (IPN) structure. Macromol. Rapid Commun. 19: 167–172.

Parvathy, K.S., N.S. Susheelamma, R.N. Tharanathan and A.K. Gaonkar. 2005. A simple non-aqueous method for carboxymethylation of galactomannans. Carbohydr. Polym. 62: 137–141.

Prabaharan, M. and J.F. Mano. 2006. Stimuli-responsive hydrogels based on polysaccharides incorporated with thermo-responsive polymers as novel biomaterials. Macromol. Biosci. 6: 991–1008.

Qiu, Y. and K. Park. 2001. Environment-sensitive hydrogels for drug delivery. Adv. Drug Deliv. Rev. 53: 321–339.

Rao, K.M., K.S.V.K. Rao, G. Ramanjaneyulu and C.-S. Ha. 2015. Curcumin encapsulated pH sensitive gelatin based interpenetrating polymeric network nanogels for anticancer drug delivery. Int. J. Pharm. 478: 788–795.

Rao, K.S.V.K., B.V.K. Naidu, M.C.S. Subha, M. Sairam and T.M. Aminabhavi. 2006. Novel chitosan-based pH-sensitive interpenetrating network microgels for the controlled release of cefadroxil. Carbohydr. Polym. 66: 333–344.

Ravikumar, M.N.V. 2000. A review of chitin and chitosan applications. React. Funct. Polym. 46: 1–27.

Ray, R., S. Maity, S. Mandal, T.K. Chatterjee and B. Sa. 2010b. Development and evaluation of a new interpenetrating network bead of sodium carboxymethyl xanthan and sodium alginate for ibuprofen release. Pharmacol. Pharm. 1: 9–17.

Ray, R., S. Maity, S. Mandal, T.K. Chatterjee and B. Sa. 2010c. Studies on the release of ibuprofen from Al³⁺ ion cross-linked homopolymeric and interpenetrating network hydrogel beads of carboxymethyl xanthan and sodium alginate. Adv. Polym. Technol. 30: 1–11.

Ray, S., S. Banerjee, S. Maiti, B. Laha, S. Barik, B. Sa et al. 2010a. Novel interpenetrating network microspheres of xanthan gum-poly(vinyl alcohol) for the delivery of diclofenac sodium to the intestine-*in vitro* and *in vivo* evaluation. Drug Deliv. 17: 508–519.

Reddy, K.M., V.R. Babu, M. Sairam, M.C.S. Subha, N.N. Mallikarjuna, P.V. Kulkarni et al. 2006. Development of chitosan-guar gum semi-interpenetrating polymer network microspheres for controlled release of cefadroxil. Des. Monomers Polym. 9: 491–501.

Reddy, K.M., V.R. Babu, K.S.V.K. Rao, M.C.S. Subha, K.C. Rao, M. Sairam et al. 2008. Temperature sensitive semi-IPN microspheres from sodium alginate and N-isopropylacrylamide for controlled release of 5-fluorouracil. J. Appl. Polym. Sci. 107: 2820–2829.

Risbud, M.V., A.A. Hardikar, S.V. Bhat and R.R. Bhonde. 2000. pH-sensitive freeze-dried chitosan–polyvinyl pyrrolidone hydrogels as controlled release system for antibiotic delivery. J. Control. Release. 68: 23–30.

Rokhade, A.P., N.B. Shelke, S.A. Patil and T.M. Aminabhavi. 2007. Novel interpenetrating network microspheres of chitosan and methylcellulose for controlled release of thephylline. Carbohydr. Polym. 69: 678–687.

Schmaljohann, D. 2006. Thermo- and pH-responsive polymers in drug delivery. Adv. Drug Deliv. Rev. 58: 1655–1670.

Sekhar, E.C., K.S.V.K. Rao and R.R. Raju. 2011. Chitosan/guargum-g-acrylamide semi IPN microspheres for controlled release studies of 5-Fluorouracil. J. Appl. Pharm. Sci. 1: 199–204.

Setty, C.M., S.S. Sahoo and B. Sa. 2005. Alginate-coated alginate–polyethyleneimine beads for prolonged release of furosemide in simulated intestinal fluid. Drug Dev. Ind. Pharm. 31: 435–446.

Sharma, K., V. Kumar, B.S. Kaith, V. Kumar, S. Som, V. Kumar, A. Pandey et al. 2015. Evaluation of a conducting interpenetrating network based on gum ghatti-g-poly(acrylic acid-aniline) as a colon-specific delivery system for amoxicillin trihydrate and paracetamol. New J. Chem. 39: 3021–3034.

Sharma, K., V. Kumar, B.S. Kaith, S. Som, V., A. Pandey et al. 2015. Synthesis of biodegradable gum ghatti based poly(methacrylic acid-aniline) conducting IPN hydrogel for controlled release of amoxicillin trihydrate. Ind. Eng. Chem. Res. 54: 1982–1991.

Shivkumar, H.N., S. Sarsija and B.G. Desai. 2006. Design and evaluation of pH-sensitive multi-particulate systems for chronotherapeutic delivery of diltiazem hydrochloride. Indian J. Pharm. Sci. 68: 781–787.

Sirajudheen, M.K., M.A. Chordiya, P.P. Naseef and K. Senthilkumaran. 2015. Development of interpenetrating polymer networks of chitosan and guar gum for propranolol hydrochloride. Sch. Acad. J. Pharm. 4: 315–323.

Soppimath, K.S., A.R. Kulkarni and T.M. Aminabhavi. 2000. Controlled release of antihypertensive drug from the interpenetrating network poly(vinyl alcohol)-guar gum hydrogel microspheres. J. Biomater. Sci. Polym. Ed. 11: 27–43.

Soppimath, K.S., T.M. Aminabhavi, A.M. Dave, S.G. Kumbar and W.E. Rudzinski. 2002. Stimulus-responsive "smart" hydrogels as novel drug delivery systems. Drug Dev. Ind. Pharm. 28: 957–974.

Sullad, A.G., L.S. Manjeshwar and T.M. Aminabhavi. 2010. Novel pH sensitive hydrogels prepared from the blends of poly(vinyl alcohol) with acrylic acid-graft-guar gum matrixes for isoniazid delivery. Ind. Eng. Chem. Res. 49: 7323–7329.

Sullad, A.G., L.S. Manjeshwar and T.M. Aminabhavi. 2011. Novel semi-interpenetrating microspheres of dextran-grafted-acrylamide and poly(vinyl alcohol) for controlled release of abacavir sulfate. Ind. Eng. Chem. Res. 50: 11778–11784.

Tang, E.S.K., L.W. Chan and P.W.S. Heng. 2005. Coating of multi-particulates for sustained release. Am. J. Drug Deliv. 3: 17–28.

Thacharodi, D. and K.P. Rao. 1993. Propranol hydrochloride release behaviour of crosslinked chitosan membranes. J. Chem. Technol. Biotechnol. 58: 177–181.

Vermonden, T., R. Censi and W.E. Hennink. 2012. Hydrogels for protein delivery. Chem. Rev. 112: 2853–2888.

Wen, C., L. Lu and X. Li. 2014. An interpenetrating network biohydrogel of gelatin and gellan gum by using a combination of enzymatic and ionic crosslinking approaches. Polym. Int. 63: 1643–1649.

Yin, L., L. Fei, F. Cui, C. Tang and C. Yin. 2007. Superporous hydrogels containing poly(acrylic acid-co-acrylamide)/O-carboxymethyl chitosan interpenetrating polymer networks. Biomaterials. 28: 1258–1266.

Zhang, J. and N.A. Peppas. 2000. Synthesis and characterization of pH- and temperature-sensitive poly(methacrylic acid)/poly(N-isopropylacrylamide) interpenetrating polymeric networks. Macromolecules. 33: 102–107.

Zhang, X.-Z., D.-Q. Wu and C.-C. Chu. 2004. Synthesis, characterization and controlled drug release of the thermosensitive IPN-PNIPAAm hydrogels. Biomaterials. 25: 3793–3805.

9

Stimuli-Responsive Hydrogels for Parenteral Drug Delivery

Gayatri C. Patel

ABSTRACT

In recent years, interest in hydrogels based on stimuli-responsive polymers is steadily increasing especially in the fields of controlled and self-regulated drug delivery systems. Stimuli-responsive, also termed as 'environmental sensitive', 'intelligent' or 'smart', these polymers are capable of returning to their initial state as soon as the trigger is removed. Stimuli may occur internally (e.g., a change in pH, temperature or in presence of specific enzymes or antigens, etc.) or externally (e.g., magnetic or electric fields, light, ultrasound, etc.). Injectable depots have been the subject of much research in the field of drug delivery. This chapter mainly focuses on the recent developments, current applications and future trends dealing with stimuli-responsive hydrogels in the field of parenteral drug delivery. This chapter also outlines injectable hydrogel materials and processing techniques used in drug delivery.

Keywords: stimuli, hydrogel, responsive, drug delivery, injectable, biopolymers, parenteral, smart

Associate Professor, Department of Pharmaceutical Technology, Ramanbhai Patel College of Pharmacy, Charotar University of Science and Technology (CHARUSAT), Changa Campus, Changa-388 421, Dist.: Anand, Gujarat, India.
Email: gayatripatel.ph@charusat.ac.in; gayatripatel26@gmail.com

List of abbreviation at the end of the text.

1. Introduction

A common misinterpretation in polymer science is the use of the terms 'gel' and 'hydrogel' synonymously. Gels are semi-solid materials made of hydrophilic polymeric systems comprising of small amounts of solids, dispersed in relatively large amounts of liquid. However, gels may appear more solid-like than liquid-like (Klech 1990). Hydrogels are also made of hydrophilic polymer strands but they are cross linked and that enables them to swell while retaining their three-dimensional structure (Gehrke and Lee 1990). Hydrogels can absorb a large amount of water or biological fluid, from 20 per cent up-to several thousand per cent, and swell without dissolving (Kamath and Park 1993). The amount of water absorbed in hydrogels is related to the presence of specific groups such as –COOH, –OH, –CONH$_2$, –CONH–, –SO$_3$H, etc. (Kamath and Park 1993) The degree of swelling is determined by the type and concentration of cross-linker and type of polymer, which makes up the network (Hatefi and Amsden 2002).

Hydrogels exhibit favourable characteristics as a carrier for injectable drug delivery, such as biocompatibility, biodegradability, hydrophilicity, self assembling, non immunogenic, tailorable properties (as release profile, mechanical strength, degradation time, controllable shape and size, etc.) and possibility to target specific sites (Patel and Dalwadi 2013) Furthermore, the soft and rubbery nature of hydrogels delivering a high degree of mobility of their surface and low interfacial tension that minimize the frictional irritation to the surrounding biological tissues make them attractive candidates as tissue engineering scaffolds (Sophie et al. 2007, Hatefi and Amsden 2002).

The hydrogels in the dried varieties are commonly referred to as Xerogel. Xerogel usually retains high porosity, enormous surface area and smaller size of pores than hydrogels. The water holding capacity of a xerogel is dependent on the number of the hydrophilic groups and cross-linking density. Higher the number of the hydrophilic groups, higher is the water holding capacity whereas with an increase in the cross-linking density, there is a decrease in the equilibrium swelling due to the decrease in the hydrophilic groups. When some drying techniques, such as freeze drying or solvent extraction drying are applied, the resulting hydrogels become extremely permeable. These porous dried hydrogels are known as Aerogels (Syed and Saphwan 2011, Wichterle 1960, Pal et al. 2009).

1.1 Classification of hydrogels

Depending on the preparation methods, ionic charges, sources, nature of swelling with changes to the environment, rate of biodegradation and nature of cross-linking, hydrogels can be classified in several ways (Fig. 1) (Dumitriu 2002, Hin 2004).

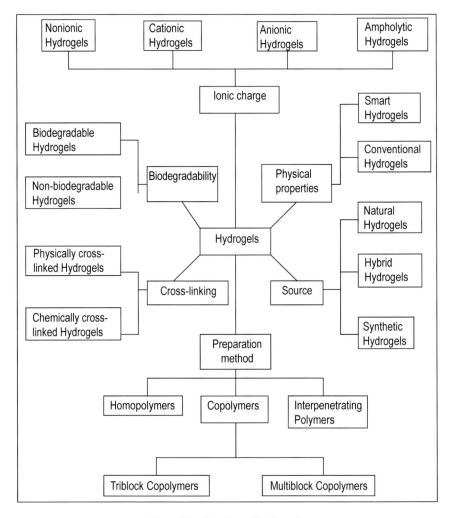

Fig. 1. Classification of hydrogels.

Based on hydrogel preparation methods, it can be classified into two categories (1) permanent or chemical hydrogels, and (2) reversible or physical hydrogels. Chemical hydrogels are formed by chemical cross-linking mechanism. Chemically crosslinked hydrogels are mechanically stronger in comparison to physically cross-linked hydrogels because the linear polymer chains are covalently bonded with each other *via.* cross-linking agent/s which provides them permanent structure. Physical hydrogels are held together by molecular entanglements, hydrogen bonds and/or ionic and hydrophobic interactions and formed by physical cross-linking mechanism. All these interactions are reversible and can be disrupted by changes in physical conditions or stress applications (Syed and Saphwan 2011, Patel and Dalwadi 2013).

Hydrogels can be classified according to the material of their origin into natural, synthetic and semi-synthetic. The natural hydrogels are based on natural polymers, for example, polypeptides, polysaccharides and polynucleotides and derived from the natural sources. For example, collagen is derived from mammals whereas chitin is derived from the exoskeleton of shellfish. Most of the semisynthetic polymers are derived from natural polymers for extension of activity. Examples of semi synthetic polymers are methyl cellulose from cellulose, chitosan from chitin, alginate from alginic acid, etc. Synthetic hydrogels are synthesized by polymerization of the different vinyl monomers. Typical examples of synthetic polymers used in hydrogel preparations are Poly lactic acid, Polycaprolactone, N-isopropylacrylamide, Polyvinyl alcohol, Polyethylene glycol, Polylacticglycolic acid, Poly(N-vinyl pyrrolidone), Polyacrylic acid, Poly(methyl methacrylate), etc. (Bindu Sri et al. 2012, Kant et al. 2011).

Further, hydrogels can be classified according to hydrogel durability into biodegradable and non-biodegradable hydrogel. Application of biodegradable hydrogels covers many areas such as pharmaceutical, biomedical, veterinary, agricultural and environmental. The use of the biodegradable system eliminates the need for the removal of the 'ghost' drug delivery system after the entire drug is released (Kamath and Park 1993, Sannino and Demitri 2009).

2. Stimuli-responsive Hydrogel

Hydrogels can be classified according to their response to environmental stimuli. The past few years have witnessed enormous advances in developing and investigating a unique class of polymer-based hydrogel drug delivery systems called 'intelligent' or 'smart hydrogels' (Gil and Hudson 2004). These are similar to hydrogels, except they exhibit a solution to gel (sol-gel) phase-transition undergoing significant volume changes in response to stimuli (Singh and Kumar 2012).

Many physical, chemical and biochemical stimuli have been applied to induce various responses of the smart hydrogel systems (Fig. 2). The physical stimuli include temperature, electric field, light, ultrasound and magnetic field, chemical stimuli include pH, ion and glucose, while biochemical stimuli include antigen, ligand and enzyme specific. Some systems have been developed to combine two stimuli-responsive mechanisms into one system, so called dual responsive systems (Qiu and Park 2012). Among all stimuli-responsive hydrogels, temperature-sensitive and pH sensitive hydrogels have gained significant attention. These two stimuli are the

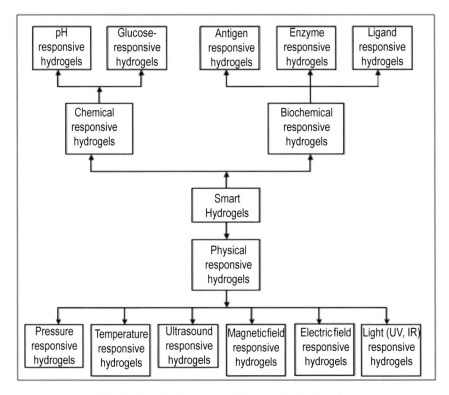

Fig. 2. Classification of stimuli-responsive hydrogels.

most relevant factors in biological systems including the human body (Masteikova and Chalupova 2003, Miyati et al. 2002).

Stimuli-responsive hydrogels have great potential in pharmaceutical applications, especially in site specific controlled drug delivery systems. The drug may be mixed with a polymer solution or polymeric hydrogel *in vitro* and the drug loaded hydrogel can form *in situ* after the *in vivo* administration, such as injection. Stimuli-responsive hydrogels have many advantages, such as ease of preparation, site-specificity, controlled/ sustained drug release, less systemic toxicity and ability to deliver both hydrophilic and hydrophobic drugs (Sophie et al. 2008, Bae and Kim 1993).

In general, changes occur to the stimuli-responsive hydrogels in response to any of the stimuli and disappear upon removal of the stimulus. Consequently, the hydrogels return to their original state in a reversible manner (Gil and Hudson 2004). The main reason for the interest in using stimuli-responsive hydrogels in drug delivery is that a good drug delivery system should respond to the physiological requirement, sense the changes and accordingly amend the drug release pattern. Stimuli are produced within the body to control the structural changes in the polymer network and to exhibit the desired drug release. Most of the time, drug release is observed during the swelling of the hydrogel (Sood et al. 2013, Soppimath et al. 2002).

2.1 Temperature responsive hydrogel

Temperature responsive hydrogels have gained considerable attention in various drug delivery and biomedical applications. The transition of polymers from sol to gel is triggered by the presence of physiological temperature as stimuli. Temperature responsive hydrogels are classified into positive temperature responsive hydrogels, negative temperature responsive hydrogels and thermally reversible gels (Peppas and Langer 1994). A positive temperature responsive hydrogel has an upper critical solution temperature (UCST). Such hydrogel contracts upon cooling below the UCST. Polymer networks of Poly(acrylic acid) (PAA) and Polyacrylamide (PAAm) and Poly(acrylamide-co-butyl methacrylate) have positive temperature dependence of swelling (Qiu and Park 2001).

Negative temperature responsive hydrogels have a lower critical solution temperature (LCST) and contract upon heating above the LCST. One of the most extensively investigated polymer that exhibit useful LCST transition is Poly(N-isopropylacrylamide)(PNIPAAm). PNIPAAm is a water soluble polymer at its low LCST, but hydrophobic above LCST, which results in precipitation of PNIPAAm from the solution at the LCST (Peppas 2000, Ruel and Leroux 2004). The most commonly used thermoreversible gels are the ones prepared from poly(ethylene oxide)-*b*-poly(propylene oxide)-*b*-poly(ethylene oxide) (PEO-PPO-PEO) (Pluronics®, Tetronics®, Poloxamer). Polymer solution is a free flowing liquid at ambient temperature and gels at body temperature. List of thermoresponsive biopolymers are given in Table 1 (Masteikova and Chalupova 2003).

2.2 pH responsive hydrogel

Another type of environmental stimuli that is most studied for sol to gel transition is pH. Polymers of this class contain pendant acidic or basic groups that either accept or release protons in response to changes in environmental pH. The polymers with a large number of ionizable groups are known as polyelectrolytes. Swelling of hydrogel increases as the external pH increases in the case of weakly acidic (anionic) groups, but decreases if polymer contains weakly basic (cationic) groups (Qiu and Park 2001, Qiu and Park 2012). Most of the anionic pH-sensitive polymers are based

Table 1. Examples of Stimuli-Responsive Biomaterials (pH, Ions & Temperature).

Types of stimuli	Responsive polymeric materials
pH	Polyvinyl sulfonic acid, Polymethacrylic acid (PMA), Poly(acrylic acid) (PAA), Poly(propylacrylic acid) (PPA), Polydiethylaminoethyl methacrylate, Polydimethylaminoethyl methacrylate, Polyvinylacetaldiethylaminoacetate (AEA), Chitosan, Poly(L-lysine) ester, Poly(ethylene glycol) (PEG) grafted poly(L-lysine), Poly(L-lysine)-g-poly(histidine), PMA grafted with PEG, etc.
Ions	Alginate, Gellan gum, Pectin, Carrageenan, Chitosan, etc.
Temperature	Poly(N-isopropylacrylamide) (PNIPAAm), N-isopropylacrylamide (NIPAAm), Poly(vinyl methyl ether) (PVME), Poly(N-vinylisobutyramide) (PNVIBA), Poly(ethylene oxide-propylene oxide-b-ethylene oxide) (PEO-PPO-PEO), Chitosan, Methyl cellulose, Hydroxypropyl methyl cellulose, etc.

on polyacrylic acid (PAA) (Carbopol®, Carbomer) and/or its derivatives (Kumar S and Himmelstein K 1995).

Hydrogels made up of crosslinked polyelectrolytes display big differences in swelling properties depending on the pH of the environment. The swelling of polyelectrolyte is mainly due to the electrostatic repulsion among charges present on the polymer chain. The swelling and pH-responsiveness of polyelectrolyte hydrogels can be adjusted by using neutral co-monomers, such as 2-hydroxyethyl methacrylate, methyl methacrylate and maleic anhydride (Gupta et al. 2002, Aikawa et al. 1998).

Hydrogels made of poly(methacrylic acid) (PMA), grafted with poly(ethylene glycol) (PEG) have unique pH-sensitive properties. As the carboxyl groups of PMA become ionized at high pH, the resulting decomplexation leads to swelling of the hydrogels. Some pH responsive polymers are listed in Table 1 (Masteikova and Chalupova 2003, Sood et al. 2013).

2.3 Ion responsive hydrogel

Some polymers may undergo sol-gel phase transition in presence of various ions. Some of the polysaccharides fall into the class of ion-sensitive ones (Bhardwaj et al. 2000). Gellan gum commercially available as Gelrite® is an anionic polysaccharide that undergoes *in situ* gelling in the presence of mono- and divalent cations, including Ca^{2+}, Mg^{2+}, K+ and Na+. Gelation of the low-methoxy pectins can be caused by divalent cations, especially Ca^{2+}. Likewise, alginic acid undergoes gelation in the presence of divalent/polyvalent cations, for example, Ca^{2+} due to the interaction with glucoronic acid block in alginate chains. Chitosan with phosphate ions for injectable solutions is also reported. The concentrations of the counter ion available under physiological conditions are usually considered as critical factor for cross-linking of the above mentioned polymers (Guo et al. 1998, Chenite et al. 2000, Cohen et al. 1997).

2.4 Glucose sensitive hydrogel

These hydrogels are glucose sensitive and show variability depending upon the presence of glucose. This class of hydrogels is very useful for the development of self-regulated insulin delivery systems and enables us to construct an artificial pancreas that can administer the necessary amount of insulin in response to the blood glucose concentration. Three types of glucose sensitive hydrogels are studied for various applications, namely, glucose oxidase-loaded hydrogel, lectin loaded hydrogels and hydrogels with phenyl boronic acid moieties (Miyata et al. 2002).

The response of these hydrogels upon changes in the environmental glucose concentration occurs too slowly. Furthermore, hydrogels do not go back to their original states fast enough after responding to the changing glucose concentration (Qiu and Park 2012). Aikawa and his group performed work using 2, 2'-azobisisobutyronitrile (AIBN) as an initiator in the presence of N, N'-218 methylene bis (acrylamide) (MBAAm) as a cross-linking agent and concluded that surface-controlled release of insulin can be achieved as the gel can form a skin layer which provides a rationale for glucose sensitive release under glucose hemostasis conditions (Aikawa et al. 1998).

2.5 Light sensitive hydrogel

Light sensitive hydrogels have potential applications in developing optical switches and various ophthalmic drug delivery devices. Since the light stimulus can be imposed instantly and delivered in specific amounts with high accuracy, light-sensitive hydrogels may possess special advantages over others (Masteikova and Chalupova 2003). The capacity for instantaneous delivery of the sol-gel stimulus makes the development of light-sensitive hydrogels important for various applications in both engineering and biochemical fields (Imran et al. 2010). Light sensitive hydrogels can be separated into UV-sensitive and visible light-sensitive hydrogels. Unlike U.V. light, visible light is readily available, inexpensive, safe, clean and easily manipulated. The UV-sensitive hydrogels were synthesized by introducing a leuco derivative molecule, bis(4-dimethyl amino) phenyl methyl leucocyanide, in to the polymer network. Visible light sensitive hydrogels were prepared by introducing a light sensitive chromophore (e.g., trisodium salt of copper chlorophyllin) to poly(N-isopropyl acrylamide) hydrogels (Mamada et al. 1990).

Matsuda developed novel tissue adhesive technology based on photocrosslinkable gelatin, which allows *in situ* drug-incorporated gelatinous gel formation on diseased tissue and sustained drug release. Limitation of this type of hydrogel while the action of stimulus (light) is instantaneous; the reaction of hydrogels in response to such action is still slow. In most cases, the conversion of light into thermal energy must precede the restructuring of polymer chains upon temperature change (Matsuda 2002).

2.6 Electrical signal sensitive hydrogel

Electric current can also be used as an environmental signal to induce responses of hydrogels. Hydrogels sensitive to electric current are usually made of polyelectrolytes, as are pH-sensitive hydrogels. Electro-sensitive hydrogels undergo shrinking or swelling in the presence of an applied electric field. Sometimes, the hydrogels show swelling on one side and deswelling on the other side, resulting in bending of the hydrogels (Ruta Masteikova and Uzana Chalupova 2003).

Ramanathan and Block 2001 evaluated and characterized the use of chitosan gels as matrices for electrically modulated drug delivery. In electrification studies, release-time profiles for neutral (hydrocortisone), anionic (benzoic acid) and cationic (lidocaine hydrochloride) drug molecules from hydrated chitosan gels were monitored in response to different milli amperages of current as a function of time. One of the advantages of electro sensitive hydrogels in drug delivery is that the drug release rate can be easily controlled simply by modulating the electric fields.

2.7 Enzyme sensitive hydrogel

Enzyme sensitive hydrogels can be prepared from biodegradable polymers that can be digested by specific enzymes. Some enzymes are used as important signals for diagnosis to monitor several physiological changes, and specific enzymes in specific organs have become useful signals for site specific drug delivery. Therefore, the enzyme sensitive hydrogels are promising candidates as enzyme sensors and enzyme-sensitive drug delivery systems (Chasin and Langer 1990). Hovgaard and Brondsted (1995) focused on the fact that microbial enzymes in the colon, such as dextranases, can degrade the polysaccharide dextran. They prepared dextran hydrogels cross-linked with diisocyanate for colon specific drug delivery. The dextran hydrogels were degraded *in vitro* by a model dextranase, as well as *in vivo* in rats and in a human colonic fermentation model. Release of a drug from the dextran hydrogels can be controlled by the presence of dextranase Akala et al. (1998) used azoaromatic bonds as cross-linking agents to prepare azoreductase-sensitive hydrogels for colon specific drug delivery. Further, dual stimuli sensitive hydrogels were prepared by combining the temperature sensitivity of PNIPAAm with enzymatic degradation (Kurisawa and Terano 1997).

2.8 Antigen sensitive hydrogel

An antibody has recognition sites to bind with a specific antigen through multiple noncovalent bonds, such as electrostatic interactions, hydrogen bonds, hydrophobic interactions, and Vander Waals interactions. Such unique features of antibodies are associated with the immune responses to protect the organism from infection. Antibodies have been employed in a variety of immunological assays which utilize their specificity and versatility in order to detect biological substances. Thus, the specific antigen recognition function of an antibody can provide the basis for constructing sensors with various uses for immunoassays and antigen sensing (Miyata et al. 2002).

Antigen sensitive hydrogels were prepared by using antigen–antibody bonds at cross-linking points in the hydrogels. For example, rabbit Immunoglobulin G (IgG), the antigen, was chemically modified by coupling it with N-succinimidylacrylate (NSA) in phosphate buffer solution to introduce vinyl groups into the rabbit IgG. The resultant vinyl rabbit IgG was mixed with the antibody, goat anti rabbit IgG (GAR IgG), to form an antigen antibody complex. The vinyl-rabbit IgG was then copolymerized with acrylamide (AAm) as co monomers an N, N 9-methylenebisacrylamide (MBAA) as a cross-linker in the presence of GAR IgG, resulting in a hydrogel containing antigen antibody bond sites (Miyata et al. 2002).

In the case of the antigen–antibody entrapment hydrogel, however, the antibody entrapped in the network leaked out of the hydrogel, while it underwent swelling in response to a specific antigen. As a result of the leak of the antibody, the antigen–antibody entrapment hydrogel did not show reversible swelling–shrinking behaviour in response to stepwise changes in the antigen concentration. Therefore, such hydrogel structures must be designed to prepare reversible antigen-sensitive hydrogels (Miyata et al. 1999).

3. Research on Stimuli-responsive Polymers in Parenteral Drug Delivery

The most reviewed research papers and patents in field of parenteral drug delivery are described in the following section. This finding suggests that the field of stimuli-responsive hydrogel has been a specialized field of research for parenteral drug delivery with relatively small sets of authors, organizations and countries.

Swatantra et al. (2016) prepared the temperature sensitive hydrogel formulation of camptothecin based on chitosan/β-Glycerophosphate/HP-β-Cyclodextrin (chitosan/β-GP/HP-β-CD) for anticancer drug delivery and studied hydrogel effectiveness on tumour cell MCF-7.

Kumar et al. (2016) formulated and evaluated the *in situ* forming dual temperature and pH responsive gelling injectable hydrogel of an anticancer drug Dacarbazine using Chitosan and concluded that optimized formulation is safe, effective, homogeneous, and stable for delivery of Dacarbazine.

Giang et al. (2016) developed a new dual pH and temperature-sensitive, biocompatible, biodegradable and injectable hydrogel based on poly(ethylene glycol)-poly(amino carbonate urethane) (PEG-PACU) copolymers for the sustained delivery of human growth hormone (hGH) and proved the prepared hydrogels to be useful biomaterials for the sustained delivery of hGH. In aqueous solutions, PEG-PACU based copolymers existed as sols at low pH and temperature (pH 6.0, 23°C), whereas they formed gels in the physiological condition (pH 7.4, 37°C).

Grijalvo et al. (2016) focused on development of cationic, neutral and anionic biopolymer based hydrogels containing liposomes, niosomes or vesicles for drug delivery and tissue engineering applications.

Sim et al. (2015) developed stimuli-sensitive injectable hydrogels, composed of biodegradable copolymers based on heparin-bearing poly(ε-caprolactone-co-lactide)-b-poly(ethylene glycol)-b-poly(ε caprolactone-co-lactide) (Hep-PCLA) as the carrier system for lysozyme. Hep-PCLA conjugates were found capable of undergoing temperature-induced sol-to-gel transitions in an aqueous solution.

Shinde et al. (2015) developed *in situ* formed thermogels of Recombinant human growth hormones (rhGH) using Poly(ethylene glycol)-poly(L-alanine-co-L-phenyl alanine) diblock copolymers (PEG–PAF) with different molecular weights of PEGs, but having a similar molecular weight ratio of hydrophobic block to hydrophilic block. Upon injection into the subcutaneous layer of rats, it formed a biocompatible stable gel.

Khodaverdi et al. (2015) prepared and characterized supramolecular hydrogels based on biodegradable poly(caprolactone)-poly(ethylene glycol)-poly(caprolactone) (PCL-PEG-PCL) triblock copolymers and γ-cyclodextrin (γ-CD) through inclusion complexation as an injectable, sustained-release vehicle for insulin.

Sindhu et al. (2014) formulated injectable *in situ* gel matrix containing metoprolol succinate using thermo-sensitive polymer Pluronic F 127 (20%) together with carbopol 934P, HPMC and Sodium CMC for controlled release.

Jiang et al. (2014) prepared thermo-sensitive hydrogels based on poly(ethylene glycol)-grafted-chitosan (PEG-g-CS) for sustained release of cyclosporine A. Degradation and drug release *in vivo* were investigated by subcutaneous injection of the hydrogel into Sprague-Dawley rats and effective drug concentration in blood for more than five weeks *in vivo*.

Huynh et al. (2008) developed poly(beta-amino ester) (PAE) as a pH sensitive moiety to conjugate to the temperature sensitive biodegradable triblock copolymer of poly(ethylene glycol)-poly(epsilon-caprolactone) (PCL-PEG-PCL) to manufacture pH/temperature sensitive injectable hydrogel of penta block copolymer PAE-PCL-PEG-PCL-PAE for controlled drug/protein delivery.

Qiao et al. (2008) synthesized thermo-sensitive PLGA-PEG-PLGA triblock copolymers with the DL-lactide/glycolide molar ratio ranging from 6/1 to 15/1 by bulk copolymerization of DL-lactide, glycolide and PEG1500 for IL-2 delivery. The resulting copolymers are soluble in water to form a free flowing fluid at room temperature but become hydrogels at body temperature. Solutions were injected subcutaneously to H22 tumour-bearing mice. IL-2 loaded copolymer hydrogel for *in vivo* use showed good anti-tumour effect.

Cappello et al. (2003) developed novel proteins polymers, Prolastins which undergoes an irreversible solution gel transition, when injected as a solution into the body. It remains at the site of injection providing adsorption times from less than one week to many months.

DesNoyer and McHugh (2003) invented a new class of injectable controlled release depots of protein which consisted of blends of poly(ethylene oxide) (PEO)/poly(propylene oxide) (PPO)/poly(ethylene oxide) (PEO) triblock copolymers (Pluronics) with poly(D,L-lactide) (PDLA)/1-methyl-2-pyrrolidinone (NMP) solutions. Some other thermo-sensitive hydrogels may also be used for parenteral administration. Ricci et al. (2002) prepared Poloxamer gels and tested for intramuscular and subcutaneous administration with the aim to develop a long acting single dose injection of lidocaine. They utilized Poloxamer 407 and additives like inorganic salts, sodium chloride and sodium carbonate, and PEG 400 for thermogelation of formulation.

Kytai and Jennifer (2002) focused on Photopolymerized hydrogels that may undergo transdermal photopolymerization after subcutaneous injection and were found to be applicable for drug release devices. It was also found that these materials were attractive for use in cell encapsulation and tissue engineering applications.

Chenite et al. (2000) formulated thermally sensitive neutral solutions based on chitosan/polyol salt for encapsulating living cells and therapeutic proteins. When injected *in vivo*, the liquid formulations turn into gel implants *in situ*.

Byeongmoon Jeong et al. (2000) developed thermo-sensitive low-molecular-weight PEG–PLGA–PEG triblock copolymers hydrogel for controlled release of drugs. Two model drugs, ketoprofen and spironolatone, which have different hydrophobicities, were studied and it was found that Ketoprofen (a model hydrophilic drug) was released over 2 wks with a first-order release profile, while spironolactone (a model hydrophobic drug) was released over 2 mon with an S-shaped release profile.

Jeong et al. (1997) reported the synthesis of thermo-sensitive biodegradable poly(ethylene oxide) and poly(L-lactic acid) hydrogel and found that on subcutaneous injection and subsequent rapid cooling to body temperature, the loaded copolymer forms a gel that can act as a sustained-release matrix for drugs.

The most referred patents in field of parenteral drug delivery are described in the following section (Table 2).

Injectable *in situ* Hydrogels were invented by Ki-Dong et al. (2014) in which introduction of two or more homogeneous or heterogeneous hydrophilic polymer bonded to each other by dehydrogenation reaction. The introduction of water soluble polymer chain as a linker between naturally occurring or synthetic polymer backbone improves not only solubility of polymers but also stability and mechanical strength.

Nair and Kulkarni (2013) have invented 'Biodegradable Hydrogel composition' which describes fast curing biodegradable polymeric hydrogel composition comprising of water soluble acrylate polymers and water soluble amine functionality polymers that form an amino ester linkage which gives gelation even at a temperature closer to human body temperature useful for medical applications such as injectable drug delivery and tissue engineering.

The invention related to the 'Injectable composition of the Hydrogel' by Robert E. Richard (2015) provides the temperature-sensitive hydrogel particles that swell and form a gel *in vivo* upon injection into the body. This composition is either in dry form or hydrated form in aqueous fluid.

A recent patent by Thorsten Steinberg et al. (2015) related to 'Bio functionalised stimulus responsive dissolvable PEG hydrogel' comprising of the matrix of PEG polymer, is modified to contain at least one multifunctional fusion protein. They have prepared stimuli-responsive hydrogels by cross-linking method which gives higher viscosity due to apparent or real increase in the molecular weight. The prepared hydrogel was issued for the treatment of lesions, in surgical dressings, for wound treating, for soft and hard tissue regeneration, for the treatment of wounds in the oral cavity, in the field of ophthalmology, in the field of periodontal defects, etc.

Brey et al. (2014) have invented 'Thermo responsive Hydrogel composition' for drug delivery. A general objective of the study is to provide hydrogel composition with thermo responsive hydrogel polymer and a biocompatible monomer. This hydrogel is thermoresponsive at a physiological temperature and can incorporate or encapsulate a treating

Table 2. List of patents on application of stimuli-responsive injectable drug delivery.

Sr. No.	Patent Number	Title	Reference
1	US7767656 B2	Blends of temperature sensitive and anionic polymers for drug delivery	Molly et al. 2010
2	US8940311 B2	*In situ* controlled release drug delivery system	Tae-Hong et al. (2010, 2015)
3	US9364545 B2	Thermosensitive injectable hydrogel for drug delivery	Hua Jing 2016
4	US20020019369 A1	Injectable drug delivery systems with cyclodextrin-polymer based hydrogels	Jun Li 2002
5	US 20130022545 A1	Drug delivery system for treatment of liver cancer based on interventional injection of temperature and ph-sensitive hydrogel	Doo et al. 2013
6	WO 2002000193 A2	Multiple stimulus reversible hydrogels	Gutowskan and Krzyminski 2002
7	US 5226902 A	Pulsatile drug delivery device using stimuli sensitive hydrogel	You H. Bae 1993
8	WO 2006047279 A3	*In situ* controlled release drug delivery system	Tae Lim et al. 2006
9	US 5904927 A	Drug delivery using pH-sensitive semi-interpenetrating network hydrogels	Mansoor M. Hamiji 1999
10	US 6586493 B1	Polysaccharide-based hydrogels and pre-gel blends for the same	Massia and Trudel 2003
11	US 7420024 B2	Partially biodegradable temperature and pH sensitive hydrogel	Chu and Zhang 2008
12	US 8586087 B2	Temperature and pH-sensitive block copolymer having excellent gel strength	Doo Sung Lee et al. 2013
13	US 20130225696 A1	pH-sensitive polymer hydrogel with dual ionic transition and use	Doo Sung Lee 2013
14	US 7066904 B2	Triggered release hydrogel drug delivery system	Rosenthal et al. 2006
15	US 20060128918 A1	Partially biodegradable temperature and pH sensitive hydrogel	Chih-Chang and Zhang (2006)
16	EP 2155165 A1	Drug delivery vehicle containing vesicles in a hydrogel base	Hirt et al. 2010
17	US 7208171 B2	Injectable and bioadhesive polymeric hydrogels as well as related methods of enzymatic preparation	Messersmith et al. 2007
18	US 8702645 B2	Implantable-glucose-responsive insulin delivery device	Xiao Yu Wu 2014

Table 2 contd. ...

...Table 2 contd.

Sr. No.	Patent Number	Title	Reference
19	WO 2014072330 A1	Glucose-responsive hydrogel comprising pba-grafted hyaluronic acid (ha)	Auzely-velty et al. 2014
20	IP 260002	Thermosensitive Neutralized Chitosan Composition Forming A Hydrogel, Lyophilizate and Processes for Producing the Same	Schuetz Yannie et al. 2014
21	US20120100103 A1	*In situ* forming hydrogel and biomedical use thereof	Dong Park et al. 2014
22	US20090053276 A1	Injectable hydrogel composition	Rechard 2015
23	WO2009146147 A3	Target responsive hydrogel	Weihong 2009
24	EP2455104 A1	Bio functionalised stimulus responsive dissolvable PEG hydrogel	Thorsten et al. 2012
25	US20120231072 A1	Thermoresponsive Hydrogel Composition	Jennifer 2012
26	US20120020932 A1	Thermosensitive hydrogel composition and method	Jian Yao 2012
27	WO2012159106 A2	pH responsive self-healing hydrogels formed by Boronate Catechol Complex	Philip B 2012
28	US8048450 B2	Aqueous dispersion of hydrogel nanoparticle with inverse thermogelling gelation	Zhibinghu 2011
29	US7658947 B2	Thermogelling composition	Yanbing Huang 2010
30	US20090117656 A1	Stimuli-responsive degradable gel	Mitsuru Akashi 2009
31	US7786220B2	pH and temperature sensitive hydrogel	Doo sung Lee 2010
32	WO2009031861 A3	Temperature and pH sensitive block copolymer having excellent safety *in vivo* and hydrogel and drug delivery system using thereof	Minh Khanh 2009

agent such as a drug, biomolecule or nanoparticle and changes to second physicochemical state that is more solid than the first physicochemical state.

A recent patent by Jian et al. (2012) related to 'Thermo-sensitive hydrogel composition and method' comprised of an extracellular matrix protein, Hyaluronic acid and thermo-sensitive biocompatible polymer methyl cellulose. Composition may be injected in the area needing treatment by therapeutic agent. The composition may form a gel at about 37°C (98.6°F) such that the gel maintains the therapeutic agent in the area of the body in need of such treatment. One advantage of the invention is that the composition is flowable liquid at ambient temperature, yet forms a gel at a temperature of about 37°C (98.6°F).

Zhibing Hu and Xiaohu Xia (2007) have invented Hydrogel nanoparticles with inverse thermogelling gelation. The present invention describes an aqueous dispersion of hydrogel nanoparticle and method of preparing it having an interpenetrating polymer network (IPN). They prepared IPN nanoparticle by polymerization of monomer and cross-linking agent with the initiator which gave first polymer nanoparticle, and this first nanoparticle was polymerized with a second combination of monomer for the IPN nanoparticles. The uniform size interpenetrating the polymeric network having inverse thermo gelation properties allows uniform distribution of medication in the liquid form of dispersion of hydrogel nanoparticle.

Yanbin et al. (2010) invented a 'Thermogelling composition' comprised of methyl cellulose and citric acid and treating agent like medicinal agent, cosmetic, adjuvant, nutritional agent and a combination thereof. This hydrogel is used to deliver agents in a controlled-release manner through body cavity, body surface and subcutaneous injection.

Shoichet et al. (2010) prepared a physical blend of an injectable hydrogel comprising thermal gelling polymers methylcellulose and hyaluronic acid and used it as a drug delivery vehicle for localized release of therapeutic agents (i.e., growth factors).

Tae-Hong et al. (2010, 2015) developed a combined system of microsphere-hydrogel in which they have employed temperature sensitive polymers for localized administration.

Hua Jing (2016) developed a thermo-sensitive injectable hydrogel based on Hyluronic acid and a copolymer of polyethylene oxide (PEO) and polypropylene oxide (PPO) for intratumoural delivery of doxorubicin.

A drug delivery system for the treatment of liver cancer that is based on interventional injection of a temperature and pH-sensitive hydrogel has been developed by Doo et al. (2013). The drug delivery system is composed of a block copolymer applicable to hepatic arterial catheterization. A therapeutic agent is loaded inside the drug delivery system, the drug delivery system is in the sol state outside, and undergoes a phase transition into the gel state inside the hepatic artery, thereby delaying or blocking blood supply of the hepatic artery, and slowly releasing the therapeutic agent during the phase transition into the gel state inside the hepatic artery.

Mansoor (1999) disclosed their drug-delivery devices and methods, which consist of a semi-interpenetrating network (semi-IPN) hydrogel comprising cationic polymer such as chitosan and a second neutral polymer such as polyethylene oxide and used as freeze-dried formulation.

Chih and Xian (2008) prepared partially biodegradable hydrogel that changes its volume and shape in response to change in pH and/or temperature by UV irradiation of composition comprising dextran-maleic acid monoester and N-isopropylacrylamide.

Philip et al. (2007) invented biomimetic gels that are prepared enzymatically, using a transglutaminase to cross-link polymer-peptide conjugates of rational design.

Auzely-velty et al. (2014) developed polymer composition comprising a mixture of PBA modified HA polymer grafted on at least a hydroxyl with a group comprising phenylboronic acid and cis-diol modified HA polymer grafted on at least a hydroxyl with a group comprising a cis-diol. Author studied injectable or implantable glucose sensitive hydrogels using this prepared polymer composition.

Schuetz Yannie et al. (2014) prepared aqueous thermosetting neutralized chitosan composition of an injectable formulation for delivering of therapeutic agent/s.

4. Commercial Technologies of Stimuli-responsive Injectable Hydrogel Systems

4.1 Regel-depot-technology

Regel is one of Macromed's proprietary drug delivery system. It is based on triblock copolymer, composed of poly(lactide-co-glycolide)-poly(ethylene glycol)-poly(lactide-co-glycolide). It is a compilation of thermally reversible gelling polymers developed for parenteral delivery. This is a field of wide range of gelation temperature, degradation rates and release characteristics as a function of molecular weight, degree of hydrophobicity and polymer concentration. After the application of the injection, the physical properties of polymer undergo a reversible phase change resulting in the formation of a water insoluble, biodegradable gel depot (Kumbhar et al. 2013, Parekh et al. 2012, Kazuhito Yamada and Mitsuaki Kuwano 2006).

4.2 Atrigel technology

The most commonly used polymers are poly(dl-lactide), lactide/glycolide copolymers, and lactide/caprolactone copolymers because of their degradation characteristics and their approval by the Food and Drug Administration (FDA). These offer the advantage that breakdown products are natural and biocompatible, hence, there is no problem of toxicity. Various rates of biodegradation can be obtained depending on the type of polymer, their combination and ratio. Polymer concentrations ranging from 10 to 80% by weight are used for preparation of Atrigel drug delivery system. The low molecular weight polymers at low polymer concentrations can be easily injected into the body using standard needles, and they can also be aerosolized for spray applications. The high molecular-weight polymers at high polymer concentrations may be used as gels or putties that can be placed into sites in the body where they solidify and provide support (Pandya et al. 2014, Dunn et al. 2013).

4.3 BST-Gel technology

Laval, Québec Canada-based Biosyntech, has developed a family of injectable thermogelling polymer solution called BST-Gel. BST-Gel is a proprietary formulation (Chenite et al. 2002) of chitosan in an aqueous solution, which allows this polymer to be used effectively for tissue regeneration and local delivery of sensitive therapeutics. BST-Gel is formulated at physiological conditions totally free from any organic cross-linker or solvent. Furthermore, its ability to remain liquid at or below the room temperature and turning into stiff gel when heated up to around 37°C, makes it an ideal candidate for designing injectable delivery systems. BST-Gel loaded with an osteogenic protein proved to be effective in promoting bone formation. Two weeks after local injection of BST-Gel containing bone morphogenetic protein onto the tibia periosteum of a rat resulted in rapid bone proliferation. The newly formed bone was detected by radiology and proved by micro-CT images. A broad IP coverage of this gel technology currently has 15 patents issued covering 15 applications (Laval and Québec 2002).

Lead products of this technology are BST-CarGel, a degradable implant for cartilage repair, BST-DermOn, a chronic-wound treatment and BST-InPod, a therapy against heel pain. It also includes BST-OssiFil, a bone consolidation material, BST-Disc, an intervertebral disc restoration treatment and Arthro-BST, an arthroscopic device used to assess the quality of cartilage. Some injectable commercial products based on above technologies are presented in Table 3.

5. Conclusion and Future Perspective

Smart hydrogels exhibit single or multiple stimuli-responsive characters which could be used in biomedical applications, including controlled drug delivery, bioengineering or tissue engineering. Stimuli like pH, temperature and dual responsive pH and temperature are monitored to attain the controlled and site specific injectable delivery and ultimately ensure achievement of better patient compliance. Over the last few years, an impressive number of stimuli-responsive injectable hydrogels based on biomaterials have been described in literature. In this chapter, the author presented various types of stimuli-responsive hydrogels with their recent developments and current applications in the field of parenteral drug

Table 3. Some injectable marketed products on *in situ* gel technologies (usfda.gov).

Sr. No.	Name	Drug	Uses	Company
1	OncoGel™	Paclitaxel	Anti-cancer therapy (in treatment of esophageal cancer)	MacroMed s.a.r.l., Lebanon
2	hGHD-1	Human growth hormone (hGH)	Human growth hormone (hGH) deficiency	MacroMed s.a.r.l., Lebanon
3	Cytoryn ™	Interleukin-2 (IL-2)	cancer immunotherapy	MacroMed s.a.r.l., Lebanon
4	Atridox®	Doxycycline hyclate	Periodontal treatment product with Sub-gingival Delivery	Tolmar Pharmaceuticals, Inc., U.S.
5	Atrisorb®-D	Doxycycline	Periodontal defects	Tolmar Pharmaceuticals, Inc., U.S.
6	Lupron depot	Leuprolide acetate	For treatment of advanced prostate cancer	Abbott Laboratories, U.S.
7	Sandostatin®	Octreotide acetate	Acromegaly	Novartis, Switzerland
8	Timoptic-XE®	Timolol Maleate	Glaucoma	Merck and Co. Inc.
9	Relday®	Risperidone	Schizophrenia and bipolar disorder	Durect, U.S.

delivery. This chapter also included injectable smart polymeric materials used in drug delivery.

The main success of the injectable stimuli-responsive hydrogel can be attained by high level of *in vitro–in vivo* correlation in their performance and ability to maintain the structural integrity in biological systems. If the achievements of the past can be extrapolated into the future, there will be a high possibility to achieve newer trend in the fields of novel drug delivery. We expect that these fundamentals and applications could help researchers in developing new stimuli-responsive injectable systems based on biomaterials which could be reliably utilized in biomedical fields.

Acknowledgement

The author is thankful to Ms. Bindu Yadav and Ms. Rutu Patel (Research Scholar) for their scientific help and writing assistance. The author acknowledges Dr. R.H. Parikh Ramanbhai Patel College of Pharmacy,

Charotar University of Science and Technology (CHARUSAT) for extended support and guidance.

Abbreviations

PMA	:	Polymethacrylic acid
PAA	:	Poly(acrylic acid)
PPA	:	Poly(propylacrylic acid)
AEA	:	Polyvinylacetal diethylaminoacetate
PNIPAAm	:	Poly(N-isopropylacrylamide)
NIPAAm	:	N-isopropylacrylamide
PNVIBA	:	Poly(N-vinylisobutyramide)
UCST	:	Upper critical solution temperature
PAAm	:	Polyacrylamide
LCST	:	Lower critical solution temperature
PEO-PPO-PEO	:	Poly(ethylene oxide)-*b*-poly(propylene oxide)-*b*-poly(ethylene oxide)
PEG	:	Poly(ethylene glycol)
AIBN	:	2, 2'-azobisisobutyronitrile
MBAAm	:	N, N'-218 methylene bis (acrylamide)
DMSO	:	Dimethyl sulfoxide
NSA	:	N- Succinimidylacrylate
GAR	:	Goat anti rabbit
PEG-PACU	:	Poly(ethylene glycol)-poly(amino carbonate urethane)
MBAA	:	N, N 9-methylenebisacrylamide
Hep-PCLA	:	Heparin-bearing poly(ε-caprolactone-co-lactide)-b-poly(ethylene glycol)-b-poly(ε caprolactone-co-lactide.
PEG–PAF	:	Poly(ethylene glycol)-poly(L-alanine-co-L-phenyl alanine) diblock copolymers
PCL-PEG-PCL	:	Poly(caprolactone)-poly(ethylene glycol)-poly(caprolactone)
γ-CD	:	γ-cyclodextrin
HPMC	:	Hydroxypropyl methyl cellulose
PEG-g-CS	:	Poly(ethylene glycol)-grafted-chitosan
PAE	:	Poly(beta-amino ester)
PCL-PEG PCL	:	Poly(ethylene glycol)-poly(epsilon-caprolactone)
PEO	:	Poly(ethylene oxide)
PPO	:	Poly(propylene oxide)
PEO	:	Poly(ethylene oxide)
PDLA	:	Poly(D,L-lactide)
NMP	:	1-methyl-2-pyrrolidinone
IPN	:	Interpenetrating polymer network

FDA   :   Food and Drug Administration
(hGH)   :   Human growth hormone
(IL-2)   :   Interleukin-2
Mon   :   months

References

Abu Bin Imran, Takahiro Seki and Yukikazu Takeoka. 2010. Recent advances in hydrogels in terms of fast stimuli responsiveness and superior mechanical performance. Polymer Journal. 42: 839–51.

Aikawa, K. et al. 1998. Drug release from pH-response polyvinylacetal diethyl aminoacetate hydrogel, and application to nasal delivery. Int. J. Pharm. 168: 181–8.

Aikawa, K., K. Matsumoto and S. Tsuchiya. 1998. Hydrogel formation of the pH response polymer polyvinylacetal diethylaminoacetate (AEA). International Journal of Pharamaceutics. 167: 97–104.

Akala, E.O., P. Kopeckova and J. Kopecek. 1998. Novel pH-sensitive hydrogels with adjustable swelling kinetics. Biomaterials. 19: 1037–47.

Alessandro Sannino and Christian Demitri. 2009. Biodegradable Cellulose-based Hydrogels: Design and Applications Materials. 2: 353–73.

Aman Kant, Suchetha Reddy and Shankraiah. 2011. *In situ* gelling system: An overview. Pharmacology Online. 2: 28–44.

Anna Gutowskan and Karol J. Krzyminski. 2002. Multiple stimulus reversible hydrogels. WO Patent # 2002000193 A2.

Arthur Rosenthal, James J. Barry and Ronald Sahatjian. 2006. Triggered release hydrogel drug delivery system US Patent# 7066904 B2.

Bhardwaj, T.R., M. Kanwar, R. Lal and A. Gupta. 2000. Natural gums and modified natural gums as sustained release carriers. Drug DevelInd Pharm. 26: 1025–38.

Bindu Sri, M., V. Ashok and Arkendu chatterjee. 2012. As a review on hydrogels as drug delivery in the pharmaceutical field. International Journal of Pharmaceutical and Chemical Science. 1: 642–61.

Brijesh Kumar, Amit K. Singh, Raj K. Prasad, Chandra S. Singh and Vivek Dwivedi. 2016. Formulation and evaluation of an injectable *in situ* forming hydrogel of dacarbazine as anticancer agent. The Pharmaceutical and Chemical Journal. 3: 100–108.

Byeongmoon Jeong, You Han Bae and Sung Wan Kim. 2000. Drug release from biodegradable injectable thermosensitive hydrogel of PEG–PLGA–PEG triblock copolymers. Journal of Controlled Release. 63: 155–163.

Capello, J., J.W. Crissman, M. Crissman, F.A. Ferrari, G. Textor, O. Wallis et al. 2003. Smart polymeric materials emerging biochemical applications. Chemistry & Biology. 10: 1161–1171.

Chasin and Langer. 1990. Biodegradable Polymers as Drug Delivery Systems. Marcel Dekker, New York.

Chenite, A., C. Chaput, D. Wang, C. Combes, M.D. Buschmann, C.D. Hoemann, J.C. Leroux, B.L. Atkinson, F. Binette and A. Selmani. 2000. Novel injectable neutral solutions of chitosan form biodegradable gels *in situ*. Biomaterials. 21(21): 2155–2161.

Chenite, Chaput, Wang, Combes, Buschmann, Hoemann et al. 2000. Novel injectable neutral solutions of chitosan form biodegradable gels *in situ*. Biomaterials. 21: 2155–2161.

Chenite, A., C. Chaput, C. Combes, A. Selmani and F. Jalal, Bio Syntech. 2002. Temperature-controlled pH-dependent formation of ionic polysaccharide gels. U.S. Patent 6,344,488.

Chih-Chang and Xian Zheng Zhang. 2006. Partially biodegradable temperature and ph sensitive hydrogel.US Patent #20060128918 A1.

Chih-Chang Chu and Xian-Zheng Zhang. 2008. Partially biodegradable temperature and pH sensitive hydrogel. U.S. Patent # 7420024 B2.

Cohen, S., E. Lobel, A. Trevgoda and Y. Peled. 1997. A novel, *In situ*-forming ophthalmic drug delivery system from alginates undergoing gelation in the eye. J. Control. Rel. 44: 201–208.

DesNoyer, J.R. and A.J. McHugh. 2003. The effect of Pluronic on the protein release kinetics of an injectable drug delivery system. J. Control Release. 86: 15–24.

Doo Sung Lee, Bong Sup KIM and Cong Truc Huynh. 2013. Drug Delivery System for Treatment of Liver Cancer Based on Interventional Injection of Temperature and Ph Sensitive Hydrogel. U.S. Patent # 20130022545 A1.

Doo Sung Lee, Bong Sup Kim and Cong Truc Huynh. 2013. ph-Sensitive Polymer Hydrogel with Dual Ionic Transition and Use Thereof. US Patent # 20130225696 A1.

Doo Sung Lee, Kasala Dayananda and Bong Sup Kim. 2013.Temperature and pH-sensitive block copolymer having excellent gel strength US Patent # 8586087 B2.

Dumitriu, S. 2002. Polymeric Biomaterials, 2nd Edition. Marcel Dekker, New York, Basel. 1184 p.

Eric Brey, Jennifer J. Kang-Mieler, Victor Perez-Luna, Bin Jiang, Pawel Drapala et al. 2014. Thermo-responsive Hydrogel Compositions. U.S. Patent # 20140065226 A1.

Gayatri C. Patel and Chintan A. Dalwadi. 2013. Recent Patents on Stimuli Responsive Hydrogel Drug Delivery System. Recent Patents on Drug Delivery & Formulation. 7: 206–215.

Gehrke, S.H. and P. Lee. 1990. Hydrogels for drug delivery systems. *In*: Specialized Drug Delivery Systems. Marcel Dekker. 333.

Giang Phan, V.H., Thavasyappan Thambi, Huu Thuy Trang Duong and Doo Sung Lee. 2016. Poly(amino carbonate urethane) based biodegradable, temperature and pH-sensitive injectable hydrogels for sustained human growth hormone delivery. Scientific Reports. 6: 1–12.

Gil, E. and S. Hudson. 2004. Stimuli-reponsive polymers and their bioconjugates. Progress in Polymer Science. 29: 1173–222.

Grijalvo, S., J. Mayr, R. Eritja and D.D. Díaz. 2016. Biodegradable liposome-encapsulated hydrogels for biomedical applications: a marriage of convenience. Biomaterials Science. 4(4): 555–574.

Guo, J.-H., G.W. Skinner, W.W. Harcum and P.E. Barnum. 1998. Pharmaceutical applications of naturally occurring water-soluble polymers. Pharm. Sci. & Technol. Today. 1: 254–61.

Hatefi, A. and B. Amsden. 2002. Biodegradable injectable *in situ* forming drug delivery systems. Journal of Controlled Release. 80: 9–28.

Hemant Ravindran Nair and Mohan G. Kulkarni. 2013. Biodegradable Polymeric Hydrogel Composition. U.S. Patent # 20130059925 A1.

Hin, T. 2004. Engineering Materials for Biomedical Applications. Singapore: World Scientific Publishing.

Hovgaard, L. and H. Brondsted. 1995. Dextran hydrogels for colon specific drug delivery. Journal of Controlled Release. 36: 159–66.

Hua Jing Jhan. 2016. Thermosensitive Injectable Hydrogel for Drug Delivery. U.S. Patent # 9364545 B2.

Huynh, D.P., M.K. Nguyen, B.S. Pi, M.S. Kim, S.Y. Chae, K.C. Lee et al. 2008. Functionalized injectable hydrogels for controlled insulin delivery. Biomaterials. 29: 2527–2534.

HyeJin Sim, Thavasyappan Thambi and Doo Sung Lee. 2015. Heparin-based temperature-sensitive injectable hydrogels for protein delivery. Journal of Materials Chemistry B Issue. 45: 1–32.

Jeong, B., Y.H. Bae, D.S. Lee and S.W. Kim. 1997. Biodegradable block copolymers as injectable drug-delivery systems. Nature. 388: 860–2.

Jian Q. Yao, Jizong Gao, Xia Huang and Sanghvi. 2012. Thermosensitive hydrogel composition and method. U.S. Patent # 20120020932 A1.

Jiang, G., J. Sun and F. Ding. 2014. PEG-g-chitosan thermosensitive hydrogel for implant drug delivery: cytotoxicity, *in vivo* degradation and drug release. Journal of Biomaterial Science Polymer Ed. 25: 241–256.

Joon B. Park and JinWhan Lee. 2006. *In situ* controlled release drug delivery system WO Patent # 2006047279 A3.

Jun Li, Hanry Yu and Kam Leong. 2002. Injectable Drug Delivery Systems with Cyclodextrin-Polymer based Hydrogels. US Patent # 20020019369.

Kala, E.O., P. Kopeckova and J. Kopecek. 1998. Novel pH-sensitive hydrogels with adjustable swelling kinetics. Biomaterials. 19: 1037–47.

Kalpana R. Kamath and Kinam Park. 1993. Biodegradable hydrogels in drug delivery. Advanced Drug Delivery Reviews. 11: 59–84.

Kazuhito Yamada and Mitsuaki Kuwano. 2006. Drug Delivery System using Subconjunctival Depot. US Patent # 20060013859 A1.

Khodaverdi, E., Z. Heidari, S.A. Tabassi, M. Tafaghodi, M. Alibolandi, F.S. Tekie et al. 2015. Injectable supramolecular hydrogel from insulin-loaded triblock PCL-PEG-PCL copolymer and γ-cyclodextrin with sustained-release property. APS PharmSciTech. 16: 140–149.

Ki-Dong Park, Yoon-K.J. and K.M. Park. 2014. *In Situ* Forming Hydrogel and Biomedical Use Thereof. U.S. Patent # 8815277 B2.

Klech, C.M. 1990. Gels and jellies. *In*: Swarbrick, J. and J.C. Boylan [eds.]. Encyclopedia of Pharmaceutical Technology Marcel Dekker. 415.

Kulwant Singh and HariKumar. 2012. Injectable *in situ* gelling controlled release drug delivery system. International Journal of Drug Development & Research. 4: 56–69.

Kumar, S. and K.J. Himmelstein. 1995. Modification of *in situ* gelling behavior of carbopol solutions by hydroxypropyl methylcellulose. Journal of Pharmaceutical Sciences. 84(3): 344–348.

Kumbhar, Amruta B., Ashwini K. Rakde and P.D. Chaudhari. 2013. *In situ* gel forming injectable drug delivery system. International Journal of Pharmaceutical Sciences and Research. 4.2: 597.

Kurisawa, M. and M. Terano. 1997. Double-stimuli-responsive degradation of hydrogels consisting of oligopeptide-terminated poly(ethylene glycol) and dextran with an interpenetrating polymer network. Journal of Biomaterial Science Polymer. 8: 691–708.

Kytai Truong Nguyen and L. Jennifer. 2002. Photopolymerizable hydrogels for tissue engineering applications. Biomaterials. 23: 4307–4314.

Laval and Québec. 2002. Thermogelling Polymer Solution for Tissue Regeneration and Delivery of Therapeutics. US # Patent 6344488.

Mamada, Tanaka and Kungwachakun. 1990. Photoinduced phase transition of gels. Macromolecules. 23: 1517–9.

Mansoor M. Hamiji. 1999. Drug Delivery using pH-sensitive Semi-interpenetrating Network Hydrogels. U.S. Patent # 5904927 A.

Matsuda, T. 2002. Device-directed therapeutic drug delivery systems. Journal of Controlled Release. 78: 125–31.

MiyataTakashi, Tadashi Uragami and Katsuhiko Nakamae. 2002. Biomolecule-sensitive hydrogels. Advanced Drug Delivery Reviews. 54: 79–98.

Molly S. Shoichet, Dimpy Gupta and Charles H. Tator. 2010. Blends of Temperature Sensitive and Anionic Polymers for Drug Delivery. U.S. Patent # 7767656 B2.

Nikhil Sood, Sahil Nagpal and Shivani Nanda. 2013. An overview on stimuli responsive hydrogels as drug delivery system. Journal of Controlled Release.

Pal, K., A.K. Banthiaand and D.K. Majumdar. 2009. Polymeric hydrogels: Characterization and biomedical applications—A mini review. Designed Monomers and Polymers. 12: 197–220.

Pandya, Yamini, Dharmesh Sisodiya and Kamlesh Dashora. 2014. ATRIGEL®, implants and controlled released drug delivery system. Int. J. Biopharmaceutics. 5.3: 208–13.

Parekh, H.B., R. Jivani, N.P. Jivani, L.D. Patel, A. Makwana and K. Sameja. 2012. Novel *in situ* polymeric drug delivery system: a review. Journal of Drug Delivery and Therapeutics. 2.

Peppas, N. and R. Langer. 1994. New challenges in biomaterials. Science. 263: 171–520.

Peppas, N.A., P. Bures, W. Leobandung and H. Ichikawa. 2000. Hydrogels in pharmaceutical formulations. Eur. J. Pharm. Biopharm.

Philip B. Messersmith, Bi-Huang Hu, Marsha and Ritter Jones. 2007. Injectable and Bioadhesive Polymeric Hydrogels as well as Related Methods of Enzymatic Preparation. U.S. Patent # 7208171 B2.

Piyush Gupta, Kavita Vermani and Sanjay Garg. 2002. Hydrogels: from controlled release to pH-responsive drug delivery. Drug Discovery Today. 7: 569–79.

Qiao, M., D. Chen, T. Hao, X. Zhao, H. Hu and X. Ma. 2008. Injectable thermosensitive PLGA-PEG-PLGA triblock copolymers-based hydrogels as carriers for interleukin-2. Pharmazie. 63: 27–30.

Qiu, Y. and K. Park. 2001. Environment-sensitive hydrogels for drug delivery. Adv. Drug Delivery. 53: 321–39.

Qiu, Y. and K. Park. 2012. Environment-sensitive hydrogels for drug delivery. Advanced Drug Delivery Reviews. 64: 49–60.

Rachel Auzely-velty, Emilie Hachet, Bogdan Catargi, Valerie Ravaine and Lea Massager. 2014. Glucose responsive hydrogel comprising pba-grafted hyaluronic acid (ha). WO Patent # 2014072330 A1.

Ramanathan, S. and LH. Block. 2001. The use of chitosan gels as matrices for electrically-modulated drug delivery. J. Control Release. 70(1-2): 109–23.

Ricci, E.J., M.V.L.B. Bentley, M. Farah, R.E.S. Bretas and J.M. Marchetti. 2002. Rheological characterization of Poloxamer 407 lidocaine hydrochloride gels. Euro. J. Pharm. Sci. 17: 161–167.

Richard L. Dunn, G. John Steven, R. Harish and Bhagya L. Chandrashekar. 2013. Polymeric Delivery Formulations of Leuprolide with Improved Efficacy. US Patent # 8486455 B2 2013.

Robert E. Richard. 2015. Multi-Component Particles for Injection and Processes for Forming the Same. U.S. Patent # 9107828 B2.

Ruel-Gariepy, E. and J.-C. Leroux. 2004. *In situ*-forming hydrogels—review of temperature-sensitive systems. European Journal of Pharmaceutics and Biopharmaceutics. 58: 409–26.

Ruta Masteikova and uzana Chalupova. 2003. Stimuli-sensitive hydrogels in controlled and sustained drug delivery. Medicina. 39: 19–24.

Schuetz Yannie, Jordan Olivier, Gorny Robert and Caratti BessonVirginie. 2014. Thermosensitive Neutralized Chitosan Composition Forming A Hydrogel, Lyophilizate and Processes for Producing the Same. IP Patent # 260002.

Sindhu, S.K., D.V. Gowda, Vishnu Datta and Siddaramaiah. 2014. Formulation and evaluation of injectable *in situ* gelling matrix system for controlled drug release. Indian Journal of Advances in Chemical Science. 2: 89–92.

Sophie, R., Van Tomme and Wim E. Hennink. 2007. Biodegradable dextran hydrogels for protein delivery applications. Expert Review of Medical Devices. 4: 147–164.

Sophie, R., Van Tomme and Gert Storm. 2008. *In situ* gelling hydrogels for pharmaceutical and biomedical applications. International Journal of Pharmaceutics. 355: 1–18.

Soppimath, K.S., T.M. Aminabhavi, A.M. Dave, S.G. Kumbar and W.E. Rudzinski. 2002. Stimulus-responsive "smart" hydrogels as novel drug delivery systems. Drug Dev. Ind. Pharm. 28: 957–74.

Stephem P. Massia and Julie Trudel. 2003. Polysaccharide-based Hydrogels and Pre-gel Blends for the Same. US Patent # 6586493 B1.

Swantantra, K.S. Kushwaha, Awani K. Rai Satyawan Singh. 2016. Thermosensitive hydrogel for controlled drug delivery of anticancer agents. Int. J. Pharm. PharmSci. 5: 547–552.

Syed Gulrez and Saphwan Assaf. 2011. Hydrogels: Methods of Preparation, Characterisation and Applications Carpi PA, editor.

Tae-Hong Lim, Joon B. Park and Jin Whan Lee. 2006. *In Situ* Controlled Release Drug Delivery System. W.O. Patent # 2006047279 A3.

Tae-Hong Lim, Joon B. Park and Jin Whan Lee. 2015. *In Situ* Controlled Release Drug Delivery System. U.S. Patent # 8940311 B2.

Takashi Miyata, N. Asami and T. Uragami. 1999. Preparation of an antigen-sensitive hydrogel using antigen–antibody bindings. Macromolecules. 32: 2082–4.

Takashi Miyata, Tadashi Uragami and Katsuhiko Nakamae. 2002. Biomolecule-sensitive hydrogels. Advanced Drug Delivery Reviews. 54: 79–98.

Thomas Hirt, Wolfgang Meier, Zhihua Lu and Xianbo Hu. 2010. Drug Delivery Vehicle containing Vesicles in a Hydrogel Base. EP Patent # 2155165 A1.

Thorsten Steinberg, Wilfried W. Raphael, Pascal Tomakidi and Dougal Laird. 2015. Bio-functionalized Stimulus-responsive Dissolvable PEG-hydrogels. U.S. Patent # 8980278 B2.

Usha P. Shinde, Hyo J. Moon, Du Y. Ko, Bo K. Jung and Byeongmoon Jeong. 2015. Control of rhGH release profile from PEG–PAF thermogel. Biomacromolecules. 16: 1461–1469.

Weihong Tan, Yang H. and L. Haipeng 2010. Target-responsive Hydrogels. WO Patent # 2009146147 A3.

Wichterle, O. 1960. Hydrophilic gels for biological use. Nature. 185: 117.

Yanbin Huang, Shu-Ping Yang and Sharon Linda Greene. 2010. Thermo-gelling Composition. U.S. Patent # 7658947 B2.

Yong Qiu and Kinam Park. 2012. Environment-sensitive hydrogels for drug delivery. Advanced Drug Delivery Reviews. 64: 49–60.

You H. Bae, Sung W. Kim and Lev I. Valuev. 1993. Pulsatile Drug Delivery Device using Stimuli Sensitive Hydrogel. US Patent #5226902 A.

You Han Bae and Sung Wan Kim. 1993. Hydrogel Delivery Systems Based on Polymer Blends, Block Co-polymers or Interpenetrating Networks. Advanced Drug Delivery Reviews. 11: 109–35.

Zhibing Hu and Xiaohu Xia. 2007. Aqueous Dispersion of Hydrogel Nanoparticles with Inverse Thermoreversible Gelation. U.S. Patent #20070116765 A1.

10

Hydrogels for Vaginal Drug Delivery

Željka Vanić[1] and *Nataša Škalko-Basnet*[2,*]

ABSTRACT

Vaginal drug delivery functionally designed for improved localized therapy of vaginal infections and inflammation, has gained momentum in past fifteen years. A well-designed vaginal formulation should be based on the vehicle (base) that enables an effective delivery of a drug to the vaginal site assuring a prolonged vaginal residence time of incorporated drug. When choosing the optimal vehicle, the physiological parameters such as vaginal anatomy, histology, microflora and secretions, as well as biodegradability and safety profile should be taken into account. The ideal vehicle should exhibit appropriate rheological and textural properties, be compatible with incorporated drug and excipients, be stable during the storage and safe for the use, without affecting the normal vaginal physiology. Gels as vaginal vehicle should maintain their viscosity when higher shear rates are applied or upon dilution with vaginal fluids and semen. The chapter provides an overview of the gels currently exploited for vaginal administration, discusses the main advantages and disadvantages of each gel-based system and summarizes the tested drugs. Specific focus is given on the nanosystems-in-hydrogels s and respective nanosystem-vehicle interactions. Finally, the formulations in clinical studies and

[1] Department of Pharmaceutical Technology, Faculty of Pharmacy and Biochemistry, University of Zagreb, A. Kovačića 1, 10 000 Zagreb, Croatia.
  Email: zvanic@pharma.hr
[2] Drug Transport and Delivery Research Group, Department of Pharmacy, Faculty of Health Sciences, University of Tromsø The Arctic University of Norway, Universitetsveien 57, 9037 Tromsø, Norway.
* Corresponding author: natasa.skalko-basnet@uit.no

perspectives are discussed in more details, especially their efficacy and safety in human subjects.

Keywords: hydrogels, vaginal therapy, nanomedicine, microbicides

1. Introduction

The vagina as a site for drug administration has been, up to now, mostly explored for a local delivery of a variety of therapeutic agents such as antimicrobials (antibacterials, antifungals, antivirals, antiprotozoals), spermicides, labour-inducing agents (prostaglandins) and sexual hormones (das Neves and Bahia 2006). Vaginal infections, particularly among women of reproductive age, are the most frequent reason for women to seek medical assistance. Local treatment of vaginal infections has been proposed as a means to achieve higher local drug concentration, reduced side effects and interference with gastrointestinal tract (Palmeira–de-Oliveira et al. 2015). Vagina as the site of drug administration/action has become especially interesting due to an urgent need for the development of efficient vaginal topical microbicides with respect to human immunodeficiency virus (HIV) infections (Yu et al. 2011). Moreover, vaginal route is an attractive site for a systemic drug delivery due to its potential to permit the absorption of various drugs while avoiding the loss of a drug in the first pass metabolism (Hussain and Ahsan 2005). It is known that the vaginal mucosa is more permeable for some molecules such as, water, 17-β-estradiol, arecoline and arecaidine (REF). Some of the reasons why vaginal drug delivery still has not been fully utilized are based on rather specific limitations that include: (i) cultural sensitivity, (ii) issue of personal hygiene, (iii) one-gender specificity, (iv) reported cases of local irritation, (v) influence of sexual intercourse on the efficacy of the therapy, and (vi) variability in the rate and extent of drug absorption (Hussain and Ahsan 2005). However, those issues could be overcome by the targeted design and development of advanced dosage forms and delivery systems that can minimize or extinguish the specific limitations. The potential of vagina as a site of drug absorption is clearly demonstrated by the anatomical and physiological advantages this site offers, such as the large surface area (rugae vaginales) and dense network of blood vessels within vagina, the possibility of avoiding first-pass metabolism, related reduction in the incidence and severity of gastrointestinal side effects, diminishing the inconvenience caused by pain, tissue damage and risk of infections associated with parenteral routes as well as the cost of treatment. Moreover, the easiness of the self-insertion and privacy of the therapy should not be neglected.

The optimal vaginal formulation should be easy to use, discreet, with possibility of reversible application if irritancy is experienced, painless to the patient upon insertion, cost-effective, widely available and safe for continuous administration. However, the stability and storage conditions need to be addressed (Vanić and Škalko-Basnet 2013). Regarding the acceptability by the users and patient compliance, the formulation should have minimal interference with the body functioning and daily life (das Neves and Bahia 2006).

A well-designed vaginal product is based on the vehicle that enables effective delivery of a drug to the desired site of action in a pattern that does not destroy the pharmacological agent and is simultaneously safe for the patient. There are a large number of vaginal medications in the market. However, most of these conventional formulations (solutions, creams, gels, suppositories and tablets) require frequent application due to their short residence time at the vaginal site, leakage and messiness. Therefore, a prolonged vaginal residence time of formulations is considered a key parameter for improved therapeutic efficacy (Justin-Temu et al. 2005). The approaches suggested for prolonging the residence time in vagina involve the use of mucoadhesive and *in situ* gelling delivery systems as well as the formulations based on the mechanical fixation. Bioadhesive gels are one of the most promising dosage forms for vaginal drug therapy. They are rather easy to manufacture, comfortable to apply from the patient's point of view and exhibit superior spreadability over the mucosal surfaces enabling intimate contact with targeted vaginal sites (Tüğcu-Demiröz et al. 2013). Additional attractiveness of bioadhesive gels is their high water content and superior rheological properties acting as hydrating and lubricating systems able to compensate for vaginal dryness at the onset of menopause (Acartürk 2009).

The specificity of vaginal anatomy, histology, microflora characteristics and secretions significantly contribute to the performance of the drug delivery and consequent efficacy of drug therapy, and should be taken into consideration when designing the optimal formulation.

2. Vagina as a Site of Drug Administration

The vagina is a slightly S-shaped fibro-muscular, tubular organ of about 6–10 cm in length and it extends from the cervix of the uterus to the vestibule. The epithelium that lines the vagina and the external surface of the cervix is multilayered, and is relatively strong and durable. Beneath this is a layer of connective tissue—the lamina propria.

Within these structures are several classes of lymphoid cell, including dendritic cells, macrophages, T lymphocytes and Langerhans cells (Fig. 1, Stone 2002). Its thickness is between 200 and 300 µm characterized by a turnover of about 10–15 layers over 7 days (Valenta 2005). The cytological changes of vaginal epithelium follow the cyclical stages in women. The epithelium is the thickest in the proliferative stage, reaching

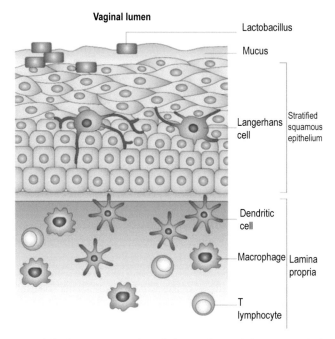

Fig. 1. Structure of the human vaginal epithelium. The multilayered epithelium and the underlying connective tissue contain several types of potential target cell for HIV. Reprinted with permission from Stone 2002. Nature Reviews Drug Discovery. 1: 977–985. Copyright@ Nature Publishing Group.

a peak at ovulation, and then diminishing with the secretory phase. The lamina propria (Fig. 1) comprises loose connective tissue containing a vast amount of elastic fibers, providing vagina the capability to distend. It is composed of fibroblasts, elastic fibers, collagen fibers, capillaries and nerves, as well as polymorphonuclear leukocytes and occasional lymph nodules. The surface of vagina is composed of numerous transverse folds known as rugae, which provide distensibility, support as well as increase surface area of vaginal wall (Husain and Ahsan 2005). In addition, rugae covering vaginal epithelium provide distensibility and support to the vaginal wall.

The vagina is a vascular organ; most importantly, the venous blood supply from the vagina does not enter the portal system and therefore, first-pass metabolism is avoided, which is of great importance for drugs prone to strong first pass effect. For example, oestradiol and progesterone, when administered orally, undergo massive inactivation due to extensive metabolism while their vaginal administration offers improved therapy (Cicinelli 2008). The vagina also contains lymphatic vessels and nerves originating from the puddental nerve and from the inferior hypogastric and uterovaginal plexus (Washington et al. 2001).

The morphology and physiology of the vulva and vagina change over a lifetime. The vaginal physiology is mainly influenced by the woman's age, hormonal balance, pregnancy, pH changes and the presence of microflora. The thickness of epithelial layer changes by about 100 μm following the estrogen level changes in the menstrual cycle. In a woman of reproductive age, the vaginal mucosa may be as thick as 45 cell layers during the first half of the menstrual cycle. However, during menopause, the thickness significantly decreases to only 3–4 cell layers, thus resulting in an increased permeability of the epithelium (Farage and Maibach 2006).

3. The Challenges Faced by a Formulation Administered at Vaginal Site

3.1 The environment at vaginal site

3.1.1 Vaginal fluid

Vagina secretes a relatively large amount of fluid, in the form of vaginal discharge, although it does not contain secretary glands. This discharge is a mixture of various components including transudates through the epithelium, cervical mucus, exfoliating epithelial cells, secretions of the Bartholin's and Skene's glands, leukocytes, endometrial and fallopian tubes' fluids. It contains enzymes, enzyme inhibitors, proteins, carbohydrates, amino acids, glycoproteins, lactic acid, acetic acid, glycerol, urea, glycogen and ions such as sodium, calcium and chlorides. Vagina also includes a wide range such as the nucleases, proteases, lysozymes and esterases (Rohan and Sassi 2009).

The amount and composition of the vaginal fluid also changes throughout the menstrual cycle and is affected by hormonal influences and the state of arousal. Women of reproductive age produce fluid at a rate of 3–4 g/4 h, while the postmenopausal women experience 50% decrease in the fluid volume. At the time of ovulation, mucus secretion increases and mucus becomes clear, thin and alkaline. During the luteal phase, in which progesterone levels are high, mucus secretion decreases and mucus is more viscous (Baloglu et al. 2009). Sexual arousal may affect the volume and composition of vaginal fluids and consequently, alter the drug release pattern from vaginal delivery system (Hussain and Ahsan 2005, Vanić and Škalko-Basnet 2013).

The mucus covering the vaginal epithelium is a viscous coating consisting mainly of water (up to 95% weight), inorganic salts, carbohydrates, lipids and glycoproteins, termed mucins. Mucins are hydrophilic and provide gel-like properties to the mucus (Serra et al. 2009). In order for mucoadhesion to take place, the wetting and swelling of mucoadhesive polymer in the formulation should enable an intimate contact with the mucosal tissue, followed by interpenetration of the polymer chains and entanglement between the polymer and mucin chains (Jøraholmen et al. 2014). It is also very important to consider the concentration of delivery system applied to vaginal tissue, as this may affect the organized structure of mucus and cause the collapsing of mucin fibers (das Neves et al. 2011). Moreover, any novel delivery system destined for administration within the vagina should exhibit a low propensity to cause genital irritation and systemic toxicity. This consideration is particularly relevant for therapy in pregnant patients (Vanić and Škalko-Basnet 2013).

3.1.2 Vaginal pH and microflora

Vaginal pH often serves as a marker for possible infections with microbial pathogens (Hainer and Gibson 2011) as well as indicator of menopausal status (Cailloutte et al. 1997). A vaginal pH of 4.5 corresponds to a premenopausal serum estradiol level and the absence of bacterial pathogens. An elevated vaginal pH between 5.0 and 6.5 either indicates the presence of bacterial pathogens or a decreased estradiol level. In the absence of bacterial pathogens, a vaginal pH of 6 to 7 is an indication of menopause. The lowest pH occurs in the middle of the cycle, whereas the higher values are obtained during the period immediately prior to or preceding menstruation. High levels of estrogen during pregnancy contribute to a thick epithelium, high level of *Lactobacilli*, and a low pH. On the contrary, estrogen deficit during menopause is manifested by an increase in the vaginal pH to up to pH 7. In addition to these clear changes related to ageing, the vaginal pH is also altered during menstruation and by the presence of semen, which is slightly alkaline (pH 7–8) (Geonnotti et al. 2005). In recent years, reports suggest that the frequent use of hygienic products and douches assist in washing away a variety of the natural vaginal defenses and can promote colonization of bacteria or alter vaginal pH, allowing pathogenic bacteria and yeast to proliferate. Vulvovaginal candidiasis and bacterial vaginosis generally increase the vaginal pH above pH 5 due to the lowering of *Lactobacilli* population (das Neves et al. 2008). Orally taken contraceptives or hormone replacement therapy may have a considerable influence on the changes in vaginal pH and membrane thickness. It has been suggested that the women on depot-medroxyprogesterone acetate therapy exhibit a decrease in the colonization of vaginal *Lactobacilli* and an increase in vaginal pH by maintaining low estradiol levels (Miller et al. 2000).

   Lactobacilli presents normal, healthy vaginal microflora, although other facultative and obligate aerobes and anaerobes reside inside vagina including *Staphylococcus, Streptococcus, Pseudomonas, Proteus, Bacteroides, Bifidobacterium, Eubacterium, Fusobacterium, Clostridium, Veillonella, Klebsiella, Enterobacter* species and *Escherichia coli*. Presence of *Lactobacilli* (Döderlein's bacilli) is crucial in the prevention of vaginal infections and pathogen control by maintaining acidic vaginal pH (3.8–4.5) and producing bactericidal compounds (i.e., hydrogen peroxide). Lactic acid, that is responsible for the acidic vaginal pH, is a product of glycogen degradation by the *Lactobacilli* proliferating near the epithelium (Fredricks et al. 2005). *Lactobacilli* also produce hydrogen peroxide, which is toxic to other microorganisms that produce little or no hydrogen peroxide-scavenging enzymes such as *Escherichia coli*, *Streptococcus B* and even human immunodeficiency virus (HIV) (Alexander et al. 2004). Therefore, an absence of hydrogen peroxide-producing *Lactobacilli* in the normal vaginal flora may result in higher risks for bacterial vaginosis, candidiasis or possibly HIV-infection.

3.2 Factors to be consider in optimizing vaginal drug delivery systems

To optimize the dosage form of delivery system destined for vaginal site, it is crucial to understand the transport kinetics of drugs and active ingredients through the vaginal tissue. In the case of localized drug therapy, both the drug and all excipients in the formulation should remain at the external vaginal surface. It is also crucial to consider that any intravaginal pharmaceutical product will be in contact with both cervical and vaginal mucosa. For example, regarding the HIV prevention, the main aim is to assure sufficient concentration of prophylactic modality at the vagina as a potential site of infection (Date and Destache 2013). However, if the aim of vaginal drug delivery is to assure the systemic drug action, it is of great importance to understand the barriers to drug absorption related to vagina as the absorption site. The secretion of cervical mucus represents a barrier to drug permeation. Enzymes such as proteases could be the prominent barrier for the absorption of intact peptide and protein drugs into the systemic circulation, which is especially interesting considering the delivery of biologicals *via* vagina as administration site. The average apparent permeability coefficient is 8×10^{-5} cm/s for fresh human cervical tissue and 7×10^{-5} cm/s for fresh human vaginal tissue, respectively (Sassi et al. 2004). The physicochemical and biopharmaceutical properties of drug including its molecular weight, solubility, acid dissociation constant (pKa), drug permeation, octanol-water partition coefficient (log P), charge and chemical characteristics affect its fate once administered vaginally (Machado et al. 2015). Most of the vaginally absorbed drugs are transported by simple diffusion (Sassi et al. 2004).

One of the absorption barriers often underestimated in the design and optimization of vaginal delivery systems is the vaginal epithelium.

The changes in the thickness of vaginal epithelium directly affect the drug permeation, particularly for hydrophilic drugs. As the vaginal epithelium becomes thin, loose and porous, the permeation rate of even larger hydrophilic drugs becomes significantly enhanced. Moreover, reduced vascularity and glycogen content connected to the vaginal dryness and an increase in the vaginal pH may also reduce drug absorption.

From pharmaceutical point of view, the characteristics of drug formulation and their effect on vaginal drug bioavailability are of special interest. Factors such as the lipophilicity of the vehicle administered to the vagina, the drug solubility within the formulation, drug release profile, spreadability/distribution of the formulation inside the vagina, the residence time, as well as final concentration of applied formulation, will affect the drug bioavailability. Many of the drugs of interest for vaginal application are poorly soluble, therefore, the use of the excipients that increases the aqueous solubility may improve drug dissolution and consequent absorption. The addition of surface active agents or encapsulation of drug into drug delivery nanosystems are interesting means to improve vaginal drug bioavailability (Wong et al. 2014). The formulations based on the hydrophilic vehicles (bases) such as hydrogels are superior to lipophilic vehicles considering the hydrophilic mucosal surface (das Neves and Bahia 2006). The optimal vaginal formulation should assure adequate spreadability throughout the vagina. The spreadability of a formulation will be dependent on the viscosity of the vehicle and should be optimized. The viscosity should also be optimized concerning the desired residence time of formulation at the site of application. Due to the self-cleansing action of the vaginal tract, the residence time of dosage forms and delivery systems will be reduced, unless the systems are especially designed to be retained at vaginal site and increase the contact time of the formulation/drug with the mucosal layer (Sassi et al. 2008). Highly saturated drug formulation will ensure that sufficient amount of drug is available throughout the intended time. However, high local drug concentration over an extended period might cause severe local irritation or adverse tissue reactions and needs to be considered as an important parameter when optimizing vaginal drug formulation. Moreover, it is essential that the natural vaginal environment is preserved, and not adversely affected by the formulation.

Various polymers forming hydrogels have the potential to be applied to mucosal surfaces, including vagina (Hoare and Kohane 2008). The most commonly used mucoadhesive polymers able to form bioadhesive hydrogels are synthetic polyacrylates, polycarbophil, chitosan, cellulose derivatives, hyaluronic acid derivatives, pectin, tragacanth, carrageenan and sodium alginate (Acartürk 2009).

4. Gels as Vaginal Drug Delivery Systems

4.1 General considerations

Among a variety of vaginal drug delivery systems currently available in the market, semi-solid formulations such as creams and particularly gels are frequently used. Their main advantages over other vaginal dosage forms and delivery systems are the easiness of administration, high acceptability by women and relatively low production cost. On the other hand, messiness and leakage during application are recognized as major limitations (Hussain and Ahsan 2005). Due to the limited residence time resulting from the self-cleansing action of the vaginal tract, many formulations fail to provide sustained drug release. Consequently, the semi-solid formulations require at least one daily dose to assure optimal therapeutic outcome (Yu et al. 2011). While vaginal creams (oil-in-water emulsion-based preparations) allow the incorporation of both hydrophilic and hydrophobic drugs in the same formulation, hydrogels are mostly prepared as vehicles for hydrophilic drugs (active ingredients) (das Neves et al. 2014).

Vaginal gels are multi-component semi-solid systems comprising a polymer network in which aqueous fluid is trapped forming a gel-matrix (Yu et al. 2011). The hydrophilicity of the polymer imparts water-attracting properties to the system. Their intrinsic water-swelling behaviour is attributed to the presence of chemical or physical cross-links, which provide a network-like structure and physical integrity to the system (Gupta et al. 2002). Due to a very high water content in the hydrogels (> 80%) and absence of emulsifiers, hydrogels can significantly increase the hydration level of the vaginal mucosa and provide higher biocompatibility, bioavailability and spreadability (das Neves et al. 2014). They commonly exhibit the non-Newtonian, pseudoplastic behaviour responsible for the formulation spreadability; an increase in the pseudoplasticity enhances the easiness of hydrogel spreadability and acceptability (Garg et al. 2002).

Hydrogels are available in various structural and chemical forms, on the basis of which they have been broadly classified in the literature (Ofner III and Klech-Gelotte 2002). Vaginal gels belong to physically bonded gel networks composed of hydrophilic polymers of synthetic, semi-synthetic or natural origin (Ofner III and Klech-Gelotte 2002, Yu et al. 2011). Depending on their rheological properties, physically bounded gels can be divided into three groups: entanglement networks, strong gels and weak gels. Entanglement networks behave as dilute solutions when diluted below their critical gelling concentrations, while strong gels have stress-strain profiles that include rupture points. Vaginal gels are considered weak gels, similar to entanglement networks; however, they undergo specific molecular interactions that increase their strength. Consequently, the rheological properties of weak gels are intermediate between the entanglement networks and strong gels. Carbomer (polyacrylic acid resin copolymerized with 0.75–2% polyalkylsucrose) and xantan gum are examples of the polymers producing weak gels. Although hyaluronic acid generally forms an entanglement network, under specific conditions, i.e., pH 2.5 and 0.15 M salt, it produces a weak gel (Ofner III and Klech-Gelotte 2002).

Design of an ideal/optimal vaginal gel with desired characteristics in terms of the safety, efficacy and patient compliance, aesthetics, acceptability to regulatory authorities and cost, requires a careful selection of the active ingredient(s) and excipients. In addition to gelling agent and water, vaginal hydrogels comprise humectants such as glycerol or propylene glycol and preservatives (benzalkonium chloride, benzenthonium chloride, benzoic acid, benzyl alcohol, cetyl pyridinium chloride, methyl- and propyl-paraben). To be compatible with vaginal mucosa, hydrogels frequently encompass appropriate amount of buffering agent or weak acids such as lactic, acetic or sorbic acid, respectively (Garg et al. 2001b).

The anatomical and physiological features of the vagina should be considered during the development and evaluation of vaginal gels. Volume, composition and pH of vaginal fluid as well as the forces the gel experiences *in vivo*, play an important role in defining rheological and drug release properties (Yu et al. 2011). These properties are strongly determined by the gel composition. The replacement of even a single constituent can lead to significantly altered rheological behaviour (Owen et al. 2001). Oscillatory or flow rheometry is usually applied in gel characterization; the oscillatory measurements are preferable because they permit a complete characterization of both the elastic and viscous components of the formulations under investigation (das Neves and Bahia 2006, das Neves et al. 2009, Vanić et al. 2014). Vaginal gels should retain their viscosity when higher shear rates are applied or upon the dilution with vaginal fluids (Garg et al. 2001a). Upon *in vivo* administration, the formulation undergoes a range of shear rates caused by the movement of the vaginal epithelial surfaces, gravity, and both steady and transient capillary flow in addition to dilution by vaginal fluids. This shearing and dilution will affect the rheological performances of the hydrogels, including their spreading and retention (Owen et al. 2000, Yu et al. 2011). Spreadability of vaginal gels is responsible for the correct dosage transfer to the target site, easiness of application, extrudability from the original package and consumer preference (Garg et al. 2002). Although vaginal gels should distribute easily over vaginal mucosa to fully cover the vaginal surface, this feature may provoke undesirable leakage thus decreasing patient compliance (das Neves et al. 2009). Once applied to the vagina, hydrogels must reside at the vaginal site for a defined period to enable controlled delivery of the incorporated drug. Therefore, to achieve maximal clinical outcome, a delicate tuning between the spreading and retention is required, emphasizing the significance of performing rheological and textural characterization (Yu et al. 2011).

Majority of the commercially available vaginal gels and those in the clinical investigations are mucoadhesive in nature. They ensure a prolonged contact between the incorporated drug/active ingredient and the vaginal mucosa, permitting the drug release over an extended period of time. The most frequently used mucoadhesive polymers for the preparation of vaginal gels are polyacrylates, polycarbophil, cellulose derivates (hydroxyethylcellulose, hydroxypropylcellulose, hydroxypropylmethylcellulose), chitosan and its thiolated derivatives, hyaluronic acid derivatives, pectin, tragacanth, carrageenan and sodium alginate (Valenta 2005). In the past decade, the environmentally responsive hydrogels (das Neves and Bahia 2006) have gained increased attention. These formulations are liquid dispersions with low viscosity and free flowing at ambient temperature, while at the body temperature they form a semi-solid gel (Khan et al. 2016). The responsiveness is of great relevance since drug containing thermo-sensitive gels have the ability to finely spread along the vagina and coat the vaginal epithelium by forming hydrogels immediately after administration. Commonly used thermoresponsive polymers include N-isopropylacrylamide, polysaccharides (chitosan, cellulose derivatives, xyloglucan) and polyethylene oxide-co-propylene oxide-co-polyethylene oxide (PEO-PPO-PEO, Poloxamer or Pluronic) (He et al. 2008). They are able to change original conformation, hydrophilic/lipophilic balance and solubility in response to the temperature change in the external environment. The polymer components are insoluble above or below a specific temperature, termed as the upper and lower critical solution temperature (UCST and LCST, respectively). The interaction forces, such as hydrogen bonding between water molecules and polymer, weakens at LCST in comparison to polymer-polymer and water-water interaction leading to the phase separation resulting in gel formation. These gels are formed by the physical reversible linkage in the chains of polymers due to temperature stimulus. By removing the stimulus, the gel returns to its solution form due to a decrease in hydrophobicity (Khan et al. 2016).

The limited residence time of the *in situ* formed hydrogels on vaginal mucosa can be enhanced by the addition of mucoadhesive polymers (e.g., polycarbophil) to the dispersion of thermoresponsive polymer. However, such multi-component gels might exhibit complex flow behaviours due to the interactions among the gel components (Chang et al. 2002).

Vaginal hydrogels have been widely applied as moisturizers, lubricants and delivery systems/vehicles for microbicides, contraceptives, labour-inducers and other active ingredients/drugs. In the majority of the preparations, the mucoadhesive poly(acrylic) acid derivatives (Carbopol 974P NF or Carbopol 934P NF) and polycarbophil (Noveol AA-1) have been used as gelling agents. Superiority of the Carbopol and polycarbophil resins lies in their ability to form gels at slightly acidic pH (pH 4–5), thus assuring favourable effect on vaginal mucosa for an extended period of time (Dittgen et al. 1997).

In the following sub-chapters, we attempt to classify the studies related to vaginal hydrogels based on their intended usage. Our intention is to provide more information on the composition and characteristics of commercially available vaginal gels and those in clinical trials as those are, in our opinion, the most relevant for the readers. Nanomedicine-based vaginal hydrogels are currently mostly in the preclinical investigations and are, therefore, discussed as a separate chapter.

4.2 *Vaginal moisturizers and lubricants*

Vaginal dryness is experienced among women of all ages; however, it is particularly common during and after the menopause as a result of the reduced estrogen levels. Since estrogen has an important role in the differentiation of epithelial cells during the menstrual cycle, it indirectly affects the production of the vaginal fluid and lubrication; its low levels lead to vaginal atrophy, thinning and inflammation of the vaginal walls and vulval tissues (Edwards and Panay 2016). Additionally, there is a substantial increase of vaginal pH from 4–5 up to pH 7 in postmenopausal females due to reduced levels of cellular glycogen which permits colonization of certain pathogens and an increase of local infections (Robinson and Bologna 1994, Sinha and Ewies 2013). Dryness is usually one of the many symptoms reported by women suffering from vaginal or vulvovaginal atrophy (VVA). The term "genitourinary syndrome of menopause" (GSM) has recently been proposed in reference to the genitourinary tract symptoms related to the menopause. The term was designed to allow the description of symptoms in a more inclusive and user friendly manner (Portman and Gass 2014). Reported prevalent rates of vaginal dryness due to VVA or GSM vary; however, it is estimated that approximately 15% of premenopausal and up to 57% of postmenopausal women experience this condition (Palacios 2009). Major signs of vaginal dryness include a discomfort caused by tight fitted clothing, burning sensation, purpulent discharge, postcoital bleeding, lack of lubrication during sexual arousal and dyspareunia (Edwards and Panay 2016, Lev-Sagie 2015). Therapy with topical vaginal estrogen reverses these changes and restores vaginal pH, the fluid volume and moisture level (Al-Baghdadi and Ewies 2009). However, many menopausal women reject the use of topical vaginal estrogen due to safety reasons and adverse publicity over recent years, an alternative for which includes the administration of vaginal lubricants and moisturizers (Sinha and Ewies 2013). Both lubricants and moisturizers reduce the friction associated with thin, dry genital tissue. The main difference between them is in their intended use; lubricants reduce discomfort during the sexual intercourse, whereas vaginal moisturizers are used as a chronic maintenance to replace normal vaginal secretions. Vaginal moisturizers are classified as Class IIa Medical Devices by the Medicines and Healthcare products Regulatory Agency, based on the intended duration of their use (vaginal moisturizers are intended to be present in the body for longer than 60 min, but a single application should not last longer than 30 days). Lubricants may or may not be classified as medical devices, depending on their individual claims (Edwards and Panay 2016).

Various vaginal moisturizers are available over the counter (OTC), such as Replens®, Summer's Eve®, Emerita®, RepHresh®, Feminize®, K-Y SILK-E®, etc. They commonly comprise mucoadhesive polymers permitting good retention on the vaginal tissue for an extended period of time. One of such product is Replens® (Anglian Pharma, Hampshire, UK), acid-buffering hydrogel (pH 3.0) and long-lasting moisturizer composed of the two mucoadhesive polymers, polycarbophil and Carbopol 934P NF, respectively (Edwards and Panay 2016). Following *in vivo* administration, the hydrogel remains adhered onto vaginal surface for up to 3 days maintaining the hydration of the epithelial cells, increasing the volume of the vaginal fluid and restoration of premenopausal pH. The superiority of the formulation has been clinically confirmed, showing that its efficiency against symptoms of VVA (itching, soreness, irritation and dyspareunia) was equivalent to topical estrogen therapy within the first week of the use (Bygdeman and Swahn 1996). Although Replens® does not entirely reverse vaginal atrophy or re-cornification, normalization of vaginal pH to values 4–5 with return of vaginal fluid volume and elasticity were shown to be sufficient to prevent vaginal infections and comfortable return of sexual function (Nachtigall 1994). Recommended regime is a single dose (2.5 g) three times per week for an initial period of 3 months (Edwards and Panay 2016). Very similar to Replens® is RepHresh® the (Anglan Pharma, Hampshire, UK), also polycarbophil and carbopol-based hydrogel for long-lasting vaginal hydration (Sinha and Ewies 2013).

Besides polyacrylic acid based polymers, some other polymers as pectin, xanthan gum and methylcellulose have also been used as gelling agents in vaginal moisturizers (e.g., Summer's Eve® by CB Fleet Company, Virginia, USA). Although the formulation was shown to be less mucoadhesive and requires daily administration, its effectiveness in removing the symptoms of vaginal dryness was comparable to Replens® but with significantly less vaginal residue (as seen in colposcopic examination) (Caswell and Kane 2002).

To improve the hydration and restoration of vaginal tissue, some moisturizers such as Hyalofemme® (Fidia Farmaceutici, Abano Terme,

Italy) contain hyaluronic acid, the natural-origin compound in the vaginal epithelium responsible for maintaining hydration levels in moisture-sensitive environment. Evaluation of the efficacy and safety of Hyalofemme® revealed significant improvement rate (84% after 10 applications, compared to 89% achieved by estriol cream) accompanied by higher safety profile (Chen et al. 2013). In another clinical study, the effect of hyaluronic acid containing moisturizer has been compared with intravaginally administered phytoestrogen genistein. A total number of 62 postmenopausal women were randomly assigned to daily receive 97 µg of genistein in a form of suppository or 5 mg of hyaluronic acid for a period of 3 months. A significant improvement was observed in genital symptoms, colposcopy scores and maturation value in both groups; however, the improvement obtained by genistein was more effective, especially regarding genital score. Both treatments did not significantly influence flow cytometry parameters, although genistein showed slight decrease in DNA ploidy, with a normalization of the aneuploid content present in some cases. These results were considered preliminary and need to be verified in larger, prospective studies (Le Donne et al. 2011).

The effectiveness of vaginal hydrogels in the treatment of VVA symptoms can be further enhanced by the addition of natural origin compounds in the gel vehicle. Thus Emerita® vaginal hydrogel (Emerita, California, USA) contain *Aloe barbadensis* leaf juice, *Chamomile matricaria*, *Calendula officinalis* and *Panax ginseng* extracts, proven to improve the healing of vaginal tissue disrupted by vaginal dryness (Tan et al. 2012). Herbal-based compounds are also included in other hydrogels used as vaginal moisturizers. For example, Yes® hydrogel (Yes Company Ltd., Alton, Hants, UK) is composed of *Linum usitatissimum* flax extract, *Aloe barbadensis* juice and a mixture of plant polymers (guar gum and locust bean gum) that coat the vaginal epithelium and release water into it. The formulation has a favourable effect on vaginal mucosa permitting moisturizing effect for up to 72 h, while the pH resembles the normal pre-menopausal vaginal pH (Tan et al. 2012).

Animal-origin compounds such as bovine colostrums, have also been shown to act on the symptoms of vaginal dryness by promoting mucosal trophic restoration and preventing from bacterial and viral infections. Zambon SpA (Bresso, Milan, Italy) has developed cellulose- and xantan gum-based hydrogel (Monurelle Biogel®) that contains a purified lyophilized bovine colostrum (2.3%, w/w), in addition to other natural substances assuring the hydrating, re-epithelizing and antioxidant properties (betaine, panthenol, sericin, vitamin E and lactic acid). Monurelle Biogel® has been proven to have beneficial effect on vaginal atrophy in ovariectoized rats, improving the vaginal hemodynamics and thickness of vaginal epithelium (Vailati et al. 2013). Recently, the formulation has been clinically tested for the efficacy, tolerability and safety in women suffering from vaginal dryness. Ninety five women of reproductive age with symptoms of vaginal dryness were allocated at random to receive either Monurelle Biogel® (5 ml) for about 23 intermenstrual days (1 or 2 times/daily intravaginally) or no treatment (lubricants on demand were allowed). Symptoms of vaginal discomfort have significantly improved after 11 days, as compared to the control group. The mean vaginal health index score was also significantly higher in the group receiving Monurelle Biogel® at the end of the study. Women reported a compliance rate of 100% for the tested formulation when administered once per day, while local tolerability was excellent or good in 82.9% of the subjects (Nappi et al. 2016).

Vaginal lubricants are used immediately before and during sexual activity to decrease the tissue irritation due to friction, and their action is temporary. They can occasionally cause irritation related to the product's osmolarity (greater osmolarity causes greater irritation) or the presence of chemically irritating or allergenic agents (Lev-Sagie 2015). Lubricants are available as water-soluble products (hydrogels), silicone-based, or oil-based; however, here we have focused only on hydrogel-based lubricants. In addition to water and gelling agent(s), excipients such as humectants, emollients and preservatives are included to achieve a proper viscosity, alter water activity, and prevent bacterial contamination (Sinha and Ewies 2013).

Numerous water-based lubricants are available in the market including K-Y Jelly®, Liquid Sylk®, Aquagel®, Astroglide®, Slippery Stuff®, Pjur Med Natural Glide Personal Lubricant® among others (Edwards and Panay 2016). For example, K-Y Jelly® (Johnson and Johnson, New Jersey, USA) is a colourless, biologically inert and pH balanced cellulose-based hydrogel (methylcellulose and carboxymethyl cellulose). It is fragrance free and has been very popular since it does not stain and can be easily cleaned. Quite similar is Liquid Sylk® (Sylk Ltd., Kingston upon Thames, UK), also cellulose based hydrogel, with the pH within 4.5–4.7 (Sinha and Ewies 2013).

Majority of personal lubricants contain glycols as humectants/emollients; among them, glycerol/glycerine and propylene glycol are the most common. To maintain the osmolality of lubricant at 51200 mOsm/kg, the World Health Organization (WHO) advises that the concentration of glycerol should not exceed 9.9% (w/w), and the concentration of propylene glycol (or a mixture of glycols) should not exceed approximately 8.3% (w/w) (Edwards and Panay 2016). However, it should be noted that the patients prone to yeast infection should avoid glycerol containing lubricants (Sinha and Ewies 2013). Regarding the pH of formulations, the preferred pH is between 4 and 5, although some marketed formulations have pH greater than 5 (Edwards and Panay 2016).

In addition to their moisturizing and lubricating effects, some of the above mentioned vaginal hydrogels (e.g., Replens®) can be also applied for normalizing the vaginal pH and prevention of vaginal infectious disorders. These acid-buffering gels generally do not contain active ingredient, but the slightly acidic pH of the formulation, hydrophilicity and appropriate mucoadhesivity enables restoration of healthy vaginal environment. Another example of acid-buffering gels is Aci-Jel Balance® (Janssen-Cilag, UK), a polycarbophyl/Carbopol 974P NF based hydrogel, buffered at pH 4 and recommended for maintaining the natural pH balance. It contains glacial acetic acid, hydroxyquinoline sulphate, ricinoleic acid (acid buffering compounds) and propyl hydroxybenzoate (preservative) (Aci-Jel 2016).

4.3 Microbicide-containing hydrogels

Microbicides are chemical agents applied vaginally/rectally for the prevention of sexually-transmitted viruses and pathogens, most commonly, human immunodeficiency virus (HIV). According to their mechanism of action, they are classified in to several categories:

- virucides (membrane disruptive agents),
- entry/fusion inhibitors,
- reverse transcriptase and integrase inhibitors, and
- dendritic cell uptake inhibitors (Nuttall et al. 2007).

Microbicides can exhibit different mechanisms of action, which require different drug targeting strategies to achieve successful delivery. Therefore, the mechanism of action of each microbicide agent will define the suitable vaginal delivery system for that product. If a microbicide substance acts by blocking the receptor or co-receptor target host cells (macrophages, T cells, dendritic cells), it is essential that the delivery system is able to deliver the drug to the site of action. Conversely, a microbicide agent that disrupts the viral membrane before the attachment of the virus to the host cell, can be delivered to the vaginal lumen without its deeper penetration into vaginal mucosa (Rohan and Sassi 2009).

An ideal vaginal microbicide should assure the following relevant and desirable features:

- safety (escaping the local and systemic toxicity, irritation of vaginal epithelium as well as fertility/fetal abnormalities, preferably during prolonged period of time),
- efficacy (prevention of HIV transmission),
- rapid and long lasting action,
- acceptability and easy placement (avoidance of leakage immediately after administration),
- simple dosage regiment (prolonged release systems are preferred),
- compatibility with male latex condom,
- low potential for resistance development,

- stability (shelf-life), and
- low-cost.

Additional desirable characteristics of microbicide products are that they should be colorless, odorless and undetectable by sexual partners (Antimisiaris and Mourtas 2015, Omar and Bergeron 2011).

A variety of vaginal dosage forms have been evaluated for microbicide delivery such as films, tablets, rings, electrospun fibers, as well as diversity of nanopharmaceuticals (Rohan et al. 2014). Almost 50% of all microbicide clinical trials included gel formulations (Agashe et al. 2012).

Surfactants/detergents (non-specific antiretroviral agents) were among the first compounds clinically tested as topical microbicides. Nonoxynol 9 was the first microbicide agent in hydrogel formulation (COL-1492) that was evaluated for the prevention of HIV transmission. Although it showed anti-HIV activity *in vitro*, the clinical results were disappointing. In the randomised, placebo-controlled trial performed on 892 female sex workers in four countries, 16% of females receiving nonoxynol 9 gel (52.5 mg nonoxynol 9) were infected by HIV, compared to 27% in placebo users. Moreover, an association between nonoxynol 9 and increased HIV seroincidence have been found when COL-1492 was used more than three times per day. Administration of nonoxynol-9 also had no significant effects on *N. gonorrhoeae* or *C. trachomatis* infections, which were considered as second endpoints of the clinical trial. Toxicity to vaginal mucosal tissue (genital ulcers) at the higher doses of nonoxynol 9 was proposed as a possible cause of increased HIV transmission among frequent users. These undesirable results ended the development of nonoxynol 9 as an anti-HIV microbicide. The experience with nonoxynol 9 also led to a greater scrutiny of the safety studies before the commencement of larger clinical trials (Van Damme et al. 2002).

Savvy® gel (C31G, Cellegy Pharmaceuticals, Quakertown, USA) is another surfactant-based microbicide product comprising cetyl betaine and myristamine oxide as active agents. It has proven *in vitro* safety and broad-spectrum activity against bacteria and viruses, including *C. trachomatis*, HSV, and especially HIV. In a Phase III placebo-controlled trial in Ghana, the effectiveness of 1% C31G microbicide hydrogel in preventing male-to-female vaginal transmission of HIV infection has been assessed on 2142 HIV-negative women. Main outcome measures were the incidence of HIV-1 and HIV-2 infections determined by detection of HIV antibodies from oral mucosal transudate specimens and adverse events. The obtained data showed no clinically significant differences in the overall frequency of adverse events, abnormal pelvic examination findings, or abnormal laboratory results between treatment groups (SAVVY® gel and placebo gel). More participants in the SAVVY group reported reproductive tract adverse events than in the placebo group (13.0% versus 9.4%, respectively). Seventeen HIV seroconversions occurred, eight in participants randomized to SAVVY and nine among participants receiving placebo. The cumulative probability of HIV infection through 12 months were 0.010 in the SAVVY group and 0.011 in the placebo group (p = 0.731), with a hazard ratio (SAVVY versus placebo) of 0.88 (95% confidence interval 0.33, 2.27). Due to a lower-than-expected HIV incidence, the required number of HIV patients (66) to obtain the desired study power was not reached (Peterson et al. 2007).

Sodium lauryl sulfate (SLS, Invisible Condom®, Universite Laval, Quebec, Canada), a surfactant-based microbicide compound, was formulated as buffered thermoreversible gel composed of 30% (w/w) poloxamer and containing 2.5% of the active agent. The formulation has been shown to be safe for rabbits following once-daily intravaginal administration for 14 days without causing significant irritations of the genital mucosa (Roy et al. 2001). The extended safety of the SLS for humans has been evaluated in a randomized, placebo-controlled Phase II clinical study in 194 healthy sexually active women from Cameroon. Invisible Condom® gel was proven to be well tolerated with no reported serious adverse events when applied twice daily for 8 weeks. The majority of reported adverse events were mild or moderate and mostly similar in all three tested groups of women, except for pelvic pain that was 10% higher in the polymer and polymer/SLS groups in comparison to placebo. Colposcopy examinations have shown neither genital ulceration nor mucosal lesions (Mbopi-Keou et al. 2010).

The second broad class of non-specific microbicides represents the acidifying agents, also known as vaginal milieu protectors. They act to maintain, restore or enhance the natural protective mechanisms within the vaginal canal, i.e., the acidic pH maintained by lactobacilli. A pH between 4 and 5.8 has been demonstrated to inactivate HIV and exert spermicidal activity, too. Therefore, the microbicide compounds in this class operate either as direct acidifying agents or as enhancers of lactobacilli production (Cutler and Justman 2008). BufferGel® (ReProtect, Baltimore, USA) and Acidform® (Amphora, Instead Inc., Dallas, USA) are examples of acidifying microbicide hydrogels that have been clinically assessed for safety and effectiveness against male-to-female HIV transmission. BufferGel®, a Carbopol 974P-based gel with a pH of 3.9, was able to buffer twice its volume of semen to a pH of 5. It was well tolerated in women at low risk for acquisition of HIV, but not effective in the prevention of HIV-1 vaginal transmission in a Phase II/IIb trial (Abdool Karim et al. 2011). Although Acidform® (alginic acid and xantan gum based gel, pH 3.5) has been demonstrated to exhibit better acid-buffering capacity than BufferGel®, no clinical trials pertaining to the prevention of HIV transmission have been reported yet (Ferguson and Rohan 2011).

In addition to the above mentioned microbicides, non-specific microbicide candidates also include so called entry inhibitors, i.e., anionic polymers such as Carraguard® gel, cellulose sulfate gel, cellulose acetate phthalate gel and PRO2000® gel (Ferguson and Rohan 2011). These agents exhibit a negative surface charge, which results in a charge interaction with the viral envelope proteins, thus interfering with attachment of virus to CD4+ cells *in vitro*. Although both Carraguard® (carrageenan based gel) and cellulose sulfate gel were proven to be safe in clinical trials, they were ineffective to prevent male-to-female vaginal transmission of HIV, gonorrhea or chlamydial infection (Halpern et al. 2008, Skoler-Karpoff et al. 2008). Similarly, disappointing results were reported for cellulose phthalate and PRO2000® gels. The Phase I trial assessing the safety and acceptability of the cellulose phthalate gel was terminated early, due to complaints of wetness and leakage after vaginal application. Upon conducting further osmolarity and rheological assessments, it was found that the formulation was hyperosmolar in comparison to vaginal fluid and upon vaginal application became hypoviscous, resulting in unfavourable events experienced by users (Lacey et al. 2010). 0.5% PRO2000® gel containing 2-naphthalenesulfonic acid as microbicide was also confirmed safe and able to decrease the risk of HIV infection by 30% in a Phase IIb trial. However, further Phase III clinical trial showed its ineffectiveness in reducing the risk of male-to-female HIV transmission (McCormack et al. 2010).

Since most of the clinical trials on non-specific microbicides (first generation) failed to show either safety or efficacy for prevention of HIV transmission, further investigations were focused on microbicide candidates that directly and specifically act against the HIV life cycle. These specific antiretroviral products include reverse transcriptase inhibitors (RTIs) comprising nucleotide and non-nucleoside RTIs, respectively (Ferguson and Rohan 2011).

Tenofovir is the clinically most studied nucleotide RTI. It exerts activity by mimicking endogenous nucleotides and once it is incorporated into the proviral DNA, the chain cannot be further extended (Nuttall et al. 2007). In a Phase IIb trial the safety and effectiveness of 1% tenofovir hydroxyethylcellulose gel (pH 4.5) has been assessed for the prevention of male-to-female HIV transmission. An overall 39% reduction in HIV-1 acquisition was associated with tenofovir gel following the insertion of the gel 12 hours before and after vaginal intercourse. Among women with high gel adherence, the tenofovir gel reduced HIV infection by 54% in comparison to placebo gel. Moreover, the formulation was well accepted by women without any significant renal, hepatic, hematologic, pregnancy or genital adverse effects (Abdool Karim et al. 2010).

Many other antiretroviral agents are under development, mostly in the preclinical investigations and early stages of clinical studies. Diarylpyirimidine TMC120 was the first non-nucleoside RTI confirmed as effective vaginal microbicide *in vivo*. TMC120 gel composed of Carbopol 940 and hydroxyethylcellulose assured 100% protection of mice inoculated with CCR5-tropic or CCYCR4-tropic viral strains (Di Fabio et al. 2003). In a dose-ranging (25, 50, 150 µM TMC120) short-term Phase I study, performed on both HIV-negative and HIV-positive female volunteers, TMC120 gel was well-tolerated in all the tested concentrations and there were no apparent differences in the safety parameters. The gel leakage was reported by 96% of participants and was rated as moderate or severe by 75% of women in placebo group and by 78% of women using TMC120 gel (Jespers et al. 2007).

Dapivirine, a second non-nucleotide RTI, was initially developed as an anti-HIV drug for oral administration; however, due to its low absorption it was proposed to be applied as vaginal microbicide. Dapivirine was evaluated in a Phase I clinical trial for safety and pharmacokinetics, following once daily vaginal administration of two different gel formulations, both containing 0.05% dapivirine, but differing in the gel composition. One formulation was prepared with 3.5% hydroxyethylcellulose, while another one additionally contained 1% hydroxypropylcellulose and 0.1% poloxamer 407. The safety of both gels was assessed in 36 healthy HIV-negative women and compared with the placebo hydroxyethylcellulose-based gel. The gels were self-administered once daily for a total of 11 days. Both tested dapivirine gel formulations were safe and well tolerated with low systemic absorption and attained dapivirine concentrations in vaginal fluids that were over 3 logs greater than plasma levels. The gel leakage after insertion was a major complain reported by a greater percentage of placebo users (92%) than dapivirine gel users (67–83%) (Nel et al. 2010).

Thiocarboxanilide UC781 is another non-nucleoside RTI with poor oral bioavailability, proposed as topical vaginal microbicide due to its ability to block cell-free and cell-associated HIV-1 transmission in a human cervical tissue-based organ culture (Zussman et al. 2003). UC781 was incorporated in three different concentrations (0.1, 0.25 and 1%) into gel composed of Carbopol 974P NF and methylcellulose and evaluated clinically. In that initial study enrolling 47 healthy and sexually abstinent women, UC781 gel was well tolerated when applied once daily for 6 days (Schwartz et al. 2008). *Ex vivo* analysis of vaginal lavage samples, collected in a phase I safety trial, revealed that the majority of UC781 was found in an insoluble fraction but was still able to inhibit HIV infection. However, further development of UC781 has been halted due to difficulties with its solubility and stability (Haaland et al. 2012).

4.4 Hydrogels for the treatment of vaginal infections

Vaginitis is a common female disorder characterized by vulvovaginal itching, burning, malodor and abnormal discharge. The most frequent causes of vaginitis are infections including bacterial vaginosis, vulvovaginal candidiasis and trichomoniasis (Quan 2010). For the local treatment of bacterial vaginosis, the hypromellose-based hydrogel containing 0.75% (w/w) metronidazole, i.e., MetroGel® (3M Pharmaceuticals, St. Paul, USA) has been developed. Several clinical trials have confirmed its safety and efficacy comparable to oral metronidazole therapy (Wain 1998). In a study comparing oral metronidazole to metronidazole vaginal gel, a total of 112 women were enrolled and randomized to receive intravaginal therapy twice a day for 5 days or 500 mg of oral metronidazole twice daily for 7 days. The results have demonstrated that both local and oral metronidazole therapy were equally effective in curing bacterial vaginosis at both the first return visit (11–17 days after initiation of therapy) and the final visit (one month following therapy). At first return visit, 84% of intravaginally treated patients and 85% of orally treated patients were considered cured. At the final visit, bacterial vaginosis was eliminated in 70.7% of the intravaginal group and 71.1% of the oral group. Recurrence rates were also similar for the both treatment groups. Although there were no differences in the efficacy of both tested formulations, gastrointestinal complains were more pronounced in the patients receiving oral metronidazole, thus confirming superiority of the topical formulation (Hanson et al. 2000).

Many studies report on design of different types of hydrogels containing antimicrobials for the treatment of vaginal infections, particularly nano-sized delivery systems; however, to the best of our knowledge, except MetroGel®, there is no other vaginal hydrogel for the treatment of vaginal infections currently available in the market.

4.5 Cervical Ripening and Labour Induction Hydrogels

Vaginal gels with prostanglandins have been used for years as efficient labour inducers. Prostin E2® gel (Pfizer, Sandwich, Kent, UK) is a colloidal silicon dioxide vaginal gel in triacetin base containing 1 or 2 mg of dinoprostone (prostaglandin E2). In a retrospective analysis, Shetty et al. (2004) compared labour outcomes among 145 consecutive women with unfavourable cervices, who received prostaglandin E2 vaginal gel (1–2 mg) for labour induction and 149 women receiving prostaglandin E2 vaginal tablet (3 mg). The results have shown that cervical dilatation in the gel group was significantly more expressed than in the tablet group. There were no significant differences between the two tested groups in the mode of delivery, in the number delivering vaginally within 24 hours of the induction (60% in the gel group versus 56% in the tablet group), in the number of doses of prostaglandin E2 administered, or in the neonatal outcomes (Shetty et al. 2004). In another study, the efficacy and safety of intracervical prostaglandin E2 gel (dinoproston, Prepidil® gel, Upjohn, Kalamazoo, USA) has been evaluated and compared to intravaginal prostaglandin E2 pessary (Cervidil®, Forest Pharmaceuticals, St. Louis, USA). Ninety patients admitted for labour were randomized to receive either 0.5 mg prostaglandin E2 intracervical gel (Prepidil®) 2 doses every 6 hours or 10 mg prostaglandin E2 slow release vaginal pessary (Cervidil®). Preinduction cervical ripening with a slow release prostaglandin E2 vaginal pessary resulted in a greater change in Bishop score than with intracervical prostaglandin E2 gel. However, there was no statistically significant difference in percent delivered in less than 24 hours between the tested formulations (Ottinger et al. 1998).

In a randomized controlled trial involving 165 pregnant women in United Kingdom, the clinical efficacy of prostaglandin E2 gel (1–2 mg) has been compared with vaginal tablet (3 mg). Both formulations were administered at 6-hour interval until the cervix was suitable for amniotomy. Prostaglandin E2 vaginal gel was found to be superior to vaginal tablet since the mean induction interval to delivery was significantly shorter in women who received the gel (1400 min, versus 1780 min for the vaginal tablet, respectively). In addition, the rate of failed induction of labour was significantly higher in women who received tablets (10%), versus gel (1%) (Taher et al. 2011).

Misoprostol, a synthetic prostanglandine E1 analog, is also used for cervical ripening and labour induction. The efficacy of misoprostol vaginal gel has been evaluated in a prospective clinical trial on 100 primigravidas at 40–42 weeks of gestation. Patients were randomized to receive 50 µg of misoprostol (every 6 h, up to 24 h), either in the form of vaginal tablet (Cytotec®, Pharmacia, Walton-on-the-Hill, UK) or extemporaneous vaginal gel prepared by incorporation of misoprostol tablet dispersion into K-Y Jelly® (Johnson & Johnson Co., New Jersey, USA). The results demonstrated that the mean interval in hours from the drug administration to the start of contractions was lower in the gel group; however, the induction to delivery interval was significantly lower in the tablet group. Although both formulations were similarly effective in inducing labour, the gel form of the drug was slower in inducing delivery, possibly a consequence of the lower doses of misoprostol administrated since the small portion of the gel was retained in the syringe after the application (Sherif and Moety 2013).

Table 1 summarizes marketed products as well as products in clinical studies.

Table 1. Examples of some currently available vaginal gels and those in clinical testing.

Use/category	Gelling agent/polymer	Product(s)	Active compound(s)	Status	Reference
Moisturizers	Polycarbophil, Carbopol 934P NF	*Replens®*	-	Market	Edwards and Panay, 2016;
	Poly(acrylic) acid, pectin, methylcellulose, xanthan gum	*Summer's Eve®*	-	Market	Caswell and Kane, 2002
	Carbomer	*Hyalofemme®*	hyaluronic acid	Market	Chen et al., 2013
	Hydroxyethylcellulose	*Emerita®*	*Aloe barbadensis* leaf juice, *Chamomile matricaria*, *Calendula officinalis* and *Panax ginseng* root extracts	Market	Tan et al., 2012
	Hydroxyethylcellulose, xantan gum	*Monurelle Biogel®*	Bovine colostrum (lyophilized)	Market	Nappi et al., 2016
Moisturizer and lubricant	Polycarbophil, Carbomer	*RepHresh®*	-	Market	Sinha and Ewies, 2013
	Guar gum, locust bean gum	*Yes®*	*Linum usitatissimum* flax extract, *Aloe barbadensis juice*	Market	Tan et al., 2012
Lubricants	Methylcellulose, carboxymethyl cellulose	*K-Y Jelly®*, *Liquid Sylk®*, *Aquagel®*, *Astroglide®*, Slippery Stuff®	-	Market	Sinha and Ewies, 2013; Edwards and Panay, 2016

Table 1 contd. ...

...*Table 2 contd.*

Use/category	Gelling agent/polymer	Product(s)	Active compound(s)	Status	Reference
Restoration of vaginal pH, prevention of infections	Polycarbophil Carbopol 934P NF	*Replens®*	-	Market	Edwards and Panay, 2016
	Polycarbophil, Carbopol 974P NF	*Aci-Jel Balance®*	Glacial acetic acid, hydroxyquinoline sulphate, ricinoleic acid	Market	Aci-Jel, 2016
Microbicides: surfactant-type	Hydroxyethylcellulose	*Savvy® gel*	Cetyl betaine, myristamine oxide	Phase III, interrupted	Peterson et al., 2007
	Poloxamer	*Invisible Condom®*	Sodium lauryl sulfate	Phase II	Mbopi-Keou et al., 2010
	Sodium carboxymethylcellulose	COL-1492	Nonoxynol-9	Phase II/III, interrupted	Van Damme et al., 2002
Microbicides: acidifying agents-type	Carbopol 974P	*BufferGel®*	Slightly acidic pH of the gel (pH =3.9)	Phase II/IIb	Abdool Karim et al., 2011
Microbicides: entry inhibitors	Carrageenan	*Carraguard®*	-	Interrupted	Skoler-Karpoff et al., 2008
	Cellulose sulfate	*Ushercell®*	-	Phase III, interrupted	Halpern et al., 2008
	Carbomer	*PRO2000®*	2-naphthalenesulfonic acid	Phase III	McCormack et al., 2010
	BufferGel® Carbopol 971P NF	*VivaGel®*	SPL7013 dendrimer	Phase I	O'Loughlin et al., 2010

Microbicides: nucleotide RTIs	Hydroxyethylcellulose	*1% tenofovir gel*	Tenofovir	Phase IIb	Abdool Karim et al., 2010
	Carbopol 940, hydroxyethylcellulose	*TMC120*	Diarylpyirimidine	Phase I	Jespers et al., 2007
Microbicides: non-nucleotide RTIs	Hydroxyethylcellulose, poloxamer 407	*0.05% dapivirine gel*	Dapivirin	Phase I	Nel et al., 2010
	Carbopol 974P NF, methylcellulose	*UC781*	Thiocarboxanilide	Phase I, interrupted	Haaland et al., 2012
Bacterial vaginosis therapy	Hypromellose	*MetroGel®*	Metronidazole	Market	Wain, 1998
	BufferGel® Carbopol 971P NF	*VivaGel®*	SPL7013 dendrimer	Phase III	Starpharma, 2016
Labor inducer	Colloidal silicon dioxide	*Prostin E2®*	Dinoprostone	Market	das Neves and Bahia, 2006

RTIs, reverse nucleotide inhibitors

5. Nanosystems-in-hydrogel Formulations

The hydrophilic nature of gels restricts incorporation of lipophilic drugs, thus limiting vaginal administration of numerous hydrophobic substances with potential to be applied vaginally for achieving either local or systemic effects. Estrogen, progesterone, diversity of antimicrobials (antivirals, antibiotics, antifungals), biologics, plant medicines, etc. are potentially interesting drugs which cannot directly be prepared in the form of hydrogels. This obstacle can be overcome by increasing the solubility of the drug (active substance) by different chemical and technological approaches including the production of more soluble drug forms (salts, insertion of hydrophilic groups, prodrugs), addition of co-solvents, amorphization, complexation, and encapsulation into different nano-sized delivery systems (nanosystems).

Vaginal drug delivery nanosystems have attracted considerable attention during the last two decades due to their abilities to encapsulate/incorporate a variety of drugs/substances acting on their solubility, stability, modulating their pharmacokinetics and improving bioavailability (Vanić and Škalko-Basnet 2014, Vanić and Škalko-Basnet 2013). Nano-sized drug delivery systems are often referred to as nanomedicines or nanopharmaceuticals (Duncan and Gaspar 2011); mostly, they are delivery systems with size ranges well below 1 μm. Nanomedicines have been proven to increase the biocompatibility and safety profiles of encapsulated/incorporated drug. Their targeting facility as well as ability to prolong and control the release of entrapped drug often results in a decrease of the dose and dosing frequency while assuring the desired therapeutic effect (Vanić and Škalko-Basnet 2013).

Various nanomedicines have been proposed for vaginal delivery of drugs including dendrimers, polymeric and lipid nanoparticles, nanofibers, liposomes, niosomes and microemulsions. Numerous investigations have proven that physico-chemical properties of nanopharmaceuticals, such as their size and surface properties play a crucial role in delivery of drug into/through the mucus (Vanić and Škalko-Basnet 2013). However, majority of nanosystems are generally liquid dispersions, which might hinder their vaginal administration due to leakage from the site of application. Therefore, their surface properties are often modified by the coating with mucoadhesive polymers to increase their retention on the vaginal mucosa or are embedded into semisolid vehicles such as gel-like bases to obtain appropriate viscosity for vaginal administration.

5.1 Liposomes-in-hydrogel

Liposomes are nanovesicles consisting of one or more phospholipid bilayer(s) enclosing inner aqueous compartments. Such a structure facilitates encapsulation/incorporation of a variety of drugs differing in physicochemical properties, i.e., lipophilic, hydrophilic and amphiphilic. Since the phospholipids are biodegradable, non-immunogenic and non-toxic, liposomes are generally recognized as physiologically acceptable nanomedicines. Although they have been explored as drug carriers for more than four decades and have the longest history in clinical use, their investigations in vaginal route of drug administration started relatively late, at the end of 1990s. In the first report on vaginal application of liposomes, progesterone liposomes were incorporated into 1% polyacrylamide gel. The progestational activity of liposomal gel was assessed by monitoring the effect on the formation of *corpora lutea*. It was demonstrated that both the liposomal and control gel (free drug in the gel) inhibited formation of corpora lutea; however, the effect of liposomal gel was found to be greater and prolonged than the control gel (Jain et al. 1997).

Liposomes-in-gel are commonly prepared with poly(acrylic) acid polymers, particularly Carbopol® 974P. Incorporation of liposomes into Carbopol gel has been proven to:

- provide the required viscosity and mucoadhesiveness of formulation,
- extend the release of the encapsulated/incorporated drug,
- protect the liposomes from acidic pH and vaginal environment, and
- preserve the original size of liposomes that is of particular interest, considering the storage stability of liposomal formulations.

Our groups have a long experience of working with Carbopol-based liposomal gels for vaginal drug delivery. Incorporation of calcein or FITC-dextrans (Mw 4.400 and 21.200) liposomes into 1% Carbopol® 974P NF gel has been shown to significantly extend the release of this hydrophilic marker as compared to control gel. This effect was found to be proportional to the molecular weight of the liposomally encapsulated marker. The slowest release was achieved for FITC-dextran Mw 21 200, while the highest amount of released marker was achieved with calcein (Mw 622.53) (Pavelić et al. 2001, Pavelić et al. 2004b). To determine the possible mechanisms of the release of the encapsulated marker (drug) from the liposomes-in-gel formulations, we have established the so-called agarose method (Fig. 2), modifying the *in vitro* model used to study the release kinetics of liposomally encapsulated material (Peschka et al. 1998). The appropriate mass of liposomes was placed on the bottom of the glass vials and covered with 2% (w/w) agarose solution to form a thin layer of inert matrix, separating the investigated gel from the receptor solution. The porosity of the agarose matrix allowed diffusion of the leaked marker/drug from liposomes inside the gel and additionally, the release of intact liposomes from the gel, which is not possible by conventional Franz-diffusion cell method (Pavelić et al. 2001, Pavelić et al. 2004b). As shown in Fig. 2, the release of the marker/drug

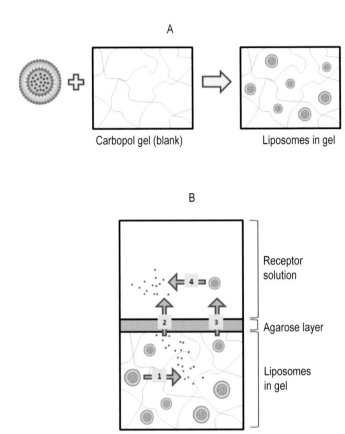

Fig. 2. Incorporation of liposomes containing a hydrophilic marker (drug) into Carbopol gel (A) and possible mechanisms of marker (drug) release (B). 1 – Leakage of the marker from liposomes inside the gel, 2 – diffusion of the marker through the agarose layer to the receptor compartment, 3 – diffusion of intact liposomes from the gel to the receptor compartment, 4 – release of the marker from liposomes inside the receptor compartment. Reprinted with permission from Vanić, Ž. and N. Škalko-Basnet. 2013. Eur. J. Pharm. Sci. 50: 29–41. Copyright@ Elsevier.

from liposomal gel comprises several interconnected mechanisms. Several studies confirmed the second pathway, i.e., diffusion of the released marker from the gel into receiver compartment, as the most dominant mechanism (Pavelić et al. 2005a, Pavelić et al. 2004a, 2005b, Vanić et al. 2014).

Due to the acidic pH, presence of proteins, enzymes and microorganisms, vaginal fluid can reduce the stability of liposomes. In this context, Carbopol gels have proven to preserve the incorporated liposomes from the unfavourable environment. Investigation of the *in vitro* stability of clotrimazole and metronidazole in conventional liposomes in the presence of vaginal fluid stimulant (pH 4.5) has shown that 57% of the originally entrapped clotrimazole or 63% of metronidazole were leaked from the liposomes after 24 hours. When the liposomes were incorporated into Carbopol 974P NF gel, the amount of the released drug was significantly reduced (33% clotrimazole, 42% metronidazole) (Pavelić et al. 2005b).

Physicochemical properties such as size, surface charge and rigidity/ elasticity of the liposome bilayers were shown to affect stability of liposomes in the vaginal fluid. In a study evaluating the stability of different surface-charged conventional liposomes with acyclovir incorporated into Carbopol gels for the treatment of genital herpes, the highest stability has been observed with positively charged vesicles (Fig. 3). This effect was a consequence of the liposome interaction with the negatively charged mucin contributing to better retention of the drug inside the vesicles (Pavelić et al. 2005a). In the case of hydrogels embedding clotrimazole or metronidazole liposomes of more elastic bilayers, increased penetration of the intact liposomes has been obtained, while the overall *in vitro* stability of liposomes in simulated vaginal conditions decreased in comparison to the corresponding conventional liposomes (Vanić et al. 2014).

This effect was a consequence of the liposome interaction with the negatively charged mucin contributing to better retention of the drug inside the vesicles (Pavelić et al. 2005a). In the case of hydrogels embedding clotrimazole- or metronidazole-containing liposomes build of more elastic bilayers, an increased penetration of the intact liposomes has been obtained, while the overall *in vitro* stability of liposomes in the simulated vaginal conditions was decreased in comparison to the corresponding conventional liposomes (Vanić et al. 2014).

In addition to improving the stability of liposomes within vaginal environment, Carbopol gels have also shown to contribute to the physical stability of liposomes. In a study investigating changes of liposomal size during the storage of acyclovir-in-liposomes-in-gel at 20 and 40°C, no significant increase in the original size distributions of liposomes has been observed during 4 weeks of storage (Pavelić et al. 2005a).

The changes in the lipid concentration and surface charge of the liposomes can affect the rheology of the gels serving as a vehicle for liposomes. While the incorporation of positively charged or sterically stabilized liposomes at lower lipid concentrations had no influence on the rheological properties of liposomal Carbopol gels, the gel viscosity significantly increased in the presence of positively charged liposomes at a 5-fold higher lipid concentration (Boulmedarat et al. 2003). In another study, the effect of liposome membrane rigidity and lipid concentration on the rheological changes of the gel was explored. While the incorporation of conventional phosphatidylcholine liposomes exhibited minimal effect on the rheological properties of Carbopol-hydroxyethyl cellulose hydrogel (even at the highest lipid concentration used), the addition of liposomes

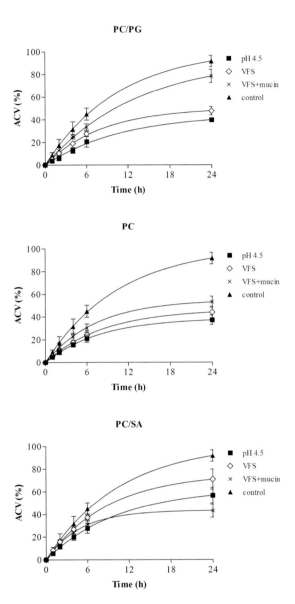

Fig. 3. *In vitro* release of negatively charged (PC/PG), neutral (PC) and positively charged (PC/SA) acyclovir (ACV) liposomes incorporated into Carbopol® 974P NF gel in different media simulating vaginal conditions: buffer, pH 4.5, vaginal fluid simulant (VFS) pH 4.5 with or without addition of mucin. Control represents the release of the solution of the free drug incorporated in the gel base in the concentration equivalent to the liposomally encapsulated drug. The values denote the average of three preparations ± S.D. PC, phosphatidylcholine; PG, phosphatidylglycerol; SA, stearylamine. Reprinted with permission from Pavelić, Ž., N. Škalko-Basnet, J. Filipović-Grčić, A. Martinac and I. Jalšenjak. 2005. J. Control. Release. 103: 34–43. Copyright@Elsevier.

with rigid (hydrogenated-phosphatidylcholine liposomes) or highly rigid (hydrogenated phosphatidylcholine/cholesterol) membranes caused significant changes in the rheological characteristics. These changes were proportional to the lipid concentration inside the gel (Mourtas et al. 2008). On the contrary, the elastic liposomes-in-Carbopol gels formulations demonstrated that membrane elasticity of liposomes had no significant effect on the rheological profiles of liposomal hydrogels. The visocosity profiles of liposomal gels containing the same concentration of lecithin, but differing in the ratio of sodium deoxycholate and propylene glycol (responsible for liposome membrane elasticity), were almost the same. Significant decrease in the viscosity was observed in simulated *in vivo* conditions, when the gels were mixed with vaginal fluid stimulant and the measurements were performed at body temperature. However, these changes were not influenced by the lipid composition as the same trend was seen also for conventional liposomes-in-gels (Vanić et al. 2014).

In addition to rheological assessments, texture analysis is another valuable technique for assessment of the mechanical properties of liposomal vaginal gels. The parameters such as the cohesiveness, hardness and adhesiveness are usually determined. Cohesiveness denotes the ability of formulation's removal from the container, while hardness relates to its easiness of administration to the application site (Hurler et al. 2012). A suitable adhesiveness of the formulation is of high importance for desired prolonged retention at the vaginal site. These three essential hydrogel features were determined and compared for both the elastic and the conventional liposomes-in-Carbopol gels, entrapping either metronidazole or clotrimazole. As shown in Fig. 4, incorporation of metronidazole- or clotrimazole-containing elastic liposomes into the hydrogel lowered the initial cohesiveness (empty hydrogel) by approximately 10% for both entrapped drugs. However, the mixing of a solution of the free drug (control gel) influenced the change in the original texture of the Carbopol hydrogel to a greater extent. Similar relationships between liposomal, control, and empty hydrogels were observed for adhesiveness and hardness (Fig. 4). The incorporation of liposomes in Carbopol hydrogels preserves the original texture of the hydrogels more than the incorporation of the drug solutions (Vanić et al. 2014).

In addition to mucoadhesive Carbopol gels, poloxamer 407 and 188-based thermo-sensitive gel were also evaluated as a vehicle for vaginal delivery of amphotericin B liposomes. Encapsulation into cationic liposomes increased the solubility of the poorly-water soluble amphotericin B, while the gel vehicle significantly sustained the drug release, increased the liposome stability and reduced the toxicity in comparison to liposomal dispersion and the control gel (Kang et al. 2010).

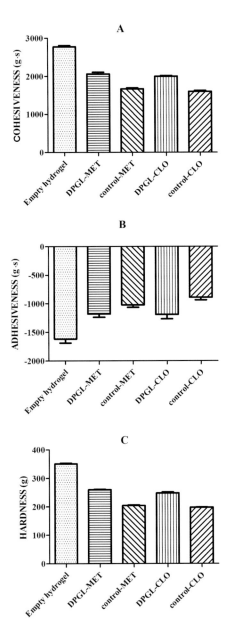

Fig. 4. The influence of deformable propylene glycol liposomes (DPGLs) on the texture properties of Carbopol® 974P NF hydrogels: cohesiveness (A), adhesiveness (B) and hardness (C). DPGL-MET and DPGL-CLO denote gel incorporating DPGLs with metronidazole (MET) or clotrimazole (CLO). Control-CLO and control-MET were hydrogels containing the solutions of free CLO or MET instead of liposomes. The values indicate the mean ± S.D (n = 5). Reprinted with permission from Vanić, Ž., J. Hurler, K. Ferdeber, P. Golja Gašparović, N. Škalko-Basnet and J. Filipović-Grčić. 2014. J. Liposome Res. 24: 27–36. Copyright@Taylor & Francis.

An interesting approach to design liposomal vaginal gels has been proposed by Li and coworkers (2012). They designed post-expansible hydroxylethyl cellulose hydrogel foam (aerosol), incorporating elastic propylene glycol liposomes containing matrine, a natural compound aimed for the treatment of vaginal/cervical inflammations. Elastic liposomes have enhanced the permeability of matrine through the vaginal mucosa, while the hydrogel foam assured the uniform and complete spreading of the liposomes inside the vaginal cavity. As a result, higher local concentrations were obtained and the residence time at the site of administration was prolonged (Li et al. 2012). Another innovative vaginal formulation, pH and temperature dual-sensitive liposome gel based on the cleavable methoxy polyethylene glycol 2000-hydrazone-cholesteryl hemisuccinate polymer inside pH-sensitive liposomes has been developed. pH-sensitive liposomes, containing natural origin compound arctigenin, possessing anti-oxidative, antitumour, anti-HIV, and anti-inflammatory activities, were designed to form a gel at body temperature and to degrade at slightly acidic vaginal conditions (pH 5), releasing the entrapped active compound. Arctigenin, encapsulated in a dual-sensitive liposome gel, was found to be more stable and less toxic than arctigenin loaded into pH-sensitive liposomes (Chen et al. 2012).

5.2 Niosomes-in-hydrogel

Niosomes are vesicular nanosystems, structurally very similar to liposomes, which, instead of phospholipids bilayers, comprise nonionic surfactants. They are characterized by better chemical stability and lower cost of membrane building constituents than liposomes. On the other hand, physiological acceptability is commonly superior with liposomes (Vanić et al. 2015).

Ning and collaborators compared the efficacy of both liposomal and niosomal gels with clotrimazole for the topical treatment of vulvovaginal candidiasis. Carbopol® 934 gel (2%, w/w) was used as a vehicle for incorporation of niosomes/liposomes. The formulations were evaluated for the drug release in vaginal fluid stimulant, storage stability, antifungal activity, and tolerability on the vaginal tissues. Both formulations were stable during one month storage at 4°C and provided extended release of clotrimazole, thus allowing reduced dosing interval. *In vivo* antifungicidal efficacy studies showed enhanced anti-Candida activities of both tested formulations in comparison to the standard ointment, the superiority atributed to the higher drug retention of liposomal/niosomal gels on vaginal mucosa. In addition, both vesicular gels were found to be safe for vaginal delivery; no morphological changes of the vaginal tissue at 24 hours post-dose were detected (Ning et al. 2005).

A thermo-sensitive gel composed of chitosan and ß-glycerophosphate has been investigated as a vehicle for incorporation of metformin hydrochloride loaded in unmodified and cationic niosomes for the vaginal treatment of polycystic ovary syndrome. The results of *in vitro* and *in vivo* studies indicate that both tested niosomal gel formulations were superior over oral administration of metformin hydrochloride solution at lower dose and dosage regimen and with less side effects (Saini et al. 2016).

5.3 *Lipid or polymeric nanoparticles-in-hydrogel*

These nanomedicines are particulate-based colloidal dispersions of lipid or polymer origin enabling incorporation, encapsulation or association of various types of drugs into nanoparticle's matrix. The nanosystems are characterized by a relatively high drug loading efficiency, ability to modify the surface properties, protection of drug from degradation, sustained drug release and long shelf life. A majority of the literature on the vaginal administration of either polymeric or lipid nanoparticles reports the use of the nanosystmes as such or incorporated into solid vehicles. There are several reports on the use of nanoparticles-in-hydrogel formulations in vaginal therapy.

Date and collaborators (2012) demonstrated the potential of antiretroviral nanoparticles-embedded into thermo-sensitve gel for long-term vaginal pre-exposure prophylaxis of HIV-1 transmission. Two microbicide agents, raltegravir and efavirenz, were loaded into poly(lactic-co-glycolic acid) (PLGA) nanoparticles and homogenously distributed into gel prepared using a combination of Pluronic F127 (20% w/v) and Pluronic F68 (1% w/v) to achieve gelation at 32.5°C. The nanoparticles were tested for inhibition of HIV-1NL4-3, whereby the obtained EC90 was lower than control microbicides solution. Rapid transfer of the nanoparticles from the gel and uptake in HeLa cells was achieved within 30 minutes. Compared to control untreated HeLa cells, the microbicides-loaded nanoparticles as well as the blank gel were not cytotoxic for 14 days (Date et al. 2012).

For the local treatment of genital herpes, Ramyadevi et al. (2016) have proposed *in situ* gelling system incorporating polyvinyl pyrrolidone-Eudragit RSPO nanoparticles containing poorly water-soluble acyclovir. Positively charged hybrid nanoparticles (approx. 100 nm-sized), embedded into 15% Pluronic F-127 gel, exhibited improved permeability through the animal vaginal mucosa. The formulation was evaluated *in vivo* in rat model for drug bioavailability and biodistribution. Following intravaginal application, acyclovir nanoparticles-in-gel maintained an average therapeutic drug level of 0.6 µg/ml in plasma for 24 hours. Significant improvement in the mean residence time of the drug was observed with a 2-fold increase in the relative bioavailability compared to that of the free drug. The tissue distribution was 2–3 folds higher in animals treated with nanoparticles-in-gel formulation compared to that of the free drug. Prolonged release of acyclovir *in vivo* was confirmed, allowing reduced frequency of the formulation administration (Ramyadevi et al. 2016).

Clotrimazole-loaded nanostructured lipid carriers embedded into thermo-sensitive and mucoadhesive gel, based on pluronic P407, were assessed for the topical treatment of vulvovaginal candidiasis. *Ex vivo* permeation studies on pig vaginal mucosa demonstrated localized effect and a low toxicity profile (HeLa cells), resulting in a cell vitality of 77% (24 hours). Interestingly, this innovative clotrimazole formulation showed 4-fold higher activity against *Candida albicans* than Fungizone® (standard topical therapy). The hydrogel as a vehicle acted as a barrier between clotrimazole and the cells, reducing the toxicity of the drug. In addition, it restricted the diffusion of clotrimazole through vaginal mucosa, and allowed a higher and intimate interaction between *Candida albicans* and the clotrimazole loaded lipid nanoparticles (Ravani et al. 2013).

5.4 Dendrimers-in-gel

Dendrimers are highly branched, star-shaped polymeric macromolecules with nanometer-scale dimensions. They consist of three components: a central core, an interior dendritic structure (the branches), and an exterior surface with functional surface groups. The unique properties of dendrimers such as uniform size, high degree of branching, water solubility, multivalency, well-defined molecular weight and available internal cavities make them attractive for drug delivery applications (Nanjwade et al. 2009).

Investigations of dendrimers for vaginal delivery are commonly focused on the prevention and treatment of infectious diseases. Currently, the most promising dendrimer is SPL7013, developed by Starpharma (Melbourne, Australia) with a specifically designed polyanionic surface (Rupp et al. 2007). Structurally, SPL7013 consists of divalent benzhydrilamine core and four generations of lysisne branches (Tyssen et al. 2010). The highly charged surface allows SPL7013 to attach to targets on viruses, blocking viral attachment and/or adsorption to cells, thereby preventing infection. In the case of HIV, SPL7013 is thought to bind gp120 proteins on the surface of the virus, through which the virus normally attaches to CD4 receptors on human cells (Rupp et al. 2007). SPL7013 is the active product in the candidate microbicide - VivaGel®, a hydrogel-based formulation containing 3% (w/w) SPL7013 in BufferGel®, and Carbopol® 971P NF-based acidic buffering gel. Among different nanomedicines for vaginal drug delivery, VivaGel® is currently the most promising nanotechnology-based formulation. A phase I clinical trial involving 37 healthy women evaluated safety of VivaGel® preparations containing SPL7013 (0.5%–3.0%

w/w) in comparison to the placebo gel. Women received either VivaGel®️ or placebo once daily intravaginally for 7 days. The results demonstrated that all SPL7013 concentrations of VivaGel®️ were safe and well tolerated as placebo (O'Loughlin et al. 2010). VivaGel®️ has also shown anti-HSV activity (Price et al. 2011) as well as antibacterial potential, and is currently evaluated in a Phase III clinical trial for the treatment and prevention of recurrent bacterial vaginosis.

In situ forming, biodegradable, dendrimer-based hydrogel for sustained release of amoxicillin has been reported by Navath et al. (2011). A poly(amido amine) (PAMAM)-based dendrimer, crosslinked with 8-arm polyethylene glycol (PEG) bearing thiol terminations, was evaluated *in vitro* and *in vivo* in a pregnant guinea pig model. The release of the drug was sustained for 240 h as compared to control gel, while the histological evaluation of the cervical tissues confirmed tolerability of the formulation. The *in vivo* results showed that the gel sufficiently covered the cervicovaginal region with a residence time of at least 72 hours. The gel was primarily retained in the maternal tissues without crossing the fetal membranes into the fetus. Moreover, the formulation was found to be stable for up to three days, followed by *in vivo* biodegradation. It should also be noted that the pH of the vagina was not altered upon application of the gel, and none of the animals aborted up to 72 hours after the formulation administration (Navath et al. 2011).

5.5 Gel-microemulsions

Microemulsions are isotropically clear dispersions of water and oil stabilized by an interfacial film of surfactant and cosurfactant, with a droplet size of typically less than 100 nm. They are characterized by high solubilizing capacity and long-term stability in comparison to conventional emulsions (Tenjarla 1999). To improve the viscosity of microemulsions for topical drug delivery, gel-microemulsions have been designed by addition of gelling agents (mucoadhesive polysaccharides, carrageenan, or xanthan gum) into the microemulsion.

Bachhav and Patarvale (2009) have designed microemulsion based gel for the vaginal delivery of fluconazole. Different polymers like sodium alginate, hydroxypropyl methylcellulose and Carbopol®️ ETD 2020 were examined for their ability to gel the microemulsion; Carbopol®️ ETD 2020 was shown to be the most promising as it effectively gelled the microemulsion without disturbing its structure. The appropriate bioadhesiveness of the formulation has been confirmed *in vitro* as well as higher anti-fungal activity as compared to that of the marketed clotrimazole formulation. Tolerability studies on a rabbit model proved the safety of the fluconazole gel-microemulsion for vaginal mucosa (Bachhav and Patravale 2009).

6. Limitations, Safety and Toxicity of Hydrogels in Vaginal Therapy

Disappointing outcomes for some of the clinical trials led to a strong focus on a better understanding of the parameters that may diminish the effectiveness of potential microbicides in drug development. For example, failure of nonoxynol-9 and cellulose sulfate gels in prophylaxis of HIV infections in Phase III microbicide effectiveness trials was, most likely, caused by a disruption of the protective genital epithelial barrier and enhanced viral replication upon repeated vaginal use (Omar and Bergeron 2011). Furthermore, for PRO2000® gel, the presence of seminal plasma was proven to diminish the efficacy of the microbicide (Patel et al. 2007). It should be noted that the adherence problems (not applying the formulation before each vaginal intercourse) in some of the Phase III trials also attributed to negative outcomes. For example, in the clinical trial with Carraguard® gel, only about 42% of enrolled women adhered to the treatment regimen (Skoler-Karpoff et al. 2008).

Vaginal gels are often associated with a messy feeling and leakage from vagina, which intensifies the non-adherence problems and may affect the bioavailability of tested formulations.

The effectiveness of the microbicide product is also influenced by the type of the applicator used for the delivery of the formulation to the site of action. Conventional applicators contain one apical hole to deliver the product to the cervix region and posterior fornix, leaving the large surface of the vaginal mucosa exposed to infection. Such design of an applicator also allows the topical microbicide product to remain in the upper vagina and cervix for more than 24 hours, resulting in the product accumulation at a specific site and possible cervical/vaginal toxicity. This may lead to inflammation and response by host defense, resulting in an increased risk of acquiring HIV, either by increasing the susceptibility to infection or by decreasing the innate protective immune response (Omar and Bergeron 2011). However, the applicators with multiple apical and lateral holes (designed for the Invisible Condom® gel) allow immediate uniform distribution of the microbicide formulation to cover the vagina, cervix and posterior fornix, thus offering the formulation to retain within the vaginal vault for 4–8 hours. This time-period following active sex offers a protection during and after sexual intercourse without the risk of prolonged accumulation (Omar et al. 2008).

In addition to the above discussed factors, the risk for potential toxicity of the microbicide product remains to be addressed. One approach in handling the toxicity could be to allow slower release and delivery of the microbicide agent. Interestingly, none of the hydrogels that failed in the Phase III clinical trials, except Invisible Condom®, exhibited a slow drug release profile. Therefore, novel strategies based on the development of nanosized delivery systems offer great potential in safe and effective microbicide delivery.

Recent reports indicate that the vaginal epithelium can secrete immune mediators able to enhance susceptibility to sexually transmitted infections upon repeated exposure to vaginal products. An additional challenge is that the animal data are often not directly correlated to human data and fail to provide a straight-forward conclusion prior to clinical testing (Cummins and Doncel 2009).

Of particular interest should be the treatment in pregnant patients, which is unfortunately often a neglected issue. Any drug therapy administered during pregnancy represents a challenge.

Currently, topical intravaginal antimicrobial agents are prescribed to treat ascending genital infections in pregnant women. However, the efficacy and prevention of recurrence associated with these therapies remains to be addressed and studied to a much greater extent (Vanić and Škalko-Basnet 2013).

7. Perspectives

Vaginal drug therapy offers much more of the therapeutic options than the current market situation indicates. However, due to unique features of vaginal tract, this therapy remains a challenging treatment modality. To fulfill the real potential of hydrogels, either as hydrogel formulations or as nanosystem-in-hydrogel formulations, the interplay between the system's features and vaginal environment requires further extensive attention. The urgent need to address sexually transmitted diseases in a more efficient manner opens up opportunity for multidisciplinary approaches in the design and development of advanced functional formulations. Understanding the mechanisms behind the interaction between vaginal environment and novel drug delivery systems should enable closer control over the optimization of delivery systems and devices destined for administration at vaginal site. Developments in polymer chemistry and nanotechnology should enable successful vaginal product development. Innovative approaches in development of advanced bioresponsive systems, both patient-friendly and efficient, possibly economically affordable, are expected to bring faster progress within the field of vaginal drug therapy. We might be able to see more of the safe and efficient products in the near future.

References

Abdool Karim, Q., S.S. Abdool Karim, J.A. Frohlich, A.C. Grobler, C. Baxter, L.E. Mansoor et al. 2010. Effectiveness and safety of tenofovir gel, an antiretroviral microbicide, for the prevention of HIV infection in women. Science. 329: 1168–1174.

Abdool Karim, S.S., B.A. Richardson, G. Ramjee, I.F. Hoffman, Z.M. Chirenje, T. Taha et al. 2011. Safety and effectiveness of BufferGel and 0.5% PRO2000 gel for the prevention of HIV infection in women. AIDS. 25: 957–966.

Acartürk, F. 2009. Mucoadhesive vaginal drug delivery systems. Recent Pat. Drug Deliv. Formul. 3: 193–205.

Aci-Jel. 2016. www.acijel.com.au/home, Accessed June 30, 2016.

Agashe, H., M. Hu and L. Rohan. 2012. Formulation and delivery of microbicides. Curr. HIV Res. 10: 88–96.

Al-Baghdadi, O. and A.A. Ewies. 2009. Topical estrogen therapy in the management of postmenopausal vaginal atrophy: an up-to-date overview. Climacteric. 12: 91–105.

Alexander, N.J., E. Baker, M. Kaptein, U. Karck, L. Miller and E. Zampaglione. 2004 Why consider vaginal drug administration? Fertil. Steril. 82: 1.

Antimisiaris, S.G. and S. Mourtas. 2015. Recent advances on anti-HIV vaginal delivery systems development. Adv. Drug Deliv. Rev. 92: 123–145.

Bachhav, Y.G. and V.B. Patravale. 2009. Microemulsion based vaginal gel of fluconazole: formulation, *in vitro* and *in vivo* evaluation. Int. J. Pharm. 365: 175–179.

Baloglu, E., Z.A. Senyingit, S.Y. Karavana and A. Bernkop-Schnürtz. 2009. Strategies to prolong the intravaginal residence time of drug delivery systems. J. Pharm. Pharmaceut. Sci. 12: 312–336.

Boulmedarat, L., J.L. Grossiord, E. Fattal and A. Bochot. 2003. Influence of methyl-beta-cyclodextrin and liposomes on rheological properties of Carbopol 974P NF gels. Int. J. Pharm. 254: 59–64.

Bygdeman, M. and M.L. Swahn. 1996. Replens versus dienoestrol cream in the symptomatic treatment of vaginal atrophy in postmenopausal women. Maturitas. 23: 259–263.

Cailloutte, J.C., C.F. Sharp, G.J. Zimmerman and S. Roy. 1997. Vaginal pH as a marker for bacterial pathogens menopausal status. Am. J. Obstet. Gynecol. 176: 1270–1277.

Caswell, M. and M. Kane. 2002. Comparison of the moisturization efficacy of two vaginal moisturizers: Pectin versus polycarbophil technologies. J. Cosmet. Sci. 53: 81–87.

Chang, J.Y., Y.K. Oh, H.G. Choi, Y.B. Kim and C.K. Kim. 2002. Rheological evaluation of thermosensitive and mucoadhesive vaginal gels in physiological conditions. Int. J. Pharm. 241: 155–163.

Chen, D., K. Sun, H. Mu, M. Tang, R. Liang, A. Wang et al. 2012. pH and temperature dual-sensitive liposome gel based on novel cleavable mPEG-Hz-CHEMS polymeric vaginal delivery system. Int. J. Nanomedicine. 7: 2621–2630.

Chen, J., L. Geng, X. Song, H. Li, N. Giordan and Q. Liao. 2013. Evaluation of the efficacy and safety of hyaluronic acid vaginal gel to ease vaginal dryness: a multicenter, randomized, controlled, open-label, parallel-group, clinical trial. J. Sex. Med. 10: 1575–1584.

Cicinelli, E. 2008. Intravaginal oestrogen and progestin administration: advantages and disadvantages. Best Pract. Res. Clin. Obstet. Gynaecol. 22: 391–405.

Cummins, Jr. J.E., and G.F. Doncel. 2009. Biomarkers of cervicovaginal inflammation for the assessment of microbicide safety. Sex. Transm. Dis. 36(3 Suppl): S84–91.

Cutler, B. and J. Justman. 2008. Vaginal microbicides and the prevention of HIV transmission. Lancet Infect. Dis. 8: 685–697.

das Neves, J. and M.F. Bahia. 2006. Gels as vaginal drug delivery. Int. J. Pharm. 318: 1–14.

das Neves, J., E. Pinto, B. Teixeira, G. Dias, P. Rocha, T. Cunha et al. 2008. Local treatment of vulvovaginal candidosis general and practical considerations. Drugs. 68: 1787–1802.

das Neves, J., M.V. da Silva, M.P. Goncalves, M.H. Amaral and M.F. Bahia. 2009. Rheological properties of vaginal hydrophilic polymer gels. Curr. Drug Deliv. 6: 83–92.

das Neves, J., M.F. Bahia, M.M. Amiji and B. Sarmento. 2011. Mucoadhesive nanomedicine: characterisation and modulation of mucoadhesion at the nanoscale. Expert Opin. Drug Deliv. 8: 1085–1104.

das Neves, J., R. Palmeira-de-Oliveira, A. Palmeira-de-Oliveira, F. Rodrigues and B. Sarmento. 2014. Vaginal mucosa and drug delivery. Mucoadhesive Materials and Drug Delivery Systems, Wiley, Chichester, pp. 99–131.

Date, A.A., A. Shibata, M. Goede, B. Sanford, K. La Bruzzo, M. Belshan et al. 2012. Development and evaluation of a thermosensitive vaginal gel containing raltegravir+efavirenz loaded nanoparticles for HIV prophylaxis. Antiviral Res. 96: 430–436.

Date, A.A. and C.J. Destache. 2013. A review of nanotechnological approaches for the prophylaxis of HIV/AIDS. Biomater. 34: 6202–6028.

Di Fabio, S., J. Van Roey, G. Giannini, G. van den Mooter, M. Spada, A. Binelli et al. 2003. Inhibition of vaginal transmission of HIV-1 in hu-SCID mice by the non-nucleoside reverse transcriptase inhibitor TMC120 in a gel formulation. AIDS. 17: 1597–1604.

Dittgen, M., M. Durrani and K. Lehmann. 1997. Acrylic polymers—A review of pharmaceutical applications. STP Pharma Sciences. 7: 403–437.

Duncan, R. and R. Gaspar. 2011. Nanomedicine(s) under the microscope. Mol. Pharm. 8: 2101–2141.

Edwards, D. and N. Panay. 2016. Treating vulvovaginal atrophy/genitourinary syndrome of menopause: how important is vaginal lubricant and moisturizer composition? Climacteric. 19: 151–161.

Farage, M. and H. Maibach. 2006. Lifetime changes in the vulva and vagina. Arch. Gynecol. Obstet. 27: 195–202.

Ferguson, L.M. and L.C. Rohan. 2011. The importance of the vaginal delivery route for antiretrovirals in HIV prevention. Ther. Deliv. 2: 1535–1550.

Fredricks, D.N., T.L. Fiedler and J.M. Marrazzo. 2005. Molecular identification of bacteria associated with bacterial vaginosis. N. Engl. J. Med. 353: 1899–1911.

Garg, A., D. Aggarwal, S. Garg and A.K. Singla. 2002. Spreading of semisolid formulations: an update. Pharm. Technol. 26: 84–105.

Garg, S., R.A. Anderson, C.J. Chany II, D.P. Waller, X.H. Diao, K. Vermani et al. 2001a. Properties of a new acid-buffering bioadhesive vaginal formulation (ACIDFORM). Contraception. 64: 67–75.

Garg, S., K.R. Tambweaker, K. Vermani, A. Garg, C.L. Kaul and L.J.D. Zaneveld. 2001b. Compendium of pharmaceutical excipients for vaginal formulations. Pharmaceutical Technology. 2001: 14–24.

Geonnotti, A.R., J.J. Peters and D.F. Katz. 2005. Erosion of microbicide formulation coating layers: Effects of contact and shearing with vaginal fluid or semen. J. Pharm. Sci. 94: 1705–1712.

Gupta, P., K. Vermani and S. Garg. 2002. Hydrogels: from controlled release to pH-responsive drug delivery. Drug Discov. Today. 7: 569–579.

Haaland, R.E., T. Evans-Strickfaden, A. Holder, C.P. Pau, J.M. McNicholl, S. Chaikummao et al. 2012. UC781 microbicide gel retains anti-HIV activity in cervicovaginal lavage fluids collected following twice-daily vaginal application. Antimicrob. Agents Chemother. 56: 3592–3596.

Hainer, B.L. and M.V. Gibson. 2011. Vaginitis: Diagnosis and treatment. Am. Family Physic. 83: 807–815.

Halpern, V., F. Ogunsola, O. Obunge, C.H. Wang, N. Onyejepu, O. Oduyebo et al. 2008. Effectiveness of cellulose sulfate vaginal gel for the prevention of HIV infection: results of a Phase III trial in Nigeria. PLoS One 3: e3784.

Hanson, J.M., J.A. McGregor, S.L. Hillier, D.A. Eschenbach, A.K. Kreutner, R.P. Galask et al. 2000. Metronidazole for bacterial vaginosis. A comparison of vaginal gel vs. oral therapy. J. Reprod. Med. 45: 889–896.

He, C., S.W. Kim and D.S. Lee. 2008. *In situ* gelling stimuli-sensitive block copolymer hydrogels for drug delivery. J. Control. Release. 127: 189–207.

Hoare, T.R. and D.S. Kohane. 2008. Hydrogels in drug delivery: Progress and challenges. Polymer. 49: 1993–2007.

Hurler, J., A. Engesland, B.P. Kermany and N. Škalko-Basnet. 2012. Improved texture analysis for hydrogel characterization: Gel cohesiveness, adhesiveness, and hardness. J. App. Polym. Sci. 125: 180–188.

Hussain, A. and F. Ahsan. 2005. The vagina as a route for systemic drug delivery. J. Control. Release. 103: 301–313.

Jain, S.K., R. Singh and B. Sahu. 1997. Development of a liposome based contraceptive system for intravaginal administration of progesterone. Drug Develop. Ind. Pharm. 23: 827–830.

Jespers, V.A., J.M. Van Roey, G.I. Beets and A.M. Buve. 2007. Dose-ranging phase 1 study of TMC120, a promising vaginal microbicide, in HIV-negative and HIV-positive female volunteers. J. Acquir. Immune Defic. Syndr. 44: 154–158.

Jøraholmen, M.W., Ž. Vanić, I. Tho and N. Škalko-Basnet. 2014. Chitosan-coated liposomes for topical vaginal therapy: Assuring localized drug effect. Int. J. Pharm. 472: 94–101.

Justin-Temu, M., F. Damian, R. Kinget and G.V.D.J. Mooter. 2004. Intravaginal gels as drug delivery systems. J. Women's Health. 13: 834–844.

Kang, J.W., E. Davaa, Y.T. Kim and J.S. Park. 2010. A new vaginal delivery system of amphotericin B: a dispersion of cationic liposomes in a thermosensitive gel. J. Drug Target. 18: 637–644.

Khan, S., A. Ullah, K. Ullah and N.-u. Rehman. 2016. Insight into hydrogels. Des. Monomers Polym. 19: 456–478.

Lacey, C.J., S. Woodhall, Z. Qi, S. Sawant, M. Cowen, S. McCormack et al. 2010. Unacceptable side-effects associated with a hyperosmolar vaginal microbicide in a phase 1 trial. Int. J. STD AIDS. 21: 714–717.

Le Donne, M., C. Caruso, A. Mancuso, G. Costa, R. Iemmo, G. Pizzimenti et al. 2011. The effect of vaginally administered genistein in comparison with hyaluronic acid on atrophic epithelium in postmenopause. Arch. Gynecol. Obstet. 283: 1319–1323.

Lev-Sagie, A. 2015. Vulvar and vaginal atrophy: Physiology, clinical presentation, and treatment considerations. Clin. Obstet. Gynecol. 58: 476–491.

Li, W.Z., N. Zhao, Y.Q. Zhou, L.B. Yang, W. Xiao-Ning, H. Bao-Hua et al. 2012. Post-expansile hydrogel foam aerosol of PG-liposomes: a novel delivery system for vaginal drug delivery applications. Eur. J. Pharm. Sci. 47: 162–169.

Machado, R.M., A. Palmeira-de-Oliveira, C. Gaspar, J. Martinez-de-Oliveira and R. Palmeira-de-Oleveira. 2015. Studies and methodologies on vaginal drug permeation Adv. Drug Deliv. Rev. 92: 14–26.

Mbopi-Keou, F.X., S. Trottier, R.F. Omar, N.N. Nkele, S. Fokoua, E.R. Mbu et al. 2010. A randomized, double-blind, placebo-controlled Phase II extended safety study of two Invisible Condom formulations in Cameroonian women. Contraception. 81: 79–85.

McCormack, S., G. Ramjee, A. Kamali, H. Rees, A.M. Crook, M. Gafos et al. 2010. PRO2000 vaginal gel for prevention of HIV-1 infection (Microbicides Development Programme 301): a phase 3, randomised, double-blind, parallel-group trial. Lancet. 376: 1329–1337.

Miller, L., D.L. Patton, A. Meier, S.S. Thwin, T.M. Hooton and D.A. Eeschenbach. 2000. Depomedroxyprogesterone-induced hypoestrogenism and changes in vaginal flora and epithelium. Obstet. Gynecol. 96: 431–439.

Mourtas, S., M. Haikou, M. Theodoropoulou, C. Tsakiroglou and S.G. Antimisiaris. 2008. The effect of added liposomes on the rheological properties of a hydrogel: a systematic study. J. Colloid Interface. Sci. 317: 611–619.

Nachtigall, L.E. 1994. Comparative-Study—Replens Versus Local Estrogen in Menopausal Women. Fertil. Steril. 61: 178–180.

Nanjwade, B.K., H.M. Bechra, G.K. Derkar, F.V. Manvi and V.K. Nanjwade. 2009. Dendrimers: emerging polymers for drug-delivery systems. Eur. J. Pharm. Sci. 38: 185–196.

Nappi, R.E., C. Benedetto, F. Campolo, S. Martella, C. Tosti, A. Cianci et al. 2016. Efficacy, tolerability and safety of a new medical device, Monurelle Biogel(R) vaginal gel, in the treatment of vaginal dryness: a randomized clinical trial in women of reproductive age. Eur. J. Obstet. Gynecol. Reprod. Biol. 203: 82–88.

Navath, R.S., A.R. Menjoge, H. Dai, R. Romero, S. Kannan and R.M. Kannan. 2011. Injectable PAMAM dendrimer-PEG hydrogels for the treatment of genital infections: formulation and *in vitro* and *in vivo* evaluation. Mol. Pharm. 8: 1209–1223.

Nel, A.M., S.C. Smythe, S. Habibi, P.E. Kaptur and J.W. Romano. 2010. Pharmacokinetics of 2 dapivirine vaginal microbicide gels and their safety vs. Hydroxyethyl cellulose-based universal placebo gel. J. Acquir. Immune Defic. Syndr. 55: 161–169.

Ning, M.Y., Y.Z. Guo, H.Z. Pan, X.L. Chen and Z.W. Gu. 2005. Preparation, *in vitro* and *in vivo* evaluation of liposomal/niosomal gel delivery systems for clotrimazole. Drug Devel. Ind. Pharm. 31: 375–383.

Nuttall, J., J. Romano, K. Douville, C. Galbreath, A. Nel, W. Heyward et al. 2007. The future of HIV prevention: prospects for an effective anti-HIV microbicide. Infect. Dis. Clin. North Am. 21: 219–239, x.

O'Loughlin, J., I.Y. Millwood, H.M. McDonald, C.F. Price, J.M. Kaldor and J.R. Paull. 2010. Safety, tolerability, and pharmacokinetics of SPL7013 gel (VivaGel): a dose ranging, phase I study. Sex. Trans. Dis. 37: 100–104.

Ofner III, C.M. and C.M. Klech-Gelotte. 2002. Gels and jellies. Encyclopedia of Pharmaceutical Technology, second edition volume 2, pp. 1327–1343.

Omar, R.F., S. Trottier, G. Brousseau, A. Lamarre, G. Alexandre and M.G. Bergeron. 2008. Distribution of a vaginal gel (Invisible Condom) before, during and after simulated sexual intercourse and its persistence when delivered by two different vaginal applicators: a magnetic resonance imaging study. Contraception. 77: 447–455.

Omar, R.F. and M.G. Bergeron. 2011. The future of microbicides. Int. J. Infect. Dis. 15: e656–660.

Ottinger, W.S., M.K. Menard and B.C. Brost. 1998. A randomized clinical trial of prostaglandin E2 intracervical gel and a slow release vaginal pessary for preinduction cervical ripening. Am. J. Obstet. Gynecol. 179: 349–353.

Owen, D.H., J.J. Peters and D.F. Katz. 2000. Rheological properties of contraceptive gels. Contraception. 62: 321–326.

Owen, D.H., J.J. Peters and D.F. Katz. 2001. Comparison of the rheological properties of Advantage-S and Replens. Contraception. 64: 393–396.

Palacios, S. 2009. Managing urogenital atrophy. Maturitas. 63: 315–318.

Palmeira-de-Oliveira, R., A. Palmeira-de-Oliveira and J. Martinez-de-Oliveira. 2015. New strategies for local treatment of vaginal infections. Adv. Drug Deliv. Rev. 92: 105–122.

Patel, S., E. Hazrati, N. Cheshenko, B. Galen, H. Yang, E. Guzman et al. 2007. Seminal plasma reduces the effectiveness of topical polyanionic microbicides. J. Infect. Dis. 196: 1394–1402.

Pavelić, Ž., N. Škalko-Basnet and R. Schubert. 2001. Liposomal gels for vaginal drug delivery. Int. J. Pharm. 219: 139–149.

Pavelić, Ž., N. Škalko-Basnet and I. Jalšenjak. 2004a. Liposomal gel with chloramphenicol: characterisation and *in vitro* release. Acta Pharm. 54: 319–330.

Pavelić, Ž., N. Škalko-Basnet, R. Schubert and I. Jalšenjak. 2004b. Liposomal gels for vaginal drug delivery. Methods Enzymol. 387: 287–299.

Pavelić, Ž., N. Škalko-Basnet, J. Filipović-Grčić, A. Martinac and I. Jalšenjak. 2005a. Development and *in vitro* evaluation of a liposomal vaginal delivery system for acyclovir. J. Control. Release. 106: 34–43.

Pavelić, Ž., N. Škalko-Basnet and I. Jalšenjak. 2005b. Characterisation and *in vitro* evaluation of bioadhesive liposome gels for local therapy of vaginitis. Int. J. Pharm. 301: 140–148.

Peschka, R., C. Dennehy and F.C., Jr. Szoka. 1998. A simple *in vitro* model to study the release kinetics of liposome encapsulated material. J. Control. Release. 56: 41–51.

Peterson, L., K. Nanda, B.K. Opoku, W.K. Ampofo, M. Owusu-Amoako, A.Y. Boakye et al. 2007. SAVVY (R) (C31G) gel for prevention of HIV infection in women: a Phase 3, double-blind, randomized, placebo-controlled trial in ghana. PLoS One. 19: e1312.

Portman, D.J. and M.L. Gass. 2014. Genitourinary syndrome of menopause: new terminology for vulvovaginal atrophy from the International Society for the Study of Women's Sexual Health and The North American Menopause Society. Climacteric. 17: 557–563.

Price, C.F., D. Tyssen, S. Sonza, A. Davie, S. Evans, G.R. Lewis et al. 2011. SPL7013 Gel (VivaGel (R)) retains Potent HIV-1 and HSV-2 inhibitory activity following vaginal administration in humans. PLoS One. 6: e24095.

Quan, M. 2010. Vaginitis: diagnosis and management. Postgrad. Med. 122: 117–127.

Ramyadevi, D., K.S. Rajan, B.N. Vedhahari, K. Ruckmani and N. Subramanian. 2016. Heterogeneous polymer composite nanoparticles loaded *in situ* gel for controlled release intra-vaginal therapy of genital herpes. Colloids Surf. B. Biointerfaces. 146: 260–270.

Ravani, L., E. Esposito, C. Bories, V.L. Moal, P.M. Loiseau, M. Djabourov et al. 2013. Clotrimazole-loaded nanostructured lipid carrier hydrogels: thermal analysis and *in vitro* studies. Int. J. Pharm. 454: 695–702.

Rohan, L.C. and A.B. Sassi. 2009. Vaginal drug delivery systems for HIV prevention. AAPS J. 11: 78–87.

Rohan, L.C., B. Devlin and H. Yang. 2014. Microbicide dosage forms. Curr. Top. Microbiol. Immunol. 383: 27–54.

Roy, S., P. Gourde, J. Piret, A. Desormeaux, J. Lamontagne, C. Haineault et al. 2001. Thermoreversible gel formulations containing sodium lauryl sulfate or n-Lauroylsarcosine as potential topical microbicides against sexually transmitted diseases. Antimicrob. Agents Chemother. 45: 1671–1681.

Rupp, R., S.L. Rosenthal and L.R. Stanberry. 2007. VivaGel (SPL7013 Gel): a candidate dendrimer—microbicide for the prevention of HIV and HSV infection. Int. J. Nanomedicine. 2: 561–566.

Saini, N., R.K. Sodhi, L. Bajaj, R.S. Pandey, U.K. Jain, O.P. Katare et al. 2016. Intravaginal administration of metformin hydrochloride loaded cationic niosomes amalgamated with thermosensitive gel for the treatment of polycystic ovary syndrome: *In vitro* and *in vivo* studies. Colloids Surf. B. Biointerfaces. 144: 161–169.

Sassi, A.B., K.D. McCullough, M.R. Cost, S.L. Hillier and L.C. Rohan. 2004. Permeability of tritiated water through human cervical and vaginal tissue. J. Pharm. Sci. 93: 2009–2016.

Sassi, A.B., C.E. Isaacs, B.J. Moncla, P. Gupta, S.L. Hillier and L.C. Rohan. 2008. Effects of physiological fluids on physical-chemical characteristics and activity of topical vaginal microbicide products. J. Pharm. Sci. 97: 3123–3139.

Schwartz, J.L., G. Kovalevsky, J.J. Lai, S.A. Ballagh, T. McCormick, K. Douville et al. 2008. A randomized six-day safety study of an antiretroviral microbicide candidate UC781, a non-nucleoside reverse transcriptase inhibitor. Sex. Transm. Dis. 35: 414–419.

Serra, L., J. Doménech and N. Peppas. 2009. Engineering design and molecular dynamics of mucoadheisve drug delivery systems as targeting agents. Eur. J. Pharm. Biopharm. 71: 519–528.

Sherif, N.A. and G.A. Moety. 2013. Vaginal misoprostol tablets versus misoprostol gel for induction of labor in post-term primigravidas. Evidence Based Womens's Health J. 3: 5–8.

Shetty, A., I. Livingston, S. Acharya and A. Templeton. 2004. Vaginal prostaglandin E2 gel versus tablet in the induction of labour at term—a retrospective analysis. J. Obstet. Gynaecol. 24: 243–246.

Sinha, A. and A.A. Ewies. 2013. Non-hormonal topical treatment of vulvovaginal atrophy: an up-to-date overview. Climacteric. 16: 305–312.

Skolei-Karpoff, S., G. Ramjee, K. Ahmed, L. Altini, M.G. Plagianos, B. Friedland et al. 2008. Efficacy of Carraguard for prevention of HIV infection in women in South Africa: a randomised, double-blind, placebo-controlled trial. Lancet. 372: 1977–1987.

Taher, S.E., J.W. Inder, S.A. Soltan, J. Eliahoo, D.K. Edmonds and P.R. Bennett. 2011. Prostaglandin E2 vaginal gel or tablets for the induction of labour at term: a randomised controlled trial. BJOG. 118: 719–725.

Tan, O., K. Bradshaw and B.R. Carr. 2012. Management of vulvovaginal atrophy-related sexual dysfunction in postmenopausal women: an up-to-date review. Menopause. 19: 109–117.

Tenjarla, S. 1999. Microemulsions: an overview and pharmaceutical applications. Crit. Rev. Ther. Drug Carrier Syst. 16: 461–521.

Tyssen, D., S.A. Henderson, A. Johnson, J. Sterjovski, K. Moore, J. La et al. 2010. Structure activity relationship of dendrimer microbicides with dual action antiviral activity. PLoS One. 5: e12309.

Vailati, S., E. Melloni, E. Riscassi, D. Behr Roussel and M. Sardina. 2013. Evaluation of the effects of a new intravaginal gel, containing purified bovine colostrum, on vaginal blood flow and vaginal atrophy in ovariectomized rat. Sex. Med. 1: 35–43.

Valenta, C. 2005. The use of mucoadhesive polymers in vaginal delivery. Adv. Drug Deliv. Rev. 57: 1692–1712.

Van Damme, L., G. Ramjee, M. Alary, B. Vuylsteke, V. Chandeying, H. Rees et al. 2002. Effectiveness of COL-1492, a nonoxynol-9 vaginal gel, on HIV-1 transmission in female sex workers: a randomized controlled trial. Lancet. 360: 971–977.

Vanić, Ž. and N. Škalko-Basnet. 2013. Nanopharmaceuticals for improved topical vaginal therapy: can they deliver? Eur. J. Pharm. Sci. 50: 29–41.

Vanić, Ž. and N. Škalko-Basnet. 2014. Mucosal nanosystems for improved topical drug delivery: vaginal route of administration. J. Drug Deliv. Sci. Tech. 24: 435–444.

Vanić, Ž., J. Hurler, K. Ferderber, P. Golja Gašparović, N. Škalko-Basnet and J. Filipović-Grčić. 2014. Novel vaginal drug delivery system: deformable propylene glycol liposomes-in-hydrogel. J. Liposome Res. 24: 27–36.

Vanić, Ž. 2015. Phospholipid vesicles for enhanced drug delivery in dermatology. J. Drug Discov. Dev. Deliv. 2: 1–9.

Wain, A.M. 1998. Metronidazole vaginal gel 0.75% (MetroGel-Vaginal): a brief review. Infect. Dis. Obstet. Gynecol. 6: 3–7.

Washington, N., S. Washington and C.G. Wilson. 2001. Vaginal and intrauterine drug delivery; pp. 271–281. *In*: Washington, N., C.M. Washington and C.G. Wilson [eds.]. Physiological Pharmaceutics: Barriers to Drug Absorption. Taylor and Francis, London.

Wong, T.W., M. Dhanawat and M.J. Rathbone. 2014. Vaginal drug delivery: strategies and concerns in polymeric nanoparticle development. Expert. Opin. Drug. Deliv. 11: 1419–1434.

Yu, T., K. Malcolm, D. Woolfson, D.J. Jones and G.P. Andrews. 2011. Vaginal gel drug delivery systems: understanding rheological characteristics and performance. Expert Opin. Drug Deliv. 8: 1309–1322.

Zussman, A., L. Lara, H.H. Lara, Z. Bentwich and G. Borkow. 2003. Blocking of cell-free and cell-associated HIV-1 transmission through human cervix organ culture with UC781. AIDS. 17: 653–661.

11

Advances in Composite Hydrogels for Ocular Drug Delivery and Biomedical Engineering Application

*Andreza Maria Ribeiro** and *Ivan Antonio Neumann*

ABSTRACT

Hydrogels have been extensively researched due to their particular properties and structures, with a wide and attractive potential for ocular applications. Various materials (ceramic, nanostructures, green polymers and polymers) have been included in the structure of some hydrogels, forming innovative composite products suitable for many ocular medical devices. The advantages of the composite hydrogels for ocular drug delivery and bioengineering applications include improvements in the hydrogel properties and significant contribution in controlled drug release. This chapter provides an overview of the current development of the design and production of composite hydrogels as vehicles for drug ocular delivery, including the main outcomes, advances, limitations and applications in ocular bioengineering. After a brief introduction about the concept of hydrogels and composites, principal polymeric materials used in hydrogel formulation are presented. Considering their structure and characteristics, the next section shows a detailed description about

Department of Engineering and Material Sciences, University of Federal of Paraná (UFPR), Curitiba, Brazil.
Email: neumann.sbs@gmail.com
* Corresponding author: ribeiroandreza@yahoo.com.br

technologies and recent modifications to improve their properties used in biomedical engineering. This is followed by reports about recent research efforts that have focused on the development of composite hydrogels for ocular drug release. Finally, new advances are presented about composite hydrogels for clinical ocular application.

Keywords: hydrogel composite, hydrogel, composite, biomaterial, ocular drug delivery, ocular bioengineering

1. Introduction

Eye diseases affect a large portion of the world population. Fortunately, with technological and medical advances, nowadays it is possible to prevent, cure and treat eye problems. Some eye diseases impair visual ability, while others may even lead to complete loss of vision. The eye can be generally classified into an anterior and posterior segment; diseases of the eye posterior segment are the major causes of irreversible blindness. This has motivated the search for new biomaterials for ocular application (Lloyd et al. 2001), which must be biocompatible, non-immunogenicity, non-toxic and provide a better life quality for the patient (Black and Hastings 2013).

Hydrogels are three-dimensional networks of hydrophilic polymers which, in contact with water, swell maintaining the structural integrity. Due to its hydrophobicity and biocompatibility, hydrogels have proved to be of great interest in the biomaterials area (Peppas 1987, Hoffman 2012). Many different formulations have been investigated with great potential to use in the treatment of ocular disorders (inflammatory, infections, hypertension), trauma and degenerative diseases. Occasionally, hydrogels do not have mechanical properties, like strength and elasticity, to satisfy the conditions necessary to use in bioengineering and some pharmaceutical areas. Thus, a significant effort is made to modulate the structural (reinforcement to the material) and physical-chemical properties of the hydrogel to improve the material's final properties (Zhao et al. 2015). In this way, with the addition of other materials to the hydrogel structure, it is possible to obtain a composite hydrogel that is more resistant (Gaharwar et al. 2014), with no loss in functionality. Thus, the incorporation of nanostructures (polymer, ceramic, calcium phosphate, bioactive glasses, hydroxyapatite, metallic), fibers (synthetic or natural), and nanotubes into hydrogels seems to be an original approach for designing innovative materials used for different functions (Kokabi et al. 2007, Tanaka et al. 2005, Sinha and Guha 2009, Ramírez et al. 2011, Sydenstricker et al. 2003, Nath and Banerjee 2013).

In recent decades, the development of a wide range of implants and biomedical devices for treatment and correction of the functional deficiencies of disease, age and ocular trauma, has increased, with the object of vision maintenance and/or recuperation (Lloyd et al. 2001, Baino et al. 2014). The challenge of improving the mechanical properties of biomaterials for ocular use without losing the biocompatibility and functionality, as well ensuring the longevity of eye health is significant for many ocular treatments (Lloyd et al. 2001). Several composite hydrogels have been explored to be used in bioengineering, medical devices and controlled drug release (Hao et al. 2014, Liu et al. 2008, Li et al. 2013, Perez et al. 1998).

2. Overview Ocular Diseases

2.1 Cataract

Clinically, cataract disease can be defined as the deterioration of vision due to an alteration of transparency in the lens. The natural aging eye is the main cause of cataract. However, some patients may develop the disease earlier for genetic reasons or related to risk factors such as use of oral corticosteroids, ocular trauma or ocular inflammation (Fraunfelder et al. 2014, Shah and Shah 2015). The disease may also be caused by diabetes, rubella, tuberculosis and toxoplasmosis (Brian and Taylor 2001, O'Neill 1998). According to the World Health Organization (WHO), cataract is responsible for 51 percent of the reasons that lead to blindness. The disease affects about 20 million people and is related to aging, which usually appears after 60 years. One treatment for cataract is to replace the opaque lens by an intraocular lens surgically (WHO 2014).

2.2 Glaucoma

Glaucoma is the name of a group of diseases characterized by distinct clinical and pathological manifestations, which have as a common denominator, the optic neuropathy. Open and closure angle are two major types of glaucoma; open angle is a chronic condition that progresses slowly over a long period of time, without the person noticing vision loss, while angle closure can appear suddenly and be painful. Glaucoma is the second leading cause of blindness in the world and it is estimated that 80 million people will be affected by 2020 (Kaur et al. 2011).

The main risk factor for glaucoma is characterized by an increase in intraocular pressure (IOP). However, it is known that there are instances when individuals with elevated IOP do not develop the disease, and that people with normal IOP, between 10–21 mm Hg, may become affected by glaucoma (Wilson et al. 1987). Elevation of intraocular pressure may affect the optic nerve due to compression of the nerve head (prolonged and/or repeated), so that cell is injured and dies; after that, the dead cells are not replaced by new ones. A consequence of untreated glaucoma can be the permanent damage of the retina optic disc, which can progress to blindness (Graham 1972). Glaucoma is not just a disease of IOP, but rather it is suggested glaucomatous optic neuropathy, which is multifactorial, or of other non-pressure dependent factors that have been considered as immunological factors, vascular diseases, genetic, myopia, diabetes mellitus and others (Weinreb 1998, Fechtner and Weinreb 1994). The most common treatment for glaucoma is topical therapy by use of eye drops, and also other forms of treatment which may include oral medicines, implants, laser therapy, surgery, and a combination of these methods (Quigley 1993, Dietlein et al. 2009).

2.3 Macular degeneration

Macular degeneration (MD) is a leading cause of visual impairment and blindness in the elderly whose etiology remains largely unknown (Haines et al. 2005). Age-related macular degeneration (AMD) is a multi-factorial disease since environmental and genetic components play a role in its development. AMD affects the macula, the central part the retina that allows the eye to see fine details. There are two forms, wet and dry AMD. Wet AMD (neovascular or exudative) is when abnormal blood vessel behind the retina starts to grow under the macula, ultimately leading to blood and fluid leakage. The wet form is rare (10 percent of the cases), severe and can progress fast. Bleeding, leaking, and scarring from these blood vessels causes damage and leads to rapid central vision loss. Dry AMD (atrophic or nonexudative) is when the macula thins overtime as part of aging process, blurring gradually central vision and generally affects both the eyes. The dry form is more common (90 percent of the cases) and can progress more slowly than the wet form. Overtime, the macula functions are impaired; consequently, the central vision of the affected eye is gradually lost and the patient may not notice the vision change. The therapies for AMD require periocular or intraocular administration of drugs (Birch and Liang 2007, CDC 2015).

2.4 Diabetic retinopathy

The Centre for Disease Control and Prevention (CDC) describes that diabetic retinopathy (DR) as a disease that affects blood vessels in the light-sensitive tissue called the retina that lines the back of the eye, usually affects both the eyes. It is characterized by progressive damage of the retinal blood vessels, the light-sensitive tissue at the back of the eye that is necessary for good vision. DR progresses through four stages, (i) nonproliferative retinopathy, (ii) mild (microaneurysms), (iii) moderate (blockage in some retinal vessels), (iv) severe, in which more vessels are blocked leading to retina deprived from blood supply leading to growing new blood vessels, and the most advanced stage called proliferative retinopathy. DR is the most common cause of vision loss among people with diabetes and the leading cause of vision impairment and blindness among working-age adults. Primary diagnosis of DR and an appropriate treatment reduces the risk of vision loss (CDC 2015, Stitt et al. 2016).

2.5 Dry eye and others ocular diseases

Dry eye is an abnormal condition of the eye surface that manifests itself when people produce insufficient tears or it is deficient in some of its components causing eye discomfort; thus, the eye is not properly moistened. The dry eye may be associated with aging and factors that make dry areas in the conjunctiva and cornea, which causes serious nuisance. Frequent symptoms of dry eye are burning, itching, photophobia, redness, irritation, blurred vision, tearing, foreign-body sensation and uncomfortableness while reading and watching television. There are several factors that can cause dry eye such as contact lenses, air conditioning, high wind, staying at high altitude environments with air conditioning system, use of cosmetics, cigarette smoke, air pollution, heat, excessive time in front of computer monitors and dry climate. Certain medicines may cause lubrication reduction in eyes such as certain decongestants, antihistamines, antidepressants, diuretics, anesthetics, anticholinergics and beta blockers. Deficiency of vitamin A and several systemic diseases are often associated with dry eye, among which are arthritis, lupus, and sarcoidosis, Sjögren Syndrome Dry Eye, thyroid, skin and Parkinson's disease among others. The treatment of dry eye should be done for the patient's well-being, to preserve the health of corneas (Lemp and Foulks 2007). The adopted dry eye treatment is done by the use of specific drops (artificial tears) (Lim et al. 2015) and tears in gel form (Wang et al. 2010c). In severe cases, it is a possible resort to occlusion of the drainage of tears, allowing them to come into contact with the eye longer. Other ways of treating it are using anti-inflammatories, antibiotics, systemic medications, topical corticosteroids and use of protective lenses (Lemp and Foulks 2007).

Besides traumas and refractive eye defects (myopia, hyperopia, presbyopia, and astigmatism), other diseases related to eyes are inflammation-based diseases, like scleritis, keratitis, uveitis, iritis, conjunctivitis, chorioretinitis, choroiditis, retinitis, retinochoroiditis (Ryan and Durand 2011), and allergic eye that is a heterogeneous group of diseases that has a common symptomatology but different pathogenesis (Manzouri et al. 2006). Fungi, bacteria, parasites and virus are capable of attacking the surface or interior of the eye, causing infections, which are difficult to treat (Mas-Coma et al. 2014, Macsai and Mojica 2013, Ryan and Durand 2011).

3. Hydrogel

Hydrogels are three dimensional (3D) networks of polymers, fully or partially hydrophilic, that swell upon contact with water and maintain their structural integrity to form insoluble polymer matrices. Hydrogels are able to absorb a large amount of water or biological fluids (Hoffman 2012, Peppas 1987). Hydrogels can be classified according to the nature of the reticulation (chemical or physical), form of network (homopolymer, copolymer, blend), presence of pores and the source of the polymers (natural or synthetic) (Hoffman 2012).

Chemical gels are those having covalent cross-links, which may be generated by direct reaction with cross-linking agents, by conversion of hydrophobic polymers to hydrophilic polymers, followed by cross-linking to form the network, or by irradiation (Hoffman 2012). The physical hydrogels, also called reversible, have chains held together by molecular matted and secondary forces including electrostatic attraction of hydrophobic forces or hydrogen bond (Hoffman 2012).

The best approach for using hydrogels in ocular bioengineering and/ or pharmaceuticals applications is to correlate the physical properties, such as absorption capacity, swelling behavior, stability, permeability, mechanical stability, optical (refractive index and high oxygen permeability) and surface properties, adhesion and bioactivity (Baino et al. 2014, Efron and Maldonado-Codina 2011). In addition, intelligent or stimuli-sensitive hydrogels have been the subject of much research (Casolaro et al. 2012, Siegel 2014). Changes in hydrogels' structure, shape and property after being exposed by external environment, such as temperature, ionic strength, pH value, salt concentration, enzymatic activity, glucose concentration, light, magnetic field, pressure, electric field and solvent composition or a combination of them have been demonstrated in a wide variety of hydrogel systems (Koetting et al. 2015, Wang et al. 2010a). The stimuli-sensitive hydrogels are expected to contribute significantly to the assessment and development of biomaterials for biological and biomedical applications, such as self-regulated drug delivery systems, sensors, transplant and site-specific drug delivery systems (Casolaro et al. 2012, Wang et al. 2010a). Hydrogels are even used as dressing of superficial and deep wounds such as pressure sores, ulcers, surgical wounds, partial thickness burns and lacerations (Caló and Khutoryanskiy 2015). In 1960, Wichterle and Lim were the first to describe the synthesis of poly(hydroxyethyl methacrylate) (PHEMA) to use as contact lenses (Wichterle and Lim 1960). Currently, there are various monomers used for the synthesis of hydrogels (Table 1) for the ocular area. In addition, hydrogels have potential applications in eye bioengineering of soft tissue replacement, artificial skin membranes, ocular device and ocular insert (Hassan 2000, Singh et al. 2011, Selvam et al. 2006, Baino et al. 2014).

Table 1. Materials used for ocular hydrogels (Mitra 2013, Doppalapudi et al. 2014, Zhao et al. 2015, Peppas et al. 2000, Lloyd et al. 2001).

Monomers	Biodegradable polymers	Materials suitable for tissue engineering
Acrylic acid (AA)	Alginic acid	Alginate
Ethylene glycol (EG)	Amino acids	Agarose
Ethylene glycol dimethacrylate (EGDMA)	Chitosan	Calcium alginate
Hydroxyethyl methacrylate (HEMA)	Collagen	Cellulose
Hydroxyethoxy ethyl methacrylate (HEEMA)	Gelatin	Chitosan
Hydroxy diethoxy ethyl methacrylate (HDEEMA)	Hyaluronic acid	Collagen
N-(2-Hydroxypropyl) methacrylamide (HPMA)	Poly(lactic acid)	Chondroitin sulphate
Methyoxyethyl methacrylate (MESMA)	Poly(L-lactic acid) (PLLA)	Fibrin
Methoxyethoxyethyl methacrylate (MEEMA)	Poli (ε-caprolactona) (PCL)	Fibroin
Methyldiethoxyethyl methacrylate (MDEEMA)	Polyglycolic acid (PGA)	Gelatin
Poly(ethylene glycol acrylate (PEGA)	Poly N-vinylpyrrolidone	Keratin
Poly(ethylene glycol methacrylate (PEGMA)	Polylactide-co-glycolide (PLGA)	Poly(epsilon-caprolactone)
Poly(ethylene glycol diacrylate (PEGDA)	Poly(alkyl cynoacrylates) (PACA)	Poly(ethylene oxide)
Poly(ethylene glycol) dimethacrylate (PEGDMA)	Polyanhydrides	Polymethacrylate s
N-isopropyl acrylamide (NIPAAm)	Poly(orthoester) (PEOs)	Poly hydroxy alkanoate
N-vinyl-2pyrrolidone (NVP)	Polysaccharides	Poly(γ-glutamic acid)
Vinyl acetate (Vac)	Proteins	Starch

3.1 Modifications to improve hydrogel properties to be used in biomedical engineering

The three-dimensional network of hydrogels (Fig. 1A) are able to absorb large amounts of water and/or other body fluids. Moreover, their porosity can be explored to be used to simulate living tissue (Caló and Khutoryanskiy 2015).

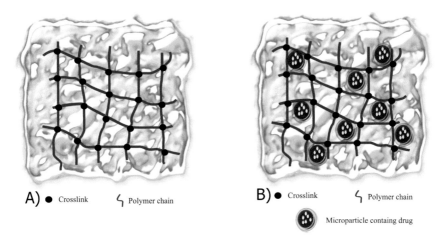

Fig. 1. (A) Swollen hydrogel structure and (B) swollen hydrogel composite structure.

Hydrogels stability is the factor used to determine what material is the most appropriate for each application. For example, the hydrogels that exhibit fast degradation can be used for immediate drug release, more stable hydrogels can be used in tissue engineering; whereas the hydrogels with low degradation rates can be used in medical devices, transplants, support cell growth and coating surfaces for antimicrobial treatment (Peppas 1987, Caló and Khutoryanskiy 2015, Vashist and Ahmad 2015). Hydrogels swelling capacity and mechanical properties are dependent on the cross-linking degree between the chains (Berger et al. 2004, Hennink and Van Nostrum 2012). One interesting approach to improve the hydrogels' properties and to include several functionalities is the incorporation of different materials or systems into hydrogels to develop composite hydrogel (Fig. 1B) (Kokabi et al. 2007, Merino et al. 2015, Biondi et al. 2015). For example, different types of nanoparticle are embedded into a hydrogel matrix (Thoniyot et al. 2015). All these properties can be widely explored in biomedical engineering (Hoffman 2012, Caló and Khutoryanskiy 2015, Vashist and Ahmad 2015).

4. Composites

Historically, the term composite material begins to be addressed in the mid-20th century, when the properties of glass fiber dispersed in polymer matrix were discovered. Material compositions were observed for thousands years, such as the construction of huts made of clay, straw and shells. However, the definition of composite material arises only with the beginning of the manufacturing of these materials, creating a new class, distinct from conventional materials as metals, polymers and ceramics (Callister and Rethwisch 2009).

Composite material is the one in which you can observe at least two phases, i.e., a named array and another backup or dispersed phase. In this structure, several materials such as plastic, metal, vitreous ceramic and natural materials may be present (Barbero 2010, Pérez et al. 2013). Composite materials have emerged due to: (i) reduction of production cost, because charges can be added to an array, thus reducing the use of raw materials; and (ii) improvement of some particular property of the material used (mechanical resistance, lightness, durability, barrier properties, among others). Composites materials are very versatile, showing immense range of applications, being used in the most diverse areas such as construction (reinforced concrete), automotive (car's tire), microelectronics (diodes and transistors), aerospace (aircraft fuselage), sports (high performance equipment very light), biomedical (implants, transport and controlled release of drugs), among others (Chawla 2012).

The development of a new composite material is time consuming and requires a lot of reviews, knowledge of each component of the material being extremely necessary, as well as the proportions that favor the desired properties, geometry, size and orientation of the dispersed phase. In this regard, nanometric particles (< 100 nm) are widely studied in the composition of nanostructured materials and nanocomposites (Whatmore 2006).

Composite materials can be divided into three types: reinforced by particles, reinforced by fibers, in which dispersed phase with high ratio between length and diameter can be neatly aligned or fully dispersed in the array, and structural composites with composition and homogeneous materials (Callister and Rethwisch 2009).

4.1 Composite materials in biomedicine

Multiple classes of materials can be used in the development of composite materials, which can be of natural or synthetic origin, inorganic and organic (Black and Hastings 2013). Polymeric materials, metallic, ceramic and glass-ceramic, natural fibers and particles can be used to compose the physical structure of the composite material, modifying its properties and expanding its range (Barbero 2010).

Composite materials feature attractive properties for the most diverse areas of biomedicine (Gaharwar et al. 2014, Zhao et al. 2015). Materials containing porous silicon particles (PSI) feature good properties for use in orthopedics (Cheng et al. 2008, Mazzocchi and Bellosi 2008, Mazzocchi et al. 2008, Anderson and Olsen 2010), oncology (Park et al. 2011, Tian et al. 2015) and ophthalmology (Cheng et al. 2008, Kashanian et al. 2010, McInnes et al.

2012). In ocular diseases polymeric matrices can be used for the transport of drugs or cell growth (McInnes et al. 2012, Irani et al. 2015).

Hyaluronic acid (HA) is present naturally in the ocular system and offers good therapeutic applications due to its excellent biocompatibility, biodegradation and viscoelasticity. HA gels and hydrogels composites can be widely applied in the controlled release of drugs into the eye system (Xu et al. 2012).

Biodegradable polymers (copolymers and blends) such as poly(L-lactic acid) (PLLA), poly(ε-caprolactone) (PCL), poly(glycolic acid) (PGA), poly(hidroxibutirate) (PHB) among others, can be used in biomedical applications as matrices for cell growth and bone, in transport and controlled release of drugs, due their excellent biocompatible and bioabsorbable property. Degradation fragments are completely absorbed by the body's metabolic routes without side effects (Södergård and Stolt 2002, He et al. 2004, Madhavan Nampoothiri et al. 2010).

Natural halloysite clay nanotubes loaded in natural polymers microspheres presents good results for drug sustained release, in addition to presenting excellent biocompatibility (Vergaro et al. 2010, Jin et al. 2016, Lvov et al. 2016); these composites can also be applied in bones as repair implants and anti-corrosion coating (Vergaro et al. 2010, Lvov et al. 2016).

Graphene oxide (GO) can be used with magnetic nanoparticles of manganese ferritic ($MnFe_2O_4$) for drugs transport, and in use with nuclear magnetic resonance, that makes it possible to monitor the absorption of these drugs by the body tissues (Kim et al. 2010, Hung et al. 2014, Wang et al. 2016).

Silver nanoparticles feature, among other physical-chemical properties, prominent antibacterial activity (Ataee-Esfahani et al. 2013, Haneda and Towata 2015, Alshehri et al. 2016). Composite materials containing silver nanoparticles can be used for loading and controlled release of drugs for the urinary tract infections treatment (Alshehri et al. 2016).

Tamarind seed gum (TSG) is a natural polysaccharide with good properties for the pharmaceutical area due to good thermal and chemical stability, mucoadhesivity and biocompatibility (Nayak et al. 2014, Priyadarshini et al. 2016). Combining TSG with other polymers materials, such as gelatin, it is possible to use it in controlled release of drugs to the treatment of *diabetes mellitus* (Nayak et al. 2014).

4.2 Biocompatible composite materials

Recent advances in composite materials provide alternative materials with attractive and potential efficiency (Butcher et al. 2014, Xu et al. 2015). Several distinct classes of polymers have been used as components of bioengineering (Hassan 2000, Drotleff et al. 2004).

Usually, a polymeric scaffold is used to provide a framework on to which cells are seeded, allowing the cells to proliferate and develop into the functional target tissue while degrading the artificial construct. Hydrogels can support cell proliferation while new tissue is formed, making them an alternative to tissue engineering scaffolds (Butcher et al. 2014). Currently, nanofiber is a very attractive system for scaffolds biomaterials, which is generally produced by electrospinning method (Li et al. 2002). Mechanical properties of nanofibrous depend on many variables of each individual fiber material, like diameter, mesh porosity, alignment and bonding between fibers. The addition of nanofibers filling meshes into their matrices can form a composite that draws from the advantages of both components. Fibrous components normally show an improvement in the hydrogels mechanical properties, with a good biocompatibility and functionality (Butcher et al. 2014). Some researchers have developed hydrogels composites filling nanofiber natural or polymeric (Kai et al. 2012, Shin et al. 2009, Cong et al. 2013, Tonsomboon and Oyen 2013).

Composite materials of PCL microfibers containing PSI, with hydride endings and oxidized surfaces, in concentrations of 6 and 20 percent (wt) were studied by Kashanian et al. The authors evaluated the links of composites with epithelial cells and carried out *in vivo* tests of biocompatibility in rats. Results showed significant linkage between composites and conjunctiva epithelial cell. After the period of 8 weeks it was found that the material did not cause inflammations, infections and did not erode the ocular surface. The authors concluded that the material can be proposed to the engineering tissue area with applications as scaffolds to controlled release of particles (Kashanian et al. 2010).

HA has a good physical property for hydrogels development like biocompatibility, viscoelasticity and biodegradability, making it an excellent material for use in ocular bioengineering (transplant, tissue engineer, medical devices, wound healing and controlled release of drugs). Latanoprost (13,14-dihydro-17-phenyl-18,19,20-trinor-prostaglandin F2 -1-isopropyl ester) is a F2 prostaglandin analogue used in the treatment of glaucoma, which acts by lowering intraocular pressure. However, latanoprost is a substance sensitive to light and heat and practically insoluble in water (Lokesh et al. 2015). Widjaja et al. had good results in controlled degradation properties and sustained release of latanaprost after including the liposomes in HA hydrogel. The cross-linking formation of composite hydrogel showed an additional resistance to latanoprost diffusion and also a potential drug release tool to use in treating eye diseases (Widjaja et al. 2014).

Chitosan is a natural polymer with good biocompatibility properties (Raemdonck et al. 2013) and the treatment with ethylene glycol increases their aqueous solubility. Mitra et al. developed chitosan glycol nanoparticles loaded with DNA plasmid for treatment of genetic disorders administered in eye retina through injections. As a result, the non-appearance of retinal toxicity after 30 days of implant was confirmed and also verified that the plasmid had maintained their original structure and released properly inside treated cells. These results were only observed in cells of the retinal epithelium pigment (EPR), which indicates that the material synthesized can be used for controlled drug release for the treatment of genetic disorders associated with the EPR, with potential use to the treatment of degenerative eye diseases (Mitra et al. 2014).

5. Recent Research Efforts that have Focused on the Development of Composite Hydrogels for Ocular Drug Release

Conventionally, topical ocular and subconjunctival administration are used in the anterior segment (cornea, conjunctiva, sclera, anterior uvea), while the intravitreal administration is used for posterior segment (retina, vitreous, choroid) (Urtti 2006). There are several potential drug delivery routes for ocular tissues, and the development of pharmaceutical formulations have a great influence on the outcome and duration of drug action. The cornea is generally considered to be an important, but not exclusive, ocular way for permeation of topically applied drugs. This is because the epithelial tissue is lipophilic and the main barrier to drug permeation into the cornea. However, the limiting step for permeation of lipophilic drugs is the partition coefficient between the epithelium and the stroma (Prausnitz and Noonan 1998). The conjunctiva is highly vascularized, has a surface area (16–18 cm^2) greater than that of cornea (1 cm^2) (Watsky et al. 1988) and depending on the drug administered, it may be 2 to 30 times more permeable (Ahmed et al. 1987, Wang et al. 1991). Another factor that may influence the permeability of drugs in cornea is the presence of protein transporters work as efflux pumps P-glycoprotein (P-gp), multidrug resistance protein (MRP) and breast cancer resistance protein (BCRP) that are expressed by the corneal epithelium (Dey et al. 2003). Vellonen et al. (2010) found MRP1 protein, MRP5 and BCRP expressed in epithelial tissues of human cornea.

In order to circumvent these drawbacks and extend the residence of drug in the precorneal area, consequently to improve ocular bioavailability, different types of systems have been investigated, such as the use of mucoadhesive solutions (Ludwig 2005), colloidal systems (Di Tommaso et al. 2011), semi-solid formulations and ocular insert devices (Luchs et al. 2010). These systems act as reservoirs, with the main goal to increase the drug remaining in the pre-corneal area. Considering all the precorneal factors, extending the contact time of the dosage form with the ocular surface is an important factor for the increased bioavailability. The use of the cyclodextrins (CD) (Loftsson and Stefansson 2007), nanocarriers (Ribeiro et al. 2013) and soft contact lenses loaded with drug (Hiratani and Alvarez-Lorenzo 2004) has been extensively proposed in order to improve the drug bioavailability and stability, and decrease the irritation caused after topical ocular administration (Davies 2000). On the other hand, recent research has been made for various filling materials, like cyclodextrins, nanocarriers, and natural fibers into hydrogel network to create composite hydrogels with superior properties and design functionalities (Merino et al. 2015, Gaharwar et al. 2014, Xu et al. 2015, Abrego Escoba et al. 2015).

Researchers developed two types of hydrophilic networks by conjugating β-cyclodextrin (β-CD), producing platforms to local release of an antimicrobial 5,6-dimethoxy-1-indanone N4-allyl thiosemicarbazone (TSC) for application in ophthalmic diseases. Poly(2-hydroxyethyl methacrylate) soft contact lenses displaying β-CD and super-hydrophilic hydrogels of directly cross-linked hydroxypropyl-β-CD were synthesized and characterized. TSC was incorporated in to the networks during polymerization and after polymer synthesis. Once TSC was incorporated, the structural parameters as a proportion of CD units, mesh size and swelling were evaluated. Both systems presented a controlled release of the antimicrobial drug for at least two weeks and also had capacity of bacterial growth inhibition against *Staphylococcus aureus* and *Pseudomonas aeruginosa* (Glisoni et al. 2013).

The soft contact lenses (SCLs) have been investigated in terms of devices for controlled release of ophthalmic drugs as they are comfortable, biocompatible and present a significant increase of drug residence in the eye. The use of these devices causes an appropriate diffusion into the target tissue. The development of SCL for drug delivery has an important role in a variety of ocular surface diseases, such as inflammation and infections (Alvarez-Lorenzo et al. 2006), and glaucoma (Xu et al. 2010). Recent studies showed that the drug is released from the SCL to the tear film between the cornea and lens, remaining there for a long time (Alvarez-Lorenzo et al. 2006, Efron and Maldonado-Codina 2011, Hiratani et al. 2005).

The main components of hydrogel lens materials are relatively hydrophilic polymers. Other monomers or materials are added to modify water content to improve the wettability, flexibility, oxygen permeability, ionicity and fluid transport of hydrogel lenses (Efron and Maldonado-Codina 2011). SCLs, made from HEMA monomers combined with NVP, are large enough to cover the whole cornea and present good oxygen permeability, ensuring more comfort for patients (Caló and Khutoryanskiy 2015). The composite hydrogel can be obtained to increase the stability of the drugs, and several methods have been developed to modify the conventional contact lenses to improve their capacity to load and to control drug release (González-Chomón et al. 2013, Malakooti et al. 2015, Ribeiro et al. 2011), which are able to modify the polymeric materials with a controlled hydrophilic/hydrophobic copolymer ratio (Hu et al. 2011), filling drug-containing nanocarriers systems and add a molecule built-in in hydrogels (Bertram et al. 2009, Ribeiro et al. 2012). Generally, the composite materials exhibit improved characteristics compared with individual components, i.e., the addition of silicone material in hydrogel synthesis is able to improve oxygen permeability and comfortable fit (Stapleton et al. 2006).

Many biological processes can develop synthetic materials with high selectivity and high potential for use by biomolecular science (Drotleff et al. 2004). In this way, molecularly imprinted polymers (MIPs) are artificial matrices and stand out for their ability to develop biomimetic recognition systems similar to antigen-antibody specific systems or enzyme-substrate (Vlatakis et al. 1993). Biomimetic materials can interact selectively with the biological microenvironment mimicking. In recent years, researchers (Venkatesh et al. 2007, Ali and Byrne 2009, Ribeiro et al. 2011) have used the MIP technique for hydrogels preparations and employed them as medicated SCLs (Hiratani et al. 2005). After making a change in the hydrogel structure, it is possible to increase loading and to control drug release in the SLCs. In the last decade, therapeutic molecules of low molecular weight (antihistamines, antibiotics, anti-glaucoma and anti-inflammatory) or proteins were used during molecular imprinting SLCs production (Hiratani and Alvarez-Lorenzo 2004, Venkatesh et al. 2007, Byrne et al. 2002, Malakooti et al. 2015). Ali et al. (2009) designed and synthesized SLCs as carrier to hyaluronic acid, which is a molecule of high molecular weight used for the dry eye treatment. Results showed that a slow release was significantly improved through biomimetic imprinting and hyaluronic acid molecule was sustained for 24 hours (Ali and Byrne 2009).

In the Patent n° US 6632457 B1, compositions and methods are provided to control the release of relatively low molecular weight therapeutic species through composite hydrogels matrices. Microparticles drug entrapped are dispersed within bioabsorbable hydrogels, so as to release the hydrosoluble therapeutic agents in a controlled form. Methods of using the compositions of the present invention in therapeutic systems can be used for topical ocular application (Sawhney 2003).

Chetone et al. developed silicone rubber hydrogel composite ocular insert. Cylindrical devices, all containing 0.8 mg oxytetracycline HCl (OXT), were prepared. Release studies using rabbits presented a prolonged release of OXT (concentration of 20–30 µg/ml) from the inserts for several days (Chetoni et al. 1998).

6. Recent Modifications to Improve Hydrogel Properties to Use in Biomedical Ocular Engineer

Biocompatible hydrogels have widely been used for the ocular tissue engineering (Vashist and Ahmad 2015), and various polymers have been used to create different types of hydrogel composite applied in the ocular surface, artificial cornea, scaffolds and transplants.

Human patients, that have a corneal perforation, are repaired with sutures, which are able to take away the infection, inflammation and vascularization (Varley and Meisler 1991). Tissue adhesives are an attractive alternative to sutures (Velazquez et al. 2004).

Hydrogels have been included in the structure of wound dressings or ocular bandage combined with various materials, to form composite products appropriate to be used on wounds. Once the ocular surface is exposed to the strange body, chemical substance and trauma, an eye bandage is indicated to the treatment. The material should have some characteristics as be transparent, easy to apply, able to load and release drugs, protect the injured eye, and be sufficiently robust to handle during a surgical proceeding. Trexler et al. synthesized a new class of cellulose fiber-reinforced hydrogel composite with the strength, transparency and biocompatibility required for ocular applications. In addition to the composite hydrogel that showed the desired curvature, size and thickness, relevant parameters as adhesive and functionalization of the materials was evaluated (Trexler et al. 2012).

Perez's research group developed methods to produce composite hydrogels (hybrid materials) made of corneal stromal tissue and a synthetic polyethylene oxide hydrogel base for corneal prostheses (Perez et al. 1998).

The potential use of bacterial cellulose (BC) as novel to artificial cornea replacement, was investigated by Wang et al. BC/poly(vinyl alcohol) (BC/PVA) hydrogel composites were synthesized utilizing freezing-thaw method. Results showed that hydrogel composites exhibited desirable properties as artificial cornea replacement biomaterial that included high water content, high visible light transmittance and suitable UV absorbance, also with increased mechanical strength and appropriate thermal properties. In addition, the authors revealed the hydrogel composites exhibited promising characteristics as artificial cornea composite material (Wang et al. 2010b).

Another research group designed an artificial cornea from a porous nano-hydroxyapatite/poly(vinyl alcohol) hydrogel (n-HA/PVA-H) skirt and a transparent center poly(vinyl alcohol) hydrogel (PVA-H). These artificial corneas were implanted in the eyes of rabbits and the corneal tissues were evaluated histologically. As a result, the material exhibited a good biocompatibility and interlocking happened between artificial cornea and host tissues, the biomaterial thus produced has potential for clinical use (Fenglan et al. 2007).

Tonsomboon and Oyen group developed an electrospun gelatin nanofiber that was infiltrated with alginate hydrogels, yielding transparent fiber-reinforced hydrogels. The developed fiber-reinforced hydrogels show great potential as mechanically robust scaffolds for corneal tissue engineering uses (Tonsomboon and Oyen 2013).

Ocular surface (OS), one of most common issues in ocular diseases, causes disorders by the limbal stem cell deficiency (LSCD), leading to an impaired vision and blindness. The main treatment modality for LSCD is the transplantation of amniotic membrane (Wright et al. 2013, Fernandes et al. 2005). The manufacturing process that combines various polymers has been used to produce different types of hydrogel applied for the tissue engineering of ocular surface, including bilayer composite hydrogel that can be used as an artificial cornea. In the case of LSCD, the reconstruction of the ocular surface with autologous stem cells inserted onto the hydrogel matrix may provide potential clinical impacts (Wright et al. 2013).

Hydrogel nanocomposites with carbon nanotubes (CNT) have been designed and characterized to evaluate their potential application as biomaterials (Cirillo et al. 2014). Hybrid composite hydrogels were synthesized using gelatin, polysaccharides or chitosan impregnated with carbon nanotubes. Mechanical strength as swelling properties of the resultant materials was evaluated. The choice of natural polymers has great importance due the advantageous physical, chemical, and biological properties, which permits an extensive range of applications in bioengineering and pharmaceutical (Chatterjee et al. 2009, Ferris 2009).

Researchers developed a hydrogel nanocomposite for use as an auto-focusing intra-ocular lens. The hydrogel scaffold was composed of a monomer-free, thiol that contained polyacrylamide (5 percent), which was allowed to gel in the presence of nanoparticles of a proteo-mimetic polyacrylamide nanogel, bovine serum albumin (BSA) and hydrophilized silica with approximately 42 nm, 6 and 3 nm respectively. Authors observed that the nanoparticle loading increased with decreased of the particle size. In addition, the elastic modulus increased with increased loading of the nanogels with BSA, and otherwise decreased with hydrophilized silica. As main features, the nanocomposite hydrogel that contained silica was the most promising class of nanocomposite hydrogels with properties equivalent to that of a young porcine lens (Ravi et al. 2005).

7. Composite Hydrogel for Ocular Clinical Application

It is possible to see that there are significant efforts of the scientific community to articulate multiple functions onto a single material to contribute for current complex ocular treatment problems, due the increase in demand for biomaterial that could perform multiple biological tasks with high efficacy. With advancement and improvement in the development of usual hydrogel materials, multifunctional materials such as hydrogel composites are obtained which are capable of forming biocompatible matrices that can be used clinically.

OcuSeal® (Beaver-Visitec International, Waltham, MA), is a two-part dendrimer-based hydrogel ocular bandage that is applied directly to the ocular surface as a liquid. The hydrogel bandage was developed to provide a barrier while stabilizing ocular wounds following surgical or non-surgical trauma or other ocular conditions. In addition, it was planned to form a low-profile, smooth, soft and transparent protective barrier film on the ocular surface. Kenyon et al. showed in their *in vitro* studies that the hydrogel can block penetration of bacterial species (*Staphylococcus aureus* or *Pseudomonas aeruginosa*) that can potentially pass through corneal incisions and cause acute endophthalmitis (Kenyon et al. 2014). Other potential applications are cataract surgery (Uy and Kenyon 2013), as an adjuvant to sutures in refractive surgery, pterygium surgery, trabeculectomy and corneal laceration (Lerit and Abaño 2012, Matossian et al. 2015).

8. Conclusion

The design of hydrogel composite for diverse applications is becoming progressively more vibrant. This innovative technology already constitutes an important part of the ocular therapeutic intervention. Moreover, the current challenges attract opportunities for the development of better and more promising hydrogel composites in the ophthalmic area, especially for the medical devices, ocular drug delivery and transplants produced by biocompatible materials.

Furthermore, the market for ophthalmic biomaterials is in expansion and researches are made to explore diverse technology solutions for the treatment of ocular disorders.

9. Conflicts of Interest

Authors have no proprietary or financial interest in the products or approaches discussed. Authors report no conflicts of interest in this work.

References

Abrego Escoba, G., H. Alvarado, E.B. Souto, B. Guevara, L. Halbaut, A. Parra et al. 2015. Biopharmaceutical profile of pranoprofen-loaded PLGA nanoparticles containing hydrogels for ocular administration. Eur. J. Pharm. Biopharm. 95: 261–270.

Ahmed, I., R.D. Gokhale, M.V. Shah and T.F. Patton. 1987. Physicochemical determinants of drug diffusion across the conjunctiva, sclera, and cornea. J. Pharm. Sci. 76: 583–586.

Ali, M. and M.E. Byrne. 2009. Controlled release of high molecular weight hyaluronic acid from molecularly imprinted hydrogel contact lenses. Pharm. Res. 26: 714–726.

Alshehri, S.M., A. Aldalbahi, A.B. Al-Hajji, A.A. Chaudhary, M.I.H. Panhuis, N. Alhokbany et al. 2016. Development of carboxymethyl cellulose-based hydrogel and nanosilver composite as antimicrobial agents for UTI pathogens. Carbohydr. Polym. 138: 229–236.

Alvarez-Lorenzo, C., H. Hiratani and A. Concheiro. 2006. Contact lenses for drug delivery. Am. J. Drug Deliver. 4: 131–151.

Anderson, M.C. and R. Olsen. 2010. Bone ingrowth into porous silicon nitride. J Biomed Mater Res A. 92A: 1598–1605.

Ataee-Esfahani, H., M. Imura and Y. Yamauchi. 2013. All-Metal Mesoporous Nanocolloids: Solution-Phase Synthesis of Core–Shell Pd@Pt Nanoparticles with a Designed Concave Surface. Angew Chem Int Ed Engl. 52: 13611–13615.

Baino, F., S. Perero, S. Ferraris, M. Miola, C. Balagna, E. Verné et al. 2014. Biomaterials for orbital implants and ocular prostheses: Overview and future prospects. Acta Biomater. 10: 1064–1087.

Barbero, E.J. 2010. Introduction to Composite Materials Design. CRC press.

Berger, J., M. Reist, J.M. Mayer, O. Felt, N. Peppas and R. Gurny. 2004. Structure and interactions in covalently and ionically crosslinked chitosan hydrogels for biomedical applications. Eur. J. Pharm. Biopharm. 57: 19–34.

Bertram, J.P., S.S. Saluja, J. Mckain and E.B. Lavik. 2009. Sustained delivery of timolol maleate from poly(lactic-co-glycolic acid)/poly(lactic acid) microspheres for over 3 months. J. Microencapsul. 26: 18–26.

Biondi, M., A. Borzacchiello, L. Mayol and L. Ambrosio. 2015. Nanoparticle-Integrated Hydrogels as Multifunctional Composite Materials for Biomedical Applications. Gels. 1: 162–178.

Birch, D.G. and F.Q. Liang. 2007. Age-related macular degeneration: a target for nanotechnology derived medicines. Int. J. Nanomedicine. 2: 65–77.

Black, J. and G. Hastings. 2013. Handbook of biomaterial properties. Berlin, Springer Science & Business Media.

Brian, G. and H. Taylor. 2001. Cataract blindness: challenges for the 21st century. Bull World Health Organ. 79: 249–256.

Butcher, A.L., G.S. Offeddu and M.L. Oyen. 2014. Nanofibrous hydrogel composites as mechanically robust tissue engineering scaffolds. Trends Biotechnol. 32: 564–570.

Byrne, M.E., K. Park and N.A. Peppas. 2002. Molecular imprinting within hydrogels. Adv. Drug Deliv. Rev. 54: 149–161.

Callister, W.D. and D.G. Rethwisch. 2009. Materials science and engineering: an introduction. USA, John Wiley & Sons Inc.

Caló, E. and V.V. Khutoryanskiy. 2015. Biomedical applications of hydrogels: A review of patents and commercial products. Eur. Polym. J. 65: 252–267.

Casolaro, M., I. Casolaro and S. Lamponi. 2012. Stimuli-responsive hydrogels for controlled pilocarpine ocular delivery. Eur. J. Pharm. Biopharm. 80: 553–561.

Cdc. 2015. Vision Health Initiative - Basics of Vision and Eye Health, Common Eye Disorders [Online]. [Accessed 22/03/2016].

Chatterjee, S., M.W. Lee and S.H. Woo. 2009. Enhanced mechanical strength of chitosan hydrogel beads by impregnation with carbon nanotubes. Carbon. 47: 2933–2936.

Chawla, K.K. 2012. Composite materials: science and engineering. Springer Science & Business Media.

Cheng, L., E. Anglin, F. Cunin, D. Kim, M.J. Sailor, I. Falkenstein et al. 2008. Intravitreal properties of porous silicon photonic crystals: a potential self-reporting intraocular drug-delivery vehicle. Br. J. Ophthalmol. 92: 705–711.

Chetoni, P., G. Di Colo, M. Grandi, M. Morelli, M.F. Saettone and S. Darougar. 1998. Silicone rubber/hydrogel composite ophthalmic inserts: preparation and preliminary *in vitro/in vivo* evaluation. Eur. J. Pharm. Biopharm. 46: 125–132.

Cirillo, G., S. Hampel, U.G. Spizzirri, O.I. Parisi, N. Picci and F. Iemma. 2014. Carbon nanotubes hybrid hydrogels in drug delivery: a perspective review. Biomed. Res. Int. 2014.

Cong, H.-P., P. Wang and S.-H. Yu. 2013. Stretchable and self-healing graphene oxide–polymer composite hydrogels: a dual-network design. Chem. Mater. 25: 3357–3362.

Davies, N.M. 2000. Biopharmaceutical considerations in topical ocular drug delivery. Clin. Exp. Pharmacol. Physiol. 27: 558–562.

Dey, S., J. Patel, B.S. Anand, B. Jain-Vakkalagadda, P. Kaliki, D. Pal et al. 2003. Molecular evidence and functional expression of P-glycoprotein (MDR1) in human and rabbit cornea and corneal epithelial cell lines. Invest. Ophthalmol. Vis. Sci. 44: 2909–2918.

Di Tommaso, C., F. Behar-Cohen, R. Gurny and M. Möller. Year. Colloidal systems for the delivery of cyclosporin A to the anterior segment of the eye. *In:* Ann. Pharm. Fr, 2011. Elsevier, 116–123.

Dietlein, T.S., M.M. Hermann and J.F. Jordan. 2009. The medical and surgical treatment of glaucoma. Dtsch Arztebl. Int. 106: 597–605.

Doppalapudi, S., A. Jain, W. Khan and A.J. Domb. 2014. Biodegradable polymers—an overview. Polym. Adv. Technol. 25: 427–435.

Drotleff, S., U. Lungwitz, M. Breunig, A. Dennis, T. Blunk, J. Teßmar et al. 2004. Biomimetic polymers in pharmaceutical and biomedical sciences. Eur. J. Pharm. Biopharm. 58: 385–407.

Efron, N. and C. Maldonado-Codina. 2011. Development of contact lenses from a biomaterial point of view—Materials, manufacture, and clinical application. *In:* Ducheyne, P. [ed.]. Comprehensive Biomaterials. Oxford: Elsevier.

Fechtner, R.D. and R.N. Weinreb. 1994. Mechanisms of optic nerve damage in primary open angle glaucoma. Surv. Ophthalmol. 39: 23–42.

Fenglan, X., L. Yubao, Y. Xiaoming, L. Hongbing and Z. Li. 2007. Preparation and *in vivo* investigation of artificial cornea made of nano-hydroxyapatite/poly(vinyl alcohol) hydrogel composite. J. Mater. Sci. Mater. Med. 18: 635–640.

Fernandes, M., M.S. Sridhar, V.S. Sangwan and G.N. Rao. 2005. Amniotic membrane transplantation for ocular surface reconstruction. Cornea. 24: 643–653.

Ferris, C.J. 2009. Conducting bio-materials based on gellan gum hydrogels. Soft Matter. 5: 3430–3437.

Fraunfelder, F.T., F.W. Jr, Fraunfelder and W.A. Chambers. 2014. Drug-Induced Ocular Side Effects: Clinical Ocular Toxicology. Elsevier Health Sciences.

Gaharwar, A.K., N.A. Peppas and A. Khademhosseini. 2014. Nanocomposite hydrogels for biomedical applications. Biotechnol. Bioeng. 111: 441–453.

Glisoni, R.J., M.J. García-Fernández, M. Pino, G. Gutkind, A.G. Moglioni, C. Alvarez-Lorenzo et al. 2013. β-Cyclodextrin hydrogels for the ocular release of antibacterial thiosemicarbazones. Carbohydr. Polym. 93: 449–457.

González-Chomón, C., A. Concheiro and C. Alvarez-Lorenzo. 2013. Soft contact lenses for controlled ocular delivery: 50 years in the making. Ther. Deliv. 4: 1141–1161.

Graham, P. 1972. Epidemiology of simple glaucoma and ocular hypertension. Br. J. Ophthalmol. 56: 223.

Haines, J.L., M.A. Hauser, S. Schmidt, W.K. Scott, L.M. Olson, P. Gallins et al. 2005. Complement factor H variant increases the risk of age-related macular degeneration. Science. 308: 419–421.

Haneda, M. and A. Towata. 2015. Catalytic performance of supported Ag nano-particles prepared by liquid phase chemical reduction for soot oxidation. Catal Today. 242: Part B: 351–356.

Hao, J., X. Wang, Y. Bi, Y. Teng, J. Wang, F. Li et al. 2014. Fabrication of a composite system combining solid lipid nanoparticles and thermosensitive hydrogel for challenging ophthalmic drug delivery. Colloids Surf. B. Biointerfaces. 114: 111–120.

Hassan, C.M. 2000. Biopolymers, PVA hydrogels, anionic polymerisation, nanocomposites. *In*: Waldmann, H. [ed.]. Advances in Polymer Science. New York: H. Waldmann.

He, A., C.C. Han and G. Yang. 2004. Preparation and characterization of PLLA/P(CL-b-LLA) blends by an *in situ* ring-opening polymerization. Polymer. 45: 8231–8237.

Hennink, W. and C.F. Van Nostrum. 2012. Novel crosslinking methods to design hydrogels. Adv. Drug Deliv. Rev. 64: 223–236.

Hiratani, H. and C. Alvarez-Lorenzo. 2004. The nature of backbone monomers determines the performance of imprinted soft contact lenses as timolol drug delivery systems. Biomaterials. 25: 1105–1113.

Hiratani, H., A. Fujiwara, Y. Tamiya, Y. Mizutani and C. Alvarez-Lorenzo. 2005. Ocular release of timolol from molecularly imprinted soft contact lenses. Biomaterials. 26: 1293–1298.

Hoffman, A.S. 2012. Hydrogels for biomedical applications. Adv. Drug Deliv. Rev. 64: 18–23.

Hu, X., L. Hao, H. Wang, X. Yang, G. Zhang, G. Wang et al. 2011. Hydrogel contact lens for extended delivery of ophthalmic drugs. Int. J. Polym. Sci. 2011: 9.

Hung, L.-Y., J.-C. Chang, Y.-C. Tsai, C.-C. Huang, C.-P. Chang, C.-S. Yeh et al. 2014. Magnetic nanoparticle-based immunoassay for rapid detection of influenza infections by using an integrated microfluidic system. Nanomedicine. 10: 819–829.

Irani, Y.D., Y. Tian, M. Wang, S. Klebe, S.J. Mcinnes, N.H. Voelcker et al. 2015. A novel pressed porous silicon-polycaprolactone composite as a dual-purpose implant for the delivery of cells and drugs to the eye. Exp. Eye Res. 139: 123–31.

Jin, Y., R. Yendluri, B. Chen, J. Wang and Y. Lvov. 2016. Composite microparticles of halloysite clay nanotubes bound by calcium carbonate. J. Colloid Interface Sci. 466: 254–260.

Kai, D., M.P. Prabhakaran, B. Stahl, M. Eblenkamp, E. Wintermantel and S. Ramakrishna. 2012. Mechanical properties and *in vitro* behavior of nanofiber–hydrogel composites for tissue engineering applications. Nanotechnol. 23: 095705.

Kashanian, S., F. Harding, Y. Irani, S. Klebe, K. Marshall, A. Loni et al. 2010. Evaluation of mesoporous silicon/polycaprolactone composites as ophthalmic implants. Acta Biomater. 6: 3566–72.

Kaur, I.P., H. Singh and S. Kakkar. 2011. Newer therapeutic vistas for antiglaucoma medicines. Crit. Rev. Ther. Drug Carrier Syst. 28.

Kenyon, K.R., L. Qiao and E. Lee. 2014. Hydrogel liquid ocular bandage (OcuSeal®) is an effective microbial barrier. Invest. Ophthalmol. Vis. Sci. 55: 2547–2547.

Kim, D.-H., D.E. Nikles and C.S. Brazel. 2010. Synthesis and characterization of multifunctional chitosan-MnFe2O4 nanoparticles for magnetic hyperthermia and drug delivery. Materials. 3: 4051.

Koetting, M.C., J.T. Peters, S.D. Steichen and N.A. Peppas. 2015. Stimulus-responsive hydrogels: Theory, modern advances, and applications. Mater. Sci. Eng. R. Rep. 93: 1–49.

Kokabi, M., M. Sirousazar and Z.M. Hassan. 2007. PVA–clay nanocomposite hydrogels for wound dressing. Eur. Polym. J. 43: 773–781.

Lemp, M.A. and G.N. Foulks. 2007. The definition and classification of dry eye disease. Ocul. Surf. 5: 75–92.

Lerit, S.J.T. and J.M.R. Abaño. 2012. Comparison of tensile strength of fibrin glue, 2-Octyl cyanoacrylate, liquid ocular bandage, and conventional nylon 10-0 sutures in corneal laceration repair in an animal model. Philipp. J. Ophthalmol. 37: 52–58.

Li, W.J., C.T. Laurencin, E.J. Caterson, R.S. Tuan and F.K. Ko. 2002. Electrospun nanofibrous structure: a novel scaffold for tissue engineering. J. Biomed. Mater. Res. 60: 613–621.

Li, X., Z. Zhang and H. Chen. 2013. Development and evaluation of fast forming nano-composite hydrogel for ocular delivery of diclofenac. Int. J. Pharm. 448: 96–100.

Lim, A., M.R. Wenk and L. Tong. 2015. Lipid-based therapy for ocular surface inflammation and disease. Trends Mol. Med. 21: 736–748.

Liu, W., M. Griffith and L. Fengfu. 2008. Alginate microsphere-collagen composite hydrogel for ocular drug delivery and implantation. J. Mater. Sci. Mater. Med. 19: 3365–3371.

Lloyd, A.W., R.G. Faragher and S.P. Denyer. 2001. Ocular biomaterials and implants. Biomaterials. 22: 769–785.

Loftsson, T. and E. Stefansson. 2007. Cyclodextrins in ocular drug delivery: theoretical basis with dexamethasone as a sample drug. J. Drug Deliv. Sci. Technol. 17: 3–9.

Lokesh, K., R. Permender and K.V.K. Vikash. 2015. Role of Prostaglandins in Glaucoma: Design and Optimization. Int. J. Clin. Toxicol. 3: 18–28.

Luchs, J.I., D.S. Nelinson, J.I. Macy and L.-S Group. 2010. Efficacy of hydroxypropyl cellulose ophthalmic inserts (LACRISERT) in subsets of patients with dry eye syndrome: findings from a patient registry. Cornea. 29: 1417–1427.

Ludwig, A. 2005. The use of mucoadhesive polymers in ocular drug delivery. Adv. Drug Deliv. Rev. 57: 1595–1639.

Lvov, Y., W. Wang, L. Zhang and R. Fakhrullin. 2016. Halloysite clay nanotubes for loading and sustained release of functional compounds. Adv. Mater. 28: 1227–1250.

Macsai, M. and G. Mojica. 2013. Medical Management of Ocular Surface Disease A2—Lee, Edward J., Holland Mark J., Mannis W. Barry. Ocular Surface Disease: Cornea, Conjunctiva and Tear Film. London: W.B. Saunders.

Madhavan Nampoothiri, K., N.R. Nair and R.P. John. 2010. An overview of the recent developments in polylactide (PLA) research. Bioresource Technology. 101: 8493–8501.

Malakooti, N., C. Alexander and C. Alvarez-Lorenzo. 2015. Imprinted contact lenses for sustained release of polymyxin B and related antimicrobial peptides. J. Pharm. Sci. 104: 3386–3394.

Manzouri, B., T.H. Flynn, F. Larkin, S.J. Ono and R. Wyse. 2006. Pharmacotherapy of allergic eye disease. Expert. Opin. Pharmacother. 7: 1191–1200.

Mas-Coma, S., V.H. Agramunt and M.A. Valero. 2014. Chapter Two—Neurological and ocular fascioliasis in humans. *In:* Rollinson, D. [ed.]. Advances in Parasitology. Academic Press.

Matossian, C., S. Makari and R. Potvin. 2015. Cataract surgery and methods of wound closure: a review. Clin. Ophthalmol. 9: 921.

Mazzocchi, M. and A. Bellosi. 2008. On the possibility of silicon nitride as a ceramic for structural orthopaedic implants. Part I: processing, microstructure, mechanical properties, cytotoxicity. J. Mater. Sci. Mater. Med. 19: 2881–7.

Mazzocchi, M., D. Gardini, P.L. Traverso, M.G. Faga and A. Bellosi. 2008. On the possibility of silicon nitride as a ceramic for structural orthopaedic implants. Part II: chemical stability and wear resistance in body environment. J. Mater. Sci. Mater. Med. 19: 2889–901.

Mcinnes, S.J.P., Y. Irani, K.A. Williams and N.H. Voelcker. 2012. Controlled drug delivery from composites of nanostructured porous silicon and poly(L-lactide). Nanomedicine. 7: 995+.

Merino, S., C. Martín, K. Kostarelos, M. Prato and E. Vázquez. 2015. Nanocomposite Hydrogels: 3D Polymer–Nanoparticle Synergies for On-Demand Drug Delivery. ACS Nano. 9: 4686–4697.

Mitra, A.K. 2013. Treatise on Ocular Drug Delivery. Bentham Science Publishers.

Mitra, R.N., Z. Han, M. Merwin, M. Al Taai, S.M. Conley and M.I. Naash. 2014. Synthesis and Characterization of Glycol Chitosan DNA Nanoparticles for Retinal Gene Delivery. ChemMedChem. 9: 189–196.

Nath, D. and P. Banerjee. 2013. Green nanotechnology–A new hope for medical biology. Environ. Toxicol. Pharmacol. 36: 997–1014.

Nayak, A.K., D. Pal and K. Santra. 2014. Tamarind seed polysaccharide–gellan mucoadhesive beads for controlled release of metformin HCl. Carbohydr. Polym. 103: 154–163.

O'neill, J.F. 1998. The ocular manifestations of congenital infection: a study of the early effect and term outcome of maternally transmitted rubella and toxoplasmosis. Trans. Am. Ophthalmol. Soc. 96: 813.

Park, J.S., J.M. Kinsella, D.D. Jandial, S.B. Howell and M.J. Sailor. 2011. Cisplatin-Loaded Porous Si Microparticles Capped by Electroless Deposition of Platinum. Small. 7: 2061–2069.

Peppas, N., P. Bures, W. Leobandung and H. Ichikawa. 2000. Hydrogels in pharmaceutical formulations. Eur. J. Pharm. Biopharm. 50: 27–46.

Peppas, N.A. 1987. Hydrogels in medicine and pharmacy. CRC press Boca Raton, FL.

Perez, E., D. Miller and E.W. Merrill. 1998. Methods for making composite hydrogels for corneal prostheses. Google Patents.

Pérez, R.A., J.-E. Won, J.C. Knowles and H.-W. Kim. 2013. Naturally and synthetic smart composite biomaterials for tissue regeneration. Adv. Drug Deliv. Rev. 65: 471–496.

Prausnitz, M.R. and J.S. Noonan. 1998. Permeability of cornea, sclera, and conjunctiva: a literature analysis for drug delivery to the eye. J. Pharm. Sci. 87: 1479–1488.

Priyadarshini, R., G. Nandi, A. Changder, S. Chowdhury, S. Chakraborty and L.K. Ghosh. 2016. Gastroretentive extended release of metformin from methacrylamide-g-gellan and tamarind seed gum composite matrix. Carbohydr. Polym. 137: 100–110.

Quigley, H.A. 1993. Open-angle glaucoma. N. Engl. J. Med. 328: 1097–1106.

Raemdonck, K., T.F. Martens, K. Braeckmans, J. Demeester and S.C. De Smedt. 2013. Polysaccharide-based nucleic acid nanoformulations. Advanced Drug Delivery Reviews. 65: 1123–1147.

Ramírez, M.G.L., K.G. Satyanarayana, S. Iwakiri, G.B. De Muniz, V. Tanobe and T.S. Flores-Sahagun. 2011. Study of the properties of biocomposites. Part I. Cassava starch-green coir fibers from Brazil. Carbohydr. Polym. 86: 1712–1722.

Ravi, N., H.A. Aliyar and P.D. Hamilton. 2005. Hydrogel nanocomposite as a synthetic intra-ocular lens capable of accommodation. *In:* Macromol Symp, 2005. Wiley Online Library. 191–202.

Ribeiro, A., F. Veiga, D. Santos, J.J. Torres-Labandeira, A. Concheiro and C. Alvarez-Lorenzo. 2011. Receptor-based biomimetic NVP/DMA contact lenses for loading/eluting carbonic anhydrase inhibitors. J. Memb. Sci. 383: 60–69.

Ribeiro, A., F. Veiga, D. Santos, J.J. Torres-Labandeira, A. Concheiro and C. Alvarez-Lorenzo. 2012. Hydrophilic acrylic hydrogels with built-in or pendant cyclodextrins for delivery of anti-glaucoma drugs. Carbohydr. Polym. 88: 977–985.

Ribeiro, A., I. Sandez-Macho, M. Casas, S. Alvarez-Pérez, C. Alvarez-Lorenzo and A. Concheiro. 2013. Poloxamine micellar solubilization of α-tocopherol for topical ocular treatment. Colloids Surf. B. Biointerfaces. 103: 550–557.

Ryan, E.T. and M. Durand. 2011. Ocular disease A2. pp. 991–1016. *In:* Richard L. Guerrant, David H. Walker and Peter F. Weller [eds.]. Tropical Infectious Diseases: Principles, Pathogens and Practice (Third Edition). Edinburgh: W.B. Saunders.

Sawhney, A.S. 2003. Composite hydrogel drug delivery systems. Google Patents.

Selvam, S., P.B. Thomas and S.C. Yiu. 2006. Tissue engineering: Current and future approaches to ocular surface reconstruction. Ocul. Surf. 4: 120–136.

Shah, M. and S. Shah. 2015. Traumatic Cataract: A Review. Studies on the Cornea and Lens. Springer.

Shin, M.K., G.M. Spinks, S.R. Shin, S.I. Kim and S.J. Kim. 2009. Nanocomposite hydrogel with high toughness for bioactuators. Adv. Mater. 21: 1712–1715.

Siegel, R.A. 2014. Stimuli sensitive polymers and self regulated drug delivery systems: A very partial review. J. Control Release. 190: 337–351.

Singh, V., S.S. Bushetti, S.A. Raju, R. Ahmad, M. Singh and M. Ajmal. 2011. Polymeric ocular hydrogels and ophthalmic inserts for controlled release of timolol maleate. J. Pharm. Bioallied Sci. 3: 280–285.

Sinha, A. and A. Guha. 2009. Biomimetic patterning of polymer hydrogels with hydroxyapatite nanoparticles. Mater. Sci. Eng. C. 29: 1330–1333.

Södergård, A. and M. Stolt. 2002. Properties of lactic acid based polymers and their correlation with composition. Prog. Polym. Sci. 27: 1123–1163.

Stapleton, F., S. Stretton, E. Papas, C. Skotnitsky and D.F. Sweeney. 2006. Silicone hydrogel contact and the ocular surface. Ocul. Surf. 4: 24–43.

Stitt, A.W., T.M. Curtis, M. Chen, R.J. Medina, G.J. Mckay, A. Jenkins et al. 2016. The progress in understanding and treatment of diabetic retinopathy. Prog. Retin. Eye Res. 51: 156–186.

Sydenstricker, T.H., S. Mochnaz and S.C. Amico. 2003. Pull-out and other evaluations in sisal-reinforced polyester biocomposites. Polym. Test. 22: 375–380.

Tanaka, Y., J.P. Gong and Y. Osada. 2005. Novel hydrogels with excellent mechanical performance. Prog. Polym. Sci. 30: 1–9.

Thoniyot, P., M.J. Tan, A.A. Karim, D.J. Young and X.J. Loh. 2015. Nanoparticle–hydrogel composites: Concept, design, and applications of these promising, multi-functional materials. Adv. Sci. 2: 1–13.

Tian, G., X. Zhang, Z. Gu and Y. Zhao. 2015. Recent Advances in Upconversion Nanoparticles-Based Multifunctional Nanocomposites for Combined Cancer Therapy. Advanced Materials. 27: 7692–7712.

Tonsomboon, K. and M.L. Oyen. 2013. Composite electrospun gelatin fiber-alginate gel scaffolds for mechanically robust tissue engineered cornea. J. Mech. Behav. Biomed. Mater. 21: 185–194.

Trexler, M.M., J.L. Graham, J.L. Breidenich, J.P. Maranchi, J.B. Patrone, M.W. Patchan et al. 2012. Wound Healing Compositions Comprising Biocompatible Cellulose Hydrogel Membranes and Methods of Use Thereof. Google Patents.

Urtti, A. 2006. Challenges and obstacles of ocular pharmacokinetics and drug delivery. Adv. Drug Deliv. Rev. 58: 1131–1135.

Uy, H.S. and K.R. Kenyon. 2013. Surgical outcomes after application of a liquid adhesive ocular bandage to clear corneal incisions during cataract surgery. J. Cataract Refract. Surg. 39: 1668–1674.

Varley, G.A. and D.M. Meisler. 1991. Complications of penetrating keratoplasty: graft infections. J. Refract. Surg. 7: 62–66.

Vashist, A. and S. Ahmad. 2015. Hydrogels in Tissue Engineering: Scope and Applications. Curr. Pharm. Biotechnol. 16: 606–620.

Velazquez, A.J., M.A. Carnahan, J. Kristinsson, S. Stinnett, M.W. Grinstaff and T. Kim. 2004. New dendritic adhesives for sutureless ophthalmic surgical procedures: *In vitro* studies of corneal laceration repair. Arch. Ophthalmol. 122: 867–870.

Vellonen, K.S., E. Mannermaa, H. Turner, M. Häkli, J.M. Wolosin, T. Tervo et al. 2010. Effluxing ABC transporters in human corneal epithelium. J. Pharm. Sci. 99: 1087–1098.

Venkatesh, S., S.P. Sizemore and M.E. Byrne. 2007. Biomimetic hydrogels for enhanced loading and extended release of ocular therapeutics. Biomaterials. 28: 717–724.

Vergaro, V., E. Abdullayev, Y.M. Lvov, A. Zeitoun, R. Cingolani, R. Rinaldi et al. 2010. Cytocompatibility and uptake of halloysite clay nanotubes. Biomacromolecules. 11: 820–826.

Vlatakis, G., L.I. Andersson, R. Müller and K. Mosbach. 1993. Drug assay using antibody mimics made by molecular imprinting. Nature. 361: 645–647.

Wang, C., A. Javadi, M. Ghaffari and S. Gong. 2010a. A pH-sensitive molecularly imprinted nanospheres/hydrogel composite as a coating for implantable biosensors. Biomaterials. 31: 4944–4951.

Wang, G., Y. Ma, L. Zhang, J. Mu, Z. Zhang, X. Zhang et al. 2016. Facile synthesis of manganese ferrite/graphene oxide nanocomposites for controlled targeted drug delivery. Journal of Magnetism and Magnetic Materials. 401: 647–650.

Wang, J., C. Gao, Y. Zhang and Y. Wan. 2010b. Preparation and *in vitro* characterization of BC/PVA hydrogel composite for its potential use as artificial cornea biomaterial. Mater. Sci. Eng. C. 30: 214–218.

Wang, T.-J., I.J. Wang, J.-D. Ho, H.-C. Chou, S.-Y. Lin and M.-C. Huang. 2010c. Comparison of the clinical effects of carbomer-based lipid-containing gel and hydroxypropyl-guar gel artificial tear formulations in patients with dry eye syndrome: A 4-week, prospective, open-label, randomized, parallel-group, noninferiority study. Clin. Ther. 32: 44–52.

Wang, W., H. Sasaki, D.-S. Chien and V.H. Lee. 1991. Lipophilicity influence on conjunctival drug penetration in the pigmented rabbit: a comparison with corneal penetration. Curr. Eye Res. 10: 571–579.

Watsky, M.A., M.M. Jablonski and H.F. Edelhauser. 1988. Comparison of conjunctival and corneal surface areas in rabbit and human. Curr. Eye Res. 7: 483–486.

Weinreb, R.N. 1998. Toward understanding the optic neuropathy of glaucoma. Arch. Ophthalmol. 116: 1102–1103.

Whatmore, R.W. 2006. Nanotechnology—what is it? Should we be worried? Occup. Med. 56: 295–299.

Who. 2014. Priority eye diseases: cataract. World Health Organization.

Wichterle, O. and D. Lim. 1960. Hydrophilic gels for biological use. Nature. 185: 117–118.

Widjaja, L.K., M. Bora, P.N.P.H. Chan, V. Lipik, T.T.L. Wong and S.S. Venkatraman. 2014. Hyaluronic acid-based nanocomposite hydrogels for ocular drug delivery applications. J. Biomed. Mater. Res. A. 102: 3056–3065.

Wilson, M.R., E. Hertzmark, A.M. Walker, K. Childs-Shaw and D.L. Epstein. 1987. A case-control study of risk factors in open angle glaucoma. Arch. Ophthalmol. 105: 1066.

Wright, B., S. Mi and C.J. Connon. 2013. Towards the use of hydrogels in the treatment of limbal stem cell deficiency. Drug Discov. Today. 18: 79–86.

Xu, J., X. Li and F. Sun. 2010. Preparation and evaluation of a contact lens vehicle for puerarin delivery. J. Biomater Sci. Polym. Ed. 21: 271–288.

Xu, S., L. Deng, J. Zhang, L. Yin and A. Dong. 2015. Composites of electrospun-fibers and hydrogels: A potential solution to current challenges in biological and biomedical field. J. Biomed. Mater. Res. B. Appl. Biomater.

Xu, X., A.K. Jha, D.A. Harrington, M.C. Farach-Carson and X. Jia. 2012. Hyaluronic acid-based hydrogels: from a natural polysaccharide to complex networks. Soft Matter. 8: 3280–3294.

Zhao, F., D. Yao, R. Guo, L. Deng, A. Dong and J. Zhang. 2015. Composites of polymer hydrogels and nanoparticulate systems for biomedical and pharmaceutical applications. Nanomater. 5: 2054–2130.

12

Hydrogels for Pulmonary Drug Delivery

Ibrahim M. El-Sherbiny,[1,*] *Mohammed Sedki,*[1] *Habiba Soliman*[1] and *Magdi H. Yacoub*[2]

ABSTRACT

Recent research has focused on pulmonary drug delivery as an alternative route of administration for the treatment of different pulmonary diseases as well as others. The pharmaceutical trend has recently been toward pulmonary delivery because of its low metabolic activity, large surface area, high vascularity, and avoidance of hepatic bypass metabolism. Recently, particulate-based drug delivery systems have emerged as innovative and promising approaches for pulmonary delivery. Several particulate-based drug delivery systems have demonstrated a great potential in pulmonary delivery due to their tremendous advantages such as overcoming pulmonary delivery barriers, providing a controlled drug release and increasing therapeutic efficiency which result in reducing dose frequency and adverse side effects. Among different particulate-based drug delivery systems, hydrogels, 3D polymeric networks, have recently been employed and investigated as drug carriers for pulmonary delivery owing to their unique physicochemical properties such as biocompatibility, biodegradability, swelling and mucoadhesive properties. This chapter provides an overview on hydrogels including synthesis methods,

[1] Nanomaterials Laboratory, Center for Materials Science, Zewail City of Science and Technology, 6th October City, 12588 Giza, Egypt.
[2] Harefield Heart Science Centre, National Heart and Lung Institute, Imperial College, London, UK.
* Corresponding author: ielsherbiny@zewailcity.edu.eg

properties, and different types of hydrogels used in the drug delivery to/through the lung. Moreover, it highlights the advantages, current applications and concerns of hydrogels in pulmonary drug delivery.

Keywords: stimuli-responsive, smart polymers, hydrogel, pH-responsive, temperature-responsive, pulmonary, drug, delivery

1. Introduction

1.1 An overview of anatomy and physiology of the respiratory tract

The respiratory system, with the help of the circulatory system, are responsible for oxygen-carbon dioxide gases exchange in cells during the respiration process, in which oxygen is inhaled to lungs and transported by blood to cells and exchanged by carbon dioxide which returns back with blood to lungs to be exhaled. The respiratory system is divided into the upper respiratory tract consisting of nose, nasal cavity and pharynx, and the lower respiratory tract consisting of larynx, trachea, bronchi, bronchioles, and alveoli. Lungs are composed of five lobes, three for the right lung and two for the left one. The gas exchange process occurs at the interface between blood capillaries and alveoli by a rate of 1 pint of inhaled air by 12–15 times per minute, for healthy lungs (El-Sherbiny et al. 2015, Paranjpe and Müller-Goymann 2014).

Alveoli are considered the main functioning parts in lung. They are coated with a layer of mucus and fluids of lipoproteins. These fluids, with a very small barrier between blood capillaries and alveoli of about 0.5 µm, facilitate a fast gas and other dissolved matter exchange with the circulatory system. Lungs have more than 300 million alveoli in a network connection with more than 250 billion capillaries with a huge surface area of about 70 m^2. This huge surface area, as well as many other unique characteristics such as the fast exchange of dissolved matter with circulatory system, high drug bioavailability and avoidance of first pass metabolism, helped pulmonary drug delivery to attract a great attention either in local delivery of drugs to lung to treat pulmonary diseases or as a non-invasive drug administration route for various diseases (McCorry 2008). Figure 1 is a schematic diagram of the upper and lower respiratory tracts (Human anatomy 2016).

2. Challenges in Pulmonary Drug Delivery

In spite of the great potential of lung as a route for drug delivery, few challenges must be considered, the first is the rapid systemic drug absorption, the second is the efficient pulmonary clearance mechanisms, and the third is the enzymatic degradation of the delivered drugs. All these effects result in low drug bioavailability and short life time, and hence, a

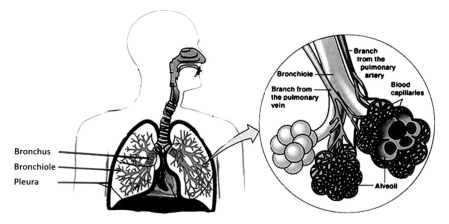

Fig. 1. A schematic diagram of the anatomy of upper and lower respiratory tracts. Reprinted with modification from (Human Anatomy 2016).

poor drug efficacy and adverse side effects (El-Sherbiny et al. 2011, Patton et al. 2010).

The rapid systemic absorption of inhaled drugs is attributed to the high surface area of alveoli-capillaries network and the good epithelial permeability as well as the solubility of drugs in pulmonary fluids. In general, absorption occurs when the inhaled drugs reach mucosa and dissolve in surfactants of tracheobronchial air passages or alveoli. This absorption depends mainly on type of inhaled molecules. For instance, hydrophobic drugs such as peptides aggregate and are cleared out after touching the airways fluids, while hydrophilic drugs of small molecular weight dissolve and get absorbed quickly (Oberdörster 1988, Olsson et al. 2011, Parkinson and Ogilvie 2001). The effect of this rapid absorption depends on the anticipated site of action. For instance, in the case of local drug delivery, rapid systemic drug absorption is an obstacle that should be overcome where drug must be deposited inside lungs and terminated over there, otherwise the drug bioavailability would be affected negatively. On the other hand, the systemic targeting would benefit from this rapid drug absorption.

The clearance mechanisms of respiratory system are of a great importance in prevention of foreign particles, including drugs, from entering the respiratory tract and hence keeping cells healthy. These mechanisms depend particularly on the deposition site of particles. For instance, when the inhaled particles are deposited in the upper airways, they may be removed by the mucociliary clearance escalator, while depositions at deep lung may be cleared by alveolar macrophages (Lohmann-Matthes et al. 1994, Sung et al. 2007). Drug particles are recognized as foreign objects, and are removed in the upper airways by the mucociliary clearance mechanism, which lowers drug bioavailability (Oberdörster 1988). Mucociliary clearance is attributed to the presence of two types of epithelial cells, ciliated cells and mucus-producing (goblet) cells in the upper airways as illustrated in Fig. 2 (Medlin Plus 2016). Mucociliary clearance mechanism starts when a foreign particle, with particle size ≥ 6 μm, enters the upper respiratory tract, where the mucus layer entraps the foreign particles, including drugs and micro-organisms, and then cilia cells push these mucus-entrapping particles back to the mouth. Actions of ciliated cells and goblet cells are in balance under normal conditions. However, this balance gets disturbed in case of respiratory inflammations or infection and accelerates the clearance of drugs, which reduces drug bioavailability and efficiency. Smaller particles of size range 1.0–5.0 μm that would escape the mucociliary escalator defense, however, face engulfment by alveolar macrophages in deep lung (Olsson et al. 2011, Ruge et al. 2013). Alveolar macrophages are phagocytic cells found abundantly in lungs as 12–13 macrophages for each alveolus to clear them from any foreign particles or micro-organisms in the above mentioned range. This defense mechanism would also inhibit the effect of inhaled aerosol drugs and shorten their half-life time in alveoli to few

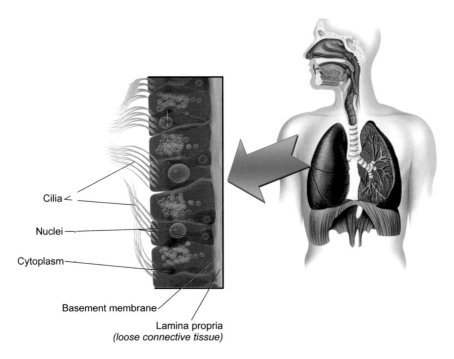

Cilia

Nuclei

Cytoplasm

Basement membrane

Lamina propria
(loose connective tissue)

Fig. 2. A schematic diagram of respiratory tract illustrating structure of cilia and goblet cells. Adapted with modification from (Medlin Plus 2016).

hours. Foreign particles with sizes smaller than 0.5 µm are deposited, by diffusion, in alveoli. However, the majority of these tiny drug particles are exhaled due to their small sizes and mass (Parkinson and Ogilvie 2001).

Metabolic activity of the small concentration of metabolic enzymes in lungs is lower than that in other organs. However, this small concentration affects the inhaled drugs and minimizes their efficiency. These metabolic enzymes act together as the detoxification defense mechanism in lungs against foreign inhaled particles. The primary acting enzymes in lungs are the P_{450} cytochrome (CYP) families which are able to degrade a wide spectrum of inhaled drugs such as ciclesonide, salmeterol, budesonide and theophylline. In addition, peptidase and protease enzymes degrade the peptide and proteins drugs such as insulin (Olsson et al. 2011, Wiedmann et al. 2000).

2.1 Carriers for pulmonary drug delivery

Drug carriers are of great importance in pulmonary drug delivery. The suitable inhalable drug carrier should satisfy some characteristics including biocompatibility, aerodynamic diameter (0.5–5.0 µm), targeted drug delivery, controlled release and the ability to escape the pulmonary clearance mechanisms. Different types of drug carriers including liposomes, nano-in-micro polymeric particles, bio-responsive carriers and hydrogels were tested and evaluated for this purpose (Zeng et al. 1995).

2.1.1 Hydrogels

Hydrogels have been used extensively over the last couple of decades in various biomedical applications including drug delivery, tissue regeneration, wound dressings, bio-implants, biosensors, contact lenses and dental materials as well as in other fields such as agriculture and waste water treatment. Hydrogels are a 3D network of crosslinked polymer chains that contain hydrophilic functional groups where water fills the space between them. They are able to swell and de-swell reversibly depending on some environmental conditions such as pH, temperature, pressure, ionic strength, electric and/or magnetic fields. They are able to absorb water from 10% to many times of their dry weight until reaching the equilibrium. First, as water is absorbed, it hydrates the hydrophilic groups and the network swells further, and this absorbed water is called primary bound water. The additional swelling exposes the hydrophobic groups which also bind some more water called secondary bound water. Together, the primary and secondary bound water, form the total bound water. Any additional water absorbed, due to the osmotic driving force, will fill the spaces between the polymer chains and is called free water. The polymer does not dissolve due to the crosslinks. As more crosslinks are formed between the polymer chains, the solution behaviour changes from Newtonian to viscoelastic and even completely elastic. Similarly, they show Newtonian behaviour at low to moderate concentration where little chain entanglements occur (Akhtar et al. 2015, Gulrez et al. 2011, Hennink and Van Nostrum 2012, Hoffman 2012).

The polymers used in the development of hydrogels are usually soft and elastic, and they can be synthetic such as PVA and PEG or natural such as chitosan, collagen, alginate and fibrin. The crosslinks can be chemical such as covalent and ionic bonds or temporary/permanent physical links such as entanglements, weak ionic interactions or hydrogen bonding. Morphology of hydrogels varies greatly as it can be amorphous, semi-crystalline or crystalline. Physical properties of hydrogel depend particularly on the type of monomer(s) used, fabrication method and the solvent used. Hydrogels can be ionic (anionic or cationic), neutral or ampholytic. When used in biomedical applications, hydrogels are designed in such a way so as to be soft, rubbery and resembling, to a great extent, living tissues, biocompatible with the immune system, having safe degradation products that can be excreted by the kidneys. Hydrogel elasticity reduces irritation to surrounding tissues and cells. In addition, their hydrophilicity reduces the tendency of proteins and cells sticking to them (Akhtar et al. 2015, Slaughter et al. 2009).

2.1.2 Synthesis methods of hydrogels

Hydrogels are prepared *via* crosslinking of synthetic, natural, or combination of both polymers through either physical interactions or the chemical linking of polymer chains.

2.1.2.1 Physical methods for hydrogels preparation

Physical interactions such as chain entanglements, ionic interactions, hydrophobic forces and/or hydrogen bonds between polymer chains can hold these chains together in the form of a hydrogel network. Physical methods usually end up with a reversible gel. The main advantage of these preparation methods is the absence of chemical cross-linking agents which could be toxic and may affect the entrapped bioactive agents. The texture of the developed hydrogels depends on many factors such as the hydrocolloid type, its concentration, pH, etc., and they are usually heterogeneous as clusters of molecular entanglements and ionic forces (Gulrez et al. 2011).

a. Hydrogen bonding

Lowering the pH of aqueous polymer solutions containing carboxyl groups, results in the protonation of these acid groups which can result in hydrogen bond formation. For example, hydrogen bonding occurred between oxygen of polyethylene glycol (PEG) and the carboxylic acid groups of the polyacrylic acid/polymethacrylic acid. In such types, the swelling extent is dependent on the pH value of the medium (Gulrez et al. 2011, Takigami et al. 2007).

b. Heating/cooling of polymer solutions

Cooling a hot aqueous mixture of gelatin and carrageenan results in gelation. This is due to helix-formation of carrageenan cooled solution. The polymer chains transform from random coil configuration at elevated temperatures to solid helical rods. Then, addition of metal ions such as Na^{1+}, K^{1+}, etc. to the helix formed chains, crosslink them more in the form of helices associations and junction zones (Funami et al. 2007) as illustrated in Fig. 3.

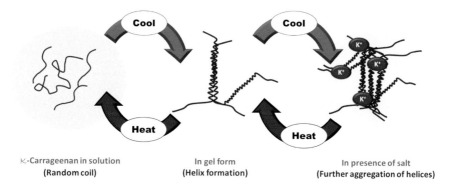

κ-Carrageenan in solution   In gel form   In presence of salt
(Random coil)   (Helix formation)   (Further aggregation of helices)

Fig. 3. Hydrogel formation after cooling of hot solution of carrageenan and addition of salts.

c. Freeze-thaw process

Freeze-thawing cycles induce the formation of microcrystals which is common in some polymeric solutions such as polyvinyl alcohol (PVA). On its own, an aqueous solution of PVA forms a weak gel, and upon subjecting to a cycle of freeze-thaw, an elastic and more tough gel is produced (Giannouli and Morris 2003).

d. Electrostatic interaction (Ionotropic gelation)

Ionic polymers (polyelectrolytes) can be crosslinked upon addition of multivalent counterions to form hydrogel beads or geli-spheres which are capable of gelation and extensive swelling. Biomolecules/drug-loaded polymeric solution is added dropwise into the counterions solution under magnetic stirring. The counterions form a 3-D lattice of ionically-crosslinked moiety by interacting with charged groups on the polymer chains. Concentration of polymer and counterions solution should be in the ratio of number of cross-linking unit. The resulting gel is called an ionotropic gel. As an example, the cross-linking of alginate chains when mixed with calcium ions as the counterions is illustrated in Fig. 4 (Bajpai et al. 2008, Zhao et al. 2009).

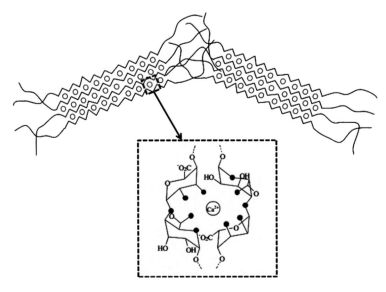

Fig. 4. Hydrogelation of alginate polymer chains upon crosslinking with Ca^{2+} counterions. Reprinted from (Gulrez et al. 2011).

e. Complex coacervation

Hydrogels can be formed by mixing a polycation with a polyanion depending on the pH, concentration and ionic strength of the mixed solutions (Fig. 5). The opposite charges stick together and form a crosslinked network, as in the case of chitosan-alginate hydrogel. The resulting hydrogel is called complex coacervates, polyion complexes, or polyelectrolyte complexes. Protein below their isoelectric point becomes positively charged and can associate with polyanion and form these kinds of hydrogel coacervates (Esteban and Severian 2000).

f. Heat-induced aggregation (maturation)

Polymers with proteinaceous groups can form a gel upon heating. This is due to the aggregation of the proteinaceous groups as it increases the molecular weight and results in a gel with improved water binding capabilities and enhanced mechanical properties. Protein in lower molecular weight fractions agglomerates to increase the concentration of larger molecular

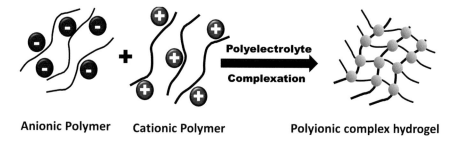

Fig. 5. Polyion complex hydrogel formation by mixing a polycation with a polyanion.

weight fractions. This has been done with gum Arabic, a carbohydrate containing 2–3% protein as well as other gums (Gulrez et al. 2011).

2.1.2.2 Chemical cross-linking of polymer chains

Chemical cross-linking produces permanent hydrogel networks with good mechanical strength. This can be achieved *via* cross-linking of two polymer chains using a suitable cross-linking agent or through the grafting of selected monomers onto the backbone of another polymer to form interpenetrating network. Hydrophobic polymers can be transformed into hydrophilic polymers *via* incorporating polar hydrophilic groups, either by hydrolysis or oxidation followed by covalent cross-linking into hydrogel. Chemically crosslinked hydrogels are usually not homogenous with clusters of high cross-linking density and low water swelling that are spread out within regions of low cross-linking density and high water swelling. This may be due to the hydrophobic aggregation of cross-linking agents. As with physical hydrogels, free end chains and chain loops are the defects found (Hoffman 2012). There are different approaches for preparation of hydrogels *via* chemical cross-linking. Some of these approaches are discussed below:

a. Using crosslinkers

This involves incorporation of other molecules between the polymer chains to form crosslinks. The selection of crosslinker and its chemical composition depends on the type of functional groups on polymer chains such as OH, COOH and NH_2. Polymers can be crosslinked through the reaction of their functional groups with that of the cross-linking agents. These reactions include, for instance, amine-carboxylic acid, isocyanate-OH/NH_2 reactions, Schiff base formation or conventional addition and condensation reactions(Akhtar et al. 2015). Aldehyde crosslinkers such as glutaraldehyde can be used with polymers that contain OH or amine groups. Polymers that have OH groups require harsh reactions conditions such as low pH, high temperature and the addition of methanol as a quencher. On the other hand, polymers that contain amine groups require milder reaction conditions and in such cases, Schiff bases are formed. This is useful in the preparation of crosslinked proteins and amine-containing polysaccharides. In spite of the wide spread use of glutaraldehyde as an efficient crosslinking agent, the main concern of its use is the cytotoxicity even at low concentrations (Hennink and Van Nostrum 2012). Figure 6 illustrates schematically the cross-linking of a hydrophilic polymer containing hydroxyl groups with glutaraldehyde.

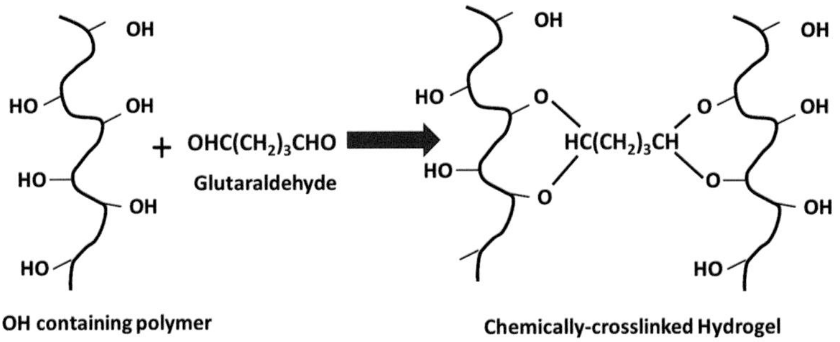

Fig. 6. A schematic representation for crosslinking between hydroxyl groups-containing polymer chains *via* glutaraldehyde crosslinker.

Other cross-linking agents react with the functional groups through addition and/or condensation reactions. For instance, polysaccharides can be crosslinked by addition of 1,6-hexanedibromide, divinylsulfone or 1,6-hexamethylenediisocyanate (Coviello et al. 1999, Simonsen et al. 1995). N,N-(3-dimethylaminopropyl)-N-ethyl carbodiimide (EDC) crosslinks polymers containing an amide group through condensation reaction. Feijen and coworkers synthesized hydrogels of gelatin using EDC. N-hydroxysuccinimide is needed to prevent possible side-reactions and better control over the cross-linking density (Kuijpers et al. 2000).

b. Grafting/free radical polymerization

Polymer chains are activated by chemical reagents and/or irradiation leading to formation of macroradicals. Then, monomers are polymerized onto the macroradical backbones resulting in branching and cross-linking. N-vinyl-2-pyrrolidone is considered one of the chemical activating reagents. High energy radiations such as X-ray, Gamma rays and electron beams produce free radicals on the polymer chain to initiate the polymerization of unsaturated monomers (Alla et al. 2012, Amin et al. 2012).

Radiation cross-linking preserves the biocompatibility of the polymers as no chemical crosslinkers are added. Radiation also sterilizes the resulting hydrogel. Additionally, in aqueous solutions, water absorbs the radiation and radiolysis takes place resulting in formation of hydroxyl radicals which also forms macroradicals by attacking polymer chains. Those macroradicals then recombine forming covalent bonds and a crosslinked structure. This reaction requires mild conditions (room temperature and physiological pH) and an inert atmosphere (nitrogen or argon) as the radicals could react with oxygen. Cross-linking density increases with increasing radiation dose and/or polymer concentration. However, since C-C crosslinks exist, the hydrogels are mostly non biodegradable. Furthermore, bioactive materials need to be added after the hydrogel formation (post loading) as they could be damaged by the radicals and/or radiation. At low concentrations, polymers exposed to radiation degrade as the chain density is too low and chains do not overlap enough to recombine and form crosslinks. In pastes, polymer concentration is high enough so that it can form free radicals directly and enough water to undergo radiolysis. Thus, there is a high concentration of polymer radicals as well as secondary polymer fragments. Cross-linking takes place *via* both radical-radical reaction and polymer-polymer reactions (Gulrez et al. 2011, Hennink and Van Nostrum 2012).

c. Enzyme cross-linking

The most commonly used enzymes in enzyme cross-linking are transglutaminase and peroxidase. Transglutaminases require mild conditions and no cofactors. They catalyze the formation of a covalent bond between the free amine group in lysine and the γ-carboxamide group in glutamine, hence, the polymer needs to be conjugated with amino acids/peptides/proteins. They are Ca^{2+} dependent and thus, gelation can be triggered, where normally, the gelation rate is quite fast (5–20 mins). However, they have a short half-life of only 11 hours, and are large and thus difficult to produce recombinantly. Horseradish peroxidase and soy bean peroxidase are the most widely used peroxidases in hydrogel synthesis. They have a very fast gelation rate, from seconds to a few minutes. As with glutaminases, polymer should be conjugated with amino acids, peptides or proteins. The main advantage of using peroxidases in cross-linking process of polymers into hydrogels is their reported nontoxicity (Hennink and Van Nostrum 2012, Teixeira et al. 2012).

2.2.2 *Advantages of hydrogel-based pulmonary drug delivery*

The airways of respiratory tract are covered with a thick layer of mucus (5–10 µm) that has some surface properties such as wettability and adhesivisity. These properties enable mucus to entrap the foreign particles that enter the lungs, followed by their removal with the aid of the mucociliary clearance mechanism. In the case of hydrogels, especially those with mucoadhesive characteristics, they adhere to mucus layer strongly and alter the viscoelastic properties of mucosal fluids which inhibit their clearance action against the administered drugs loaded into the hydrogel particles. In this way, a longer contact time between drug-releasing hydrogel and the respiratory system is achieved (Shahiwala and Misra 2005). However, there are many concerns about the increase of viscoelastic properties of mucus and also the inhibition of mucociliary clearance mechanism (Yang et al. 2009). Another important clearance mechanism of the respiratory system is the alveolar phagocytosis of foreign particulates with an aerodynamic diameter of 0.5–5.0 µm, and hence, a loss in pharmacological effects of inhaled drug particulates (Balasubramanian et al. 2013, Mahmud and Discher 2011). Some research articles discussed the delivery of drugs in nano-carriers to evade the macrophages and diffuse to alveolar cells, but this is countered by the direct exhalation of these small particles (Beck-Broichsitter et al. 2009, Grenha et al. 2005, Todoroff and Vanbever 2011). Powder hydrogels are prepared in a dried form with aerodynamic sizes suitable for settlement into deep lung to ensure a high absorption of drugs and then they swell, when they touch the moisture of airways fluids, to larger sizes that cannot be engulfed by alveolar macrophages (El-Sherbiny and Smyth 2010, Selvam et al. 2011). The effect of mucoadhesion of hydrogels on inhibition of mucociliary clearance has been tested *in vivo* in few cases (Hwang et al. 2008, Sakagami et al. 2002, Surendrakumar et al. 2003). However, the timescale renewal of mucus and the negative effects of inhibiting the mucociliary escalator are still considerable limitations. On the other hand, the remarkable swelling properties of hydrogels can avoid the macrophage uptake either chemically or physically. Chemically, the highly hydrated polymers show a significant stealth effect against macrophages, as in the case of using polyethylene glycol (PEG). In recent studies, the use of PEG (PEGylation) became a common step to avoid phagocytosis. Physically, particles swell and enlarge to the extent that macrophages cannot uptake them. Swelling level of hydrogels depend on the degree of cross-linking, application environment conditions, and the type of polymer itself (Chen et al. 2011, González-Alvarez and Bermejo 2013, Guvendiren et al. 2010). The tunable mechanical property is another advantage of hydrogel particle where it can be controlled and engineered as required by controlling the level of cross-linking. In general, increasing degree of cross-linking results in stronger but brittle hydrogels (Das 2013, Shetye and Bhilegaokar 2015).

2.2.3 Types of hydrogels used for pulmonary drug delivery

Hydrogels are classified generally into many categories according to different bases such as physical appearance, polymeric composition, charge, source of polymers, configuration and type of cross-linking (Shetye et al. 2015).

  i. According to source of polymers, hydrogels are classified into natural and synthetic ones.
 ii. Regarding their physical appearance, hydrogels appear as film, matrix or sphere, and this depends particularly on the preparation method.
iii. According to the net charge located on the crosslinked polymer chains, hydrogels can be neutral, ionic (cationic or anionic) or ampholytic (amphoteric) electrolyte with both basic and acidic groups.
 iv. Regarding their polymeric composition, hydrogels are classified into homopolymeric, where the building monomers/polymers are of the same species, and copolymeric, where the building monomers/polymers are of two different species and at least one of them is hydrophilic, multi-polymer interpenetrating polymeric hydrogel (IPN), which is a highly important class of polymers.
  v. Depending on their crystalline configuration, hydrogels may be crystalline, semi-crystalline or amorphous (non-crystalline).
 vi. According to the cross-linking between polymer chains, hydrogels are classified into chemically crosslinked and physically crosslinked.

On the other hand, hydrogels applied in pulmonary drug delivery could be summarized in four categories depending on their mode of drug release and way of assembly or composition. These categories and their most recent applications in pulmonary drug delivery are discussed in detail below.

2.2.3.1 Swellable hydrogels

To meet the requirements of pulmonary drug delivery mentioned above, such swellable hydrogel micro particles were developed by El-Sherbiny et al. (El-Sherbiny and Smyth 2010, El-Sherbiny et al. 2010) using chitosan, PEG and pluronic F108. Chitosan was used as it is a non-toxic, biocompatible and biodegradable natural polymer. It also aids drug absorption in the lungs as it helps in preventing enzymatic degradation and opens tight junctions between epithelial cells (Park et al. 2006). However, chitosan displays some characteristics of hydrophobicity and thus needs to be grafted with a hydrophilic polymer. PEG was the polymer of choice due to its hydrophilicity, biodegradability and desired biocompatibility. Furthermore, coating chitosan with PEG reduces macrophage clearance. Pluronics are biocompatible triblock copolymers that contain both hydrophilic poly(ethylene oxide) and hydrophobic poly(propylene oxide) blocks arranged in an A-B-A pattern, and hence they can also act as surfactants and solvate hydrophobic drugs in aqueous media. The hydrogel microparticles were prepared *via* cryomilling of the dried graft copolymers under mild conditions. Three variations were produced: PEG grafted onto chitosan, PEG grafted onto chitosan derivative, N-phythaloyl chitosan (NPHCs) and both in combination of pluronic. They were crosslinked by amphiphilic interaction between the copolymer chains and the copolymers and/or the pluronics (Fig. 7). The dry and swelled sizes of the developed hydrogel particles as well as their swelling patterns were assessed as they

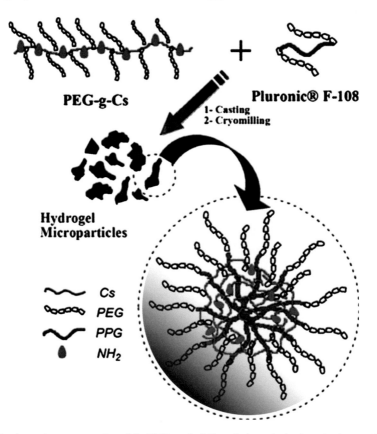

Fig. 7. A schematic representation of the PEG-grafted-Cs and pluronics hydrogel microparticles. Reprinted from (El-Sherbiny et al. 2010).

needed to have a respirable size when dry and then swell after depositing in the deep lungs. The synthesized particles had irregular shapes and their volume median diameters were in the range of 10–13.7 μm, and it was noted that those with NPHCs were smaller. Likewise, increasing the percentage of pluronic resulted in a smaller size. Swelling of the obtained hydrogel particles in simulated body fluids resulted in an increase of size between 700–1300%. Both the PEG-chitosan and the PEG-chitosan-pluronic showed fast swelling within the first 30 mins. The rest showed a relative gradual increase over the course of 1 hour. This is due to the osmotic driving force and the hydrophilicity of the hydrogel. Swelling is then opposed by the crosslinks which may force some of the swelling fluid to leave. All of this is dependent on the crosslink density, and equilibrium is achieved when a balance between the osmotic forces and the cohesive forces is reached. At equilibrium, those that contained NPHCS had significantly lower degrees of swelling. This may be due to the hydrophobic phythaloyl group whose hydrophobicity slows down water entering the matrix. It was noticed that decreasing the percentage of the pluronic increases the swelling degree at equilibrium but in a statistically insignificant manner. This may be due to an increase in cross-linking density due to the extra amphiphilic interaction (El-Sherbiny and Smyth 2010, El-Sherbiny et al. 2010).

Degradation and release studies were performed to determine the system's potential as a drug carrier. Degradation study was performed using the enzyme, lysozyme which is present in saliva, tears, mucus (even in airways), primary and secondary granules of neutrophils and granules of mononuclear phagocytes (Ganz 2002). Degradation started within the first hour, and those that contained pluronic showed less degradation. This may be attributed to the swelling behaviour mentioned above, where those with pluronics exhibited less swelling which would slow down the diffusion of enzymes. Particles that contain NPHCs were less degradable than those with chitosan due to the hydrophobicity and/or the steric hindrance of the bulky phythaloyl group. The release study was performed with the hydrophilic model drug, sodium fluorescein, and the release profile goes as follows: an initial burst within the first 30 mins followed by a slow sustained release for up to 10 days, during which a faster release was observed due to particle degradation (El-Sherbiny and Smyth 2010).

Continuing their previous work, the same group has developed a carrier where swellable hydrogel system encapsulates nanoparticles (NPs) since earlier studies had shown that NPs stay in the lungs once deposited. They are not cleared up by the phagocytosis or ciliary action (Kawaguchi et al. 1986, Günter Oberdörster 2000, Rudt and Müller 1992). Thus, encapsulating NPs into a swellable hydrogel carrier system is promising as it could prevent their exhalation. Sodium alginate, a poly anionic, biodegradable, biocompatible and non-toxic polymer was selected to be used for the outer hydrogel microspheres while PEG grafted onto NPHCS (PEG-g-NPHCS) was selected for the inner NPs. The microspheres were prepared by spray drying of sodium alginate solution containing the NPs and cross-linking was performed by ionotropic gelation using calcium ions.

As with their prior work, the particle size, swelling, degradation and drug release were measured to assess the suitability of the developed nano-in-micro swellable hydrogel system as a drug carrier. The size of the obtained NPs was 206.4 ± 34.8 nm. The microspheres were 1.02–2.63 µm in aerodynamic diameter. The developed hydrogel carrier particles showed a fast initial swelling during the first 2 mins from 4 µm when dry to 23.6, 26.0 and 48.1 µm depending on the weight composition, alginate vs NPs. Swelling increased regularly for the next 20 mins reaching 84.1, 66.3 and 84.2 µm. Increasing percentage of alginate decreases size at equilibrium; as with the pervious situation, this may be due to a higher cross-linking density. Increasing percent by weight of NPs decreased degradation rate. In congruence with the pervious study, there was also an initial burst of release which could be due to the fast initial swelling. Afterwards, there was a sustained release of drug in the microsphere for the following 4 days. This was followed by a period of slower release (a second phase of drug release from the NPs). Moreover, the preliminary *in-vitro* aerosolization study using a dry-powder, breath-activated inhaler device has shown that the hydrogel microspheres are suitable for pulmonary drug delivery (El-Sherbiny and Smyth 2010). These results were followed by another study also based on a nano-in-micro carrier system but with the PEG-chitosan graft as hydrogel microparticles while the NPs were made from poly(lactic-co-glycolic acid), PLGA. This study involved the pulmonary delivery of curcumin with enhancing its bioavailability. Curcumin, a good anti-inflammatory and antioxidant with tumour inhibiting properties, has potential in the treatment of asthma and COPDs (Egan et al. 2004, Huang et al. 1997, Reddy and Lokesh 1994, Sethi et al. 2009). However, it is chemically unstable in the gastro intestinal tract (GIT) and has low water solubility (Cheng et al. 2001, Dhillon et al. 2008). As such, a carrier system based on encapsulation of curcumin loaded PLGA NPs in PEG-chitosan hydrogel microparticles has been developed to increase curcumin's therapeutic potential through sustained release, higher dosage and delivery not just to the alveoli but also to the lumen. Its swelling capabilities, degradation, release and encapsulation were also assessed. The curcumin loaded PLGA NPs were synthesized by the single emulsion–solvent evaporation method. The hydrogel microparticles were prepared by spray-drying of a homogenous solution containing the NPs of either the PEG-chitosan graft copolymer or chitosan alone. The developed plain and curcumin-loaded NPs had an average radius (R) of 221.9 ± 16.6 and 243.4 ± 34.8 nm, respectively. Volume median diameter (VMD) of curcumin containing microsphere was between 3.1 and 3.9 µm while those without curcumin had VMD between 3.1 and 3.9. Increasing the percentage of PLGA NPs increased particle size in a statistically insignificant manner. As with the above mentioned studies, there was a fast initial swelling followed by a continuous swelling regularly for the next 20 mins. Increasing PLGA content decreased particle size at equilibrium which may be due to the hydrophobicity of PLGA. Degradation of the microparticles by lysozyme started within the first few hours. Carriers with grafted PEG showed less degradation. Similarly, lowering the percentage of PLGA reduced degradation. Entrapment efficiency of curcumin was from 89.6 to 94.4 and was unaffected by particle composition. There was an initial burst release of drug within the first hour which could be due to the fast initial swelling followed by a relatively slow release. Increasing PLGA content decreased amount of curcumin released. Based on the obtained results, this nano-in-swellable hydrogel microparticles system was deemed suitable for pulmonary drug delivery (El-Sherbiny and Smyth 2010).

2.2.3.2 Stimuli-responsive hydrogels

Stimuli-responsive or smart hydrogels would change their physical or chemical properties in response to an external stimulus such as pH, temperature, magnetic field, electric field, enzyme, etc. Scientists worked thoroughly on this type of hydrogels and used it in different applications including pulmonary drug delivery (Stocke et al. 2015). Using various building monomers, different types of crosslinkers and adjusting synthesis conditions, properties of hydrogels could be tuned in a variety of controlled manners involving size shrinkage/swelling, changing permeability or even degradation of the whole network, and hence a control in the drug release (De et al. 2002, Ghandehari et al. 1997, Hickey and Mansour 2009, Secret et al. 2014, Soppimath et al. 2002). Liquid aerosols of stimuli-responsive nano and microparticles of hydrogels suspensions were also tested using nebulizers and metered dose inhalers (Farhat et al. 2009, Selvam et al. 2011). In addition, the *in vivo* study of applying 220 nm hydrogel NPs in pulmonary drug delivery showed a sustained release of some peptide, thereby highlighting their potential in pulmonary drug delivery (Lee et al. 2012).

a. pH-responsive hydrogels

pH-responsive hydrogels are of great importance as drug carriers and have been widely studied because of the large variation in body physiological pH in different sites in both normal and pathological conditions (Gupta et al. 2002). Many research articles have introduced different types of pH-responsive hydrogel nano/microparticles as drug delivery systems in different human organs. However, this was the first time to introduce a strong promising study by Stocke et al. (2015) as pH-responsive hydrogel

NPs (HNPs) for pulmonary drug delivery. In this work, the HNPs were prepared by polymerization of methacrylic acid (MAA) with poly(ethylene glycol) (n = 400) diacrylate (PEG400DA) as the crosslinker. Two different particle sizes were prepared and evaluated for their hydrodynamic diameters, under effect of different pH values with the aid of dynamic light scattering (DLS). One particle size was selected to be formulated in a powder composite for spray drying. and the aerodynamic characteristics were evaluated for the inhalable dried particles. The pH response of the MAA-HNPs depends on the chemical behaviour of MAA (Halacheva et al. 2013). At low pHs (acidic medium), the carboxylic groups of MAA are protonated, negative charges are reduced and more H-bonds are formed, resulting in size shrinkage of HNPs, while at higher pH values (alkaline medium), the carboxylic groups are deprotonated, more negative charges, and so repulsion forces and less H-bonds are formed, resulting in swelling of HNPs, and hence an increase in particle size (Fig. 8).

These HNPs were prepared in two different sizes, 270 and 120 nm at their highest swelling state, referred to as HNPs270 and HNPs120, respectively. Diameters of HNPs270 and HNPs120 were reduced to 115 nm and 80 nm when they agglomerated at lower pH values. The interesting part in this point is the particles agglomeration at higher pHs for smaller particle sizes, which means we can tune the particle size by controlling the initial particle size and composition to precipitate at deep lungs and also escape phagocytosis. The positively charged anticancer drug, cisplatin was loaded to these HNPs by electrostatic interactions to be released in lower pH values at tumour sites in lungs (Zhou et al. 2015).

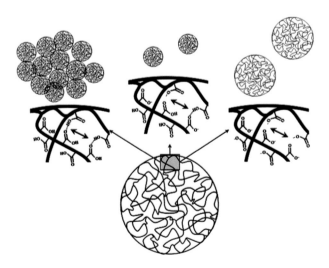

Fig. 8. A schematic diagram of pH-responsive hydrogel NPs at high pH (right) and low pH (left). Reprinted from (Stocke et al. 2015).

b. Enzyme-responsive hydrogels

Enzymes are very specific as they catalyze the reaction of only certain substrates (and/or substrate mimics) into specific products. Briefly, the substrate/substrate mimic binds to the enzyme forming an enzyme-substrate complex. Then, a chemical transformation takes place in the form of whether making or breaking chemical bonds in the complex. Incorporating enzyme substrates/substrate mimics in hydrogels has a very high potential for targeted therapy as enzymes are very selective and vary in distribution between different tissues, cell types, development stage, phase in the cell cycle, disease, disease stage, etc. (Ulijn 2006, Yang and Xu 2006). Researchers have synthesized systems where disease-specific enzymes initiate drug or prodrug release from the hydrogel. One method used enzyme-triggered gel dissolution in which the drug was not conjugated using any linkers but was rather held freely within the polymer matrix. The pharmacokinetics and release profile could be controlled *via* the polymer design (Ulijn et al. 2007). An additional novel technique involves the use of substrate that is converted into a hydrogelator by the enzyme catalyzed reaction, consequently inducing hydrogel formation. Another way is to conjugate the drug to a specific enzyme-cleavable linker. Access to these linkers by the enzyme can also be controlled by other stimuli such as change in temperature or pH. It is also possible that the linkers are made of peptides which can be designed to be enzyme specific or have the peptide itself incorporated within the polymer chains (Plunkett et al. 2005). This is the main trend for using enzyme-responsive hydrogels for pulmonary drug delivery, as illustrated in Fig. 9.

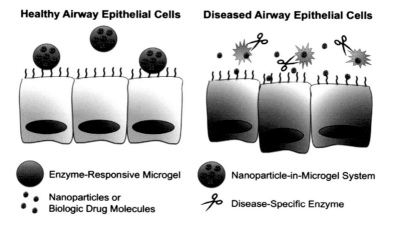

Fig. 9. A schematic diagram of the enzyme-responsive hydrogels for pulmonary drug delivery. Reprinted from (Wanakule et al. 2012).

Enzyme-responsive PEG-based HNPs have been developed for pulmonary drug delivery by emulsion polymerization. These incorporate collagenase, a metalloproteinase, and specific peptides within the polymer backbone *via* a coupling reaction, as illustrated in Fig. 10. Metalloproteinases are proteases overexpressed in pulmonary diseases such as TB, COPD and lung cancer, where the metalloproteinase-2 up to 17 fold in lung carcinoma samples compared to healthy controls. The peptide was a trimer with the sequence Gly-Leu-Lys, The Gly-Leu bond for cleavage by the enzyme while the lysine was added to provide an extra amine group for the coupling reaction. To show that these particles are indeed enzyme-responsive, they were dispersed and incubated with collagenase. After 24 hours, they were completely degraded by the enzyme at the enzyme concentrations higher than 6 µg/ml, and showed some degradation at 2 µg/ml. Particles not containing the peptide were degraded at the same rate as those in PBS solution. To test for the specificity of the peptide, the particles were incubated with another activated metalloproteinase called MMP2, and these were not degraded. It should also be noted that the degradation rate was affected by the molecular weight of the PEG used and whether it was PEG or PEG-diacrylate (PEGDA).

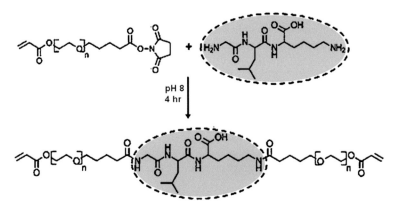

Fig. 10. Coupling reaction between peptide and PEG precursor. Adapted with modification from (Secret et al. 2014).

To increase enzyme sensitivity, a second peptide containing nine amino acids with the sequence Gly-Pro-Gln-Gly-Ile-Phe-Gly-Gln-Lys (GPQGIFGQK) was used. Particles were completely degraded at collagenase concentration of 0.6 µg/ml indicating that the longer peptide has a higher affinity for it. They were also able to be degraded by MMP-2 (Law et al. 2006, Secret et al. 2014). Continuing work, the cytotoxicity of particles containing the long peptide was assessed using a lactate dehydrogenase (LDH) assay and a live/dead assay on healthy lung fibroblasts (IMR-90) and lung carcinoma cells (A549). The particles were biocompatible in both cell lines. Furthermore, a release study for three drugs, hydrophilic, hydrophobic and a protein drug was performed. The drug was added to the polymer solution before emulsion to encapsulate it, resulting in the drug being physically entrapped within the polymer matrix. In the absence of collagenase, only 15–17% of the either drug was released while at concentrations of 0.6 and 3 mg/ml of collagenase, 100% of the drug was released rapidly within 24 hours. The hydrophobic drug had a slower release than the hydrophilic drug (5 hours vs. 1 hour at the same enzyme concentration) and required higher, but still clinically relevant, enzyme concentration. In the presence of the enzyme, the release profile of the protein was similar to that of the hydrophobic drug. Thus, by editing the sequence and/or length of peptide chain, different enzymes could potentially be targeted (Secret et al. 2015).

3. Future Perspectives

Hydrogels have opened new promising channels in pulmonary drug delivery, either for local or systemic purposes. The recent *in vitro* studies, at this point, highlights the ability of hydrogels to deliver many kinds of therapeutic agents such as small molecules, proteins, peptides and even genes successfully to deep lung which broadens the scope of their application as drug carriers. In addition, hydrogels' unique properties of tunable sizes by swelling/deswelling which enable them to escape the respiratory clearance mechanisms, mucoadhesion which increases exposure time and decreases mucociliary escalator action, and the stimuli-responsive characters enabled them to achieve the controlled release manner and the targeted delivery of therapeutics, which lowers drug doses and frequencies and decreases drug side effects. All the above mentioned advantages of hydrogels entitle them to be excellent candidates for pulmonary drug delivery. However, there is still a huge gap between lab (*in vitro*) studies level and the clinical applications due to the huge challenges regarding deep lung delivery, low immunological response, long-term safety of these newly introduced materials, variation in physiological conditions of lungs between different pulmonary diseases, etc. Therefore, further studies on both levels of *in vitro* and *in vivo* are still needed to enhance the applicability of hydrogels in pulmonary drug delivery.

References

Akhtar, M.F., M. Hanif and N.M. Ranjha. 2015. Methods of synthesis of hydrogels. A review. SPJ.
Alla, S.G.A., M. Sen and A.W.M. El-Naggar. 2012. Swelling and mechanical properties of superabsorbent hydrogels based on Tara gum/acrylic acid synthesized by gamma radiation. Carbohydr. Polym. 89(2): 478–485.

Amin, M.C.I.M., N. Ahmad, N. Halib and I. Ahmad. 2012. Synthesis and characterization of thermo- and pH-responsive bacterial cellulose/acrylic acid hydrogels for drug delivery. Carbohydr. Polym. 88(2): 465–473.

Bajpai, A., S.K. Shukla, S. Bhanu and S. Kankane. 2008. Responsive polymers in controlled drug delivery. Prog. Polym. Sci. 33(11): 1088–1118.

Balasubramanian, S.K., K.-W. Poh, C.-N. Ong, W.G. Kreyling, W.-Y. Ong and E.Y. Liya. 2013. The effect of primary particle size on biodistribution of inhaled gold nano-agglomerates. Biomaterials. 34(22): 5439–5452.

Beck-Broichsitter, M., J. Gauss, C.B. Packhaeuser, K. Lahnstein, T. Schmehl, W. Seeger et al. 2009. Pulmonary drug delivery with aerosolizable nanoparticles in an *ex vivo* lung model. Int. J. Pharm. 367(1): 169–178.

Chen, K., Q.S. Zhang and L. Chen. 2011. Effect of cross-linking degree on hydrogels using surfactant detergent as template. Paper Presented at the Adv. Mat. Res.

Cheng, A.-L., C.-H. Hsu, J.-K. Lin, M.-M. Hsu, Y.-F. Ho, T.-S. Shen et al. 2001. Phase I clinical trial of curcumin, a chemopreventive agent, in patients with high-risk or pre-malignant lesions. Anticancer Res. 21(4B): 2895–2900.

Coviello, T., M. Grassi, G. Rambone, E. Santucci, M. Carafa, E. Murtas et al. 1999. Novel hydrogel system from scleroglucan: synthesis and characterization. J. Control. Release. 60(2): 367–378.

Das, N. 2013. Preparation methods and properties of hydrogel: a review. Int. J. Pharm. Sci. 5: 112–117.

De, S.K., N. Aluru, B. Johnson, W. Crone, D.J. Beebe and J. Moore. 2002. Equilibrium swelling and kinetics of pH-responsive hydrogels: Models, experiments, and simulations. J. Microelectromech. Syst. 11(5): 544–555.

Dhillon, N., B.B. Aggarwal, R.A. Newman, R.A. Wolff, A.B. Kunnumakkara, J.L Abbruzzese et al. 2008. Phase II trial of curcumin in patients with advanced pancreatic cancer. Clin. Cancer Res. 14(14): 4491–4499.

Egan, M.E., M. Pearson, S.A. Weiner, V. Rajendran, D. Rubin, J. Glöckner-Pagel et al. 2004. Curcumin, a major constituent of turmeric, corrects cystic fibrosis defects. Science. 304(5670): 600–602.

El-Sherbiny, I.M. and H.D. Smyth. 2010a. Poly(ethylene glycol)–carboxymethyl chitosan-based pH-responsive hydrogels: photo-induced synthesis, characterization, swelling, and *in vitro* evaluation as potential drug carriers. Carbohydr. Res. 345(14): 2004–2012.

El-Sherbiny, I.M., S. McGill and H.D. Smyth. 2010b. Swellable microparticles as carriers for sustained pulmonary drug delivery. J. Pharm. Sci. 99(5): 2343–2356.

El-Sherbiny, I. and H. Smyth. 2010. Novel cryomilled physically cross-linked biodegradable hydrogel microparticles as carriers for inhalation therapy. J. Microencapsul. 27(8): 657–668.

El-Sherbiny, I.M., D.G. Villanueva, D. Herrera and H.D. Smyth. 2011. Overcoming lung clearance mechanisms for controlled release drug delivery. pp. 101–126. *In*: Controlled pulmonary drug delivery, Springer.

El-Sherbiny, I.M., N.M. El-Baz and M.H. Yacoub. 2015. Inhaled nano-and microparticles for drug delivery. Glob. Cardiol. Sci. Pract. 2015.

Esteban, C. and D. Severian. 2000. Polyionic hydrogels based on xanthan and chitosan for stabilising and controlled release of vitamins, Vol. WO0004086 (A1).

Farhat, A., Y. Holloway, T. Jones, S. Taylor, S. Britland and D. Eagland. 2009. Towards improved pulmonary delivery of budesonide using a nebulisable nanoparticulate hydrogel. Paper Presented at the J. Pharm. Pharmacol.

Funami, T., M. Hiroe, S. Noda, I. Asai, S. Ikeda and K. Nishinari. 2007. Influence of molecular structure imaged with atomic force microscopy on the rheological behavior of carrageenan aqueous systems in the presence or absence of cations. Food Hydrocoll. 21(4): 617–629.

Ganz, T. 2002. Antimicrobial polypeptides in host defense of the respiratory tract. The J. Clin. Invest. 109(6): 693–697.

Gehrke, S.H., L.H. Uhden and J.F. McBride. 1998. Enhanced loading and activity retention of bioactive proteins in hydrogel delivery systems. J. Control. Release. 55(1): 21–33.

Ghandehari, H., P. Kopečková and J. Kopecek. 1997. *In vitro* degradation of pH-sensitive hydrogels containing aromatic azo bonds. Biomaterials. 18(12): 861–872.

Giannouli, P. and E. Morris. 2003. Cryogelation of xanthan. Food Hydrocoll. 17(4): 495–501.

González-Alvarez, M., I. González-Alvarez and M. Bermejo. 2013. Hydrogels: an interesting strategy for smart drug delivery. Ther. Deliv. 4(2): 157–160.

Grenha, A., B. Seijo and C. Remunán-López. 2005. Microencapsulated chitosan nanoparticles for lung protein delivery. Eur. J. Pharm. Sci. 25(4): 427–437.

Gulrez, S.K., G.O. Phillips and S. Al-Assaf. 2011. Hydrogels: methods of preparation, characterisation and applications: INTECH Open Access Publisher.

Gupta, P., K. Vermani and S. Garg. 2002. Hydrogels: from controlled release to pH-responsive drug delivery. Drug Discov. Today. 7(10): 569–579.

Guvendiren, M., J.A. Burdick and S. Yang. 2010. Kinetic study of swelling-induced surface pattern formation and ordering in hydrogel films with depth-wise crosslinking gradient. Soft Matter. 6(9): 2044–2049.

Halacheva, S.S., T.J. Freemont and B.R. Saunders. 2013. pH-responsive physical gels from poly(meth) acrylic acid-containing crosslinked particles: the relationship between structure and mechanical properties. J. Mater. Chem. B. 1(33): 4065–4078.

Hennink, W. and C.F. Van Nostrum. 2012. Novel crosslinking methods to design hydrogels. Adv. Drug Deliv. Rev. 64: 223–236.

Hickey, A.J. and H.M. Mansour. 2009. Delivery of drugs by the pulmonary route. Modern Pharmaceutics. 2: 191–220.

Hoffman, A.S. 2012. Hydrogels for Biomedical Applications. Adv. Drug Deliv. Rev. 64: 18–23.

Huang, M.T., H.L. Newmark and K. Frenkel. 1997. Inhibitory effects of curcumin on tumorigenesis in mice. J. Cell. Biochem. 67(S27): 26–34.

Human Anatomy Pictures-Structure of The Lower Respiratory Tract. February 11, 2016. Available at: http://anatomypicture.us/structure-of-the-lower-respiratory-tract/.

Hwang, S., D. Kim, S. Chung and C. Shim. 2008. Delivery of ofloxacin to the lung and alveolar macrophages *via* hyaluronan microspheres for the treatment of tuberculosis. J. Control. Release. 129(2): 100–106.

Kawaguchi, H., N. Koiwai, Y. Ohtsuka, M. Miyamoto and S. Sasakawa. 1986. Phagocytosis of latex particles by leucocytes. I. Dependence of phagocytosis on the size and surface potential of particles. Biomaterials. 7(1): 61–66.

Kuijpers, A., P. Van Wachem, M. Van Luyn, G. Engbers, J. Krijgsveld, S. Zaat et al. 2000. *In vivo* and *in vitro* release of lysozyme from cross-linked gelatin hydrogels: a model system for the delivery of antibacterial proteins from prosthetic heart valves. J. Control. Release. 67(2): 323–336.

Law, B., R. Weissleder and C.-H. Tung. 2006. Peptide-based biomaterials for protease-enhanced drug delivery. Biomacromolecules. 7(4): 1261–1265.

Lee, J., C. Lee, T.H. Kim, E.S. Lee, B.S. Shin, S.-C. Chi et al. 2012. Self-assembled glycol chitosan nanogels containing palmityl-acylated exendin-4 peptide as a long-acting anti-diabetic inhalation system. J. Control. Release. 161(3): 728–734.

Lohmann-Matthes, M., C. Steinmuller and G. Franke-Ullmann. 1994. Pulmonary macrophages. Eur. Respir. J. 7(9): 1678–1689.

Mahmud, A. and D.E. Discher. 2011. Lung vascular targeting through inhalation delivery: insight from filamentous viruses and other shapes. IUBMB Life. 63(8): 607–612.

McCorry, L.K. 2008. Essentials of human physiology for pharmacy: CRC Press.

Medlin Plus-Respiratory cilia. September 3, 2016. Available at:https://medlineplus.gov/ency/imagepages/19533.htm.

Oberdörster, G. 1988. Lung clearance of inhaled insoluble and soluble particles. J. Aerosol. Med. 1(4): 289–330.

Oberdörster, G. 2000. Pulmonary effects of inhaled ultrafine particles. Int. Arch. Occup. Environ. Health. 74(1): 1–8.

Olsson, B., E. Bondesson, L. Borgström, S. Edsbäcker, S. Eirefelt, K. Ekelund et al. 2011. Pulmonary drug metabolism, clearance, and absorption. pp. 21–50. *In*: Hugh D.C. Smyth and Anthony J. Hickey [eds.]. Controlled Pulmonary Drug Delivery. Springer.

Paranjpe, M. and C.C. Müller-Goymann. 2014. Nanoparticle-mediated pulmonary drug delivery: a review. Int. J. Mol. Sci. 15(4): 5852–5873.

Park, J.H., S. Kwon, M. Lee, H. Chung, J.-H. Kim, Y.-S. Kim et al. 2006. Self-assembled nanoparticles based on glycol chitosan bearing hydrophobic moieties as carriers for doxorubicin: *in vivo* biodistribution and anti-tumor activity. Biomaterials. 27(1): 119–126.

Parkinson, A. and B.W. Ogilvie. 2001. Biotransformation of xenobiotics: McGraw-Hill New York.

Patton, J.S., J.D. Brain, L.A. Davies, J. Fiegel, M. Gumbleton, K.-J. Kim et al. 2010. The particle has landed—characterizing the fate of inhaled pharmaceuticals. Int. J. Mol. Sci. and Pulm. Drug Deliv. 23(S2): S-71–S-87.

Plunkett, K.N., K.L. Berkowski and J.S. Moore. 2005. Chymotrypsin responsive hydrogel: application of a disulfide exchange protocol for the preparation of methacrylamide containing peptides. Biomacromolecules. 6(2): 632–637.

Reddy, A.C.P. and B. Lokesh. 1994. Effect of dietary turmeric (Curcuma longa) on iron-induced lipid peroxidation in the rat liver. Food Chem. Toxicol. 32(3): 279–283.

Rudt, S. and R. Müller. 1992. *In vitro* phagocytosis assay of nano-and microparticles by chemiluminescence. I. Effect of analytical parameters, particle size and particle concentration. J. Control. Release. 22(3): 263–271.

Ruge, C.A., J. Kirch and C.-M. Lehr. 2013. Pulmonary drug delivery: from generating aerosols to overcoming biological barriers—therapeutic possibilities and technological challenges. Lancet Respir. Med. 1(5): 402–413.

Sakagami, M., W. Kinoshita, K. Sakon, J.-i. Sato and Y. Makino. 2002. Mucoadhesive beclomethasone microspheres for powder inhalation: their pharmacokinetics and pharmacodynamics evaluation. J. Control. Release. 80(1): 207–218.

Secret, E., S.J. Kelly, K.E. Crannell and J.S. Andrew. 2014. Enzyme-responsive hydrogel microparticles for pulmonary Drug Delivery. ACS Appl. Mater. Interfaces. 6(13): 10313–10321.

Secret, E., K.E. Crannell, S.J. Kelly, M. Villancio-Wolter and J.S. Andrew. 2015. Matrix metalloproteinase-sensitive hydrogel microparticles for pulmonary drug delivery of small molecule drugs or proteins. J. Mater. Chem. B. 3(27): 5629–5634.

Selvam, P., I.M. El-Sherbiny and H.D. Smyth. 2011. Swellable hydrogel particles for controlled release pulmonary administration using propellant-driven metered dose inhalers. J Aerosol Med. Pulm. Drug Deliv. 24(1): 25–34.

Sethi, G., B. Sung and B.B. Aggarwal. 2009. The role of curcumin in modern medicine. pp. 97–113. *In*: Herbal Drugs: Ethnomedicine to modern medicine. Springer.

Shahiwala, A. and A. Misra. 2005. A preliminary pharmacokinetic study of liposomal leuprolide dry powder inhaler: a technical note. AAPS PharmSciTech. 6(3): E482–E486.

Shetye, S.P., A.G. Shilpa and P.G. Bhilegaokar. 2015. Hydrogels: Introduction, preparation, characterization and applications. Int. J. Soc. Res. Meth. 1(1): 47–71.

Simonsen, L., L. Hovgaard, P.B. Mortensen and H. Brøndsted. 1995. Dextran hydrogels for colon-specific drug delivery. V. Degradation in human intestinal incubation models. Eur. J. Pharm. Sci. 3(6): 329–337.

Slaughter, B.V., S.S. Khurshid, O.Z. Fisher, A. Khademhosseini and N.A. Peppas. 2009. Hydrogels in regenerative medicine. Adv. Mater. 21(32-33): 3307–3329.

Soppimath, K., T. Aminabhavi, A. Dave, S. Kumbar and W. Rudzinski. 2002. Stimulus-responsive "smart" hydrogels as novel drug delivery systems. Drug Dev. Ind. Pharm. 28(8): 957–974.

Stocke, N.A., S.M. Arnold and J.Z. Hilt. 2015. Responsive hydrogel nanoparticles for pulmonary delivery. Journal of Drug Delivery Science and Technology. 29: 143–151.

Sung, J.C., B.L. Pulliam and D.A. Edwards. 2007. Nanoparticles for drug delivery to the lungs. Trends Biotechnol. 25(12): 563–570.

Surendrakumar, K., G. Martyn, E. Hodgers, M. Jansen and J. Blair. 2003. Sustained release of insulin from sodium hyaluronate based dry powder formulations after pulmonary delivery to beagle dogs. J. Control. Release. 91(3): 385–394.

Takigami, M., H. Amada, N. Nagasawa, T. Yagi, T. Kasahara, S. Takigami et al. 2007. Preparation and properties of CMC gel. Transactions-Materials Research Society of Japan. 32(3): 713.

Teixeira, L.S.M., J. Feijen, C.A. van Blitterswijk, P.J. Dijkstra and M. Karperien. 2012. Enzyme-catalyzed crosslinkable hydrogels: emerging strategies for tissue engineering. Biomaterials. 33(5): 1281–1290.

Todoroff, J. and R. Vanbever. 2011. Fate of nanomedicines in the lungs. Curr. Opin. Colloid Interface Sci. 16(3): 246–254.

Ulijn, R.V. 2006. Enzyme-responsive materials: a new class of smart biomaterials. J. Mater. Chem. 16(23): 2217–2225.

Ulijn, R.V., N. Bibi, V. Jayawarna, P.D. Thornton, S.J. Todd, R.J. Mart et al. 2007. Bioresponsive hydrogels. Mater. Today. 10(4): 40–48.

Wanakule, P., G.W. Liu, A.T. Fleury and K. Roy. 2012. Nano-inside-micro: disease-responsive microgels with encapsulated nanoparticles for intracellular drug delivery to the deep lung. J. Control. Release. 162(2): 429–437.

Wiedmann, T., R. Bhatia and L. Wattenberg. 2000. Drug solubilization in lung surfactant. J. Control. Release. 65(1): 43–47.

Yang, Y., N. Bajaj, P. Xu, K. Ohn, M.D. Tsifansky and Y. Yeo. 2009. Development of highly porous large PLGA microparticles for pulmonary drug delivery. Biomaterials. 30(10): 1947–1953.

Yang, Z. and B. Xu. 2006. Using enzymes to control molecular hydrogelation. Adv. Mater. 18(22): 3043–3046.

Zeng, X.M., G.P. Martin and C. Marriott. 1995. The controlled delivery of drugs to the lung. Int. J. Pharm. 124(2): 149–164.

Zhao, Q.S., Q.X. Ji, K. Xing, X.Y. Li, C.S. Liu and X.G. Chen. 2009. Preparation and characteristics of novel porous hydrogel films based on chitosan and glycerophosphate. Carbohydr. Polym. 76(3): 410–416.

Zhou, Z., Y. Hu, X. Shan, W. Li, X. Bai, P. Wang et al. 2015. Revealing Three Stages of DNA-Cisplatin Reaction by a Solid-State Nanopore. Scientific Reports. 5.

Index

B

bioconjugate 88–90, 93, 99, 106
biomaterial 304, 305, 308, 313, 317–319
biopolymers 239, 244
bovine serum albumin 157, 160, 187

C

cancer therapeutics 113, 142
carbohydrates 113, 114, 119, 130, 134, 141
chitosan 199, 200, 210, 212–217, 219, 225
composite 303–305, 310–319
controlled release 113, 130, 134, 140, 143
cryogels 173, 181, 182
cyclodextrins 52–54, 59–61

D

delivery 327–329, 331, 338, 339, 342–346
drug 327–331, 333, 338–347
drug delivery 1–4, 6–8, 10, 11, 14–18, 24–27,
    29–38, 40–45, 65, 66, 69, 74, 77, 79, 82,
    84, 197–201, 204, 206, 209, 211, 212, 217,
    219, 220, 223–225, 227, 228, 234, 235,
    237–239, 241–244, 246–252

G

gellan gum 199, 200, 209, 211, 212
glutaraldehyde 208, 225
graft copolymers 205

H

hydrogel 1–18, 64–66, 69–84, 88–106,
    113–118, 127–144, 197–199, 201, 202,
    211, 214, 216–219, 226–228, 234–252,
    259, 266–276, 279, 284, 287, 289–296,
    303–305, 308–310, 312–319, 327, 328,
    331–345, 347
hydrogel composite 310, 316, 317, 319

I

injectable 235, 241, 244–252
insulin 157, 159, 160, 162–165, 167, 168, 175,
    176, 180, 185
interpenetrating network 197–199, 215, 228

L

locust bean gum 199, 200, 220
lysozyme 158, 160, 185, 187

M

macroporous hydrogels 169, 170, 174
micelles 52–54, 57–59
microbicides 260, 269, 274–277, 282, 283,
    292, 295
molecular imprinting 70, 84
multi-component hydrogels 57

N

nanocomposite hydrogel 24–26, 29, 44, 45
nanomedicine 270, 284, 285, 292, 293

O

ocular administration 79
ocular bioengineering 303, 308, 313
ocular drug delivery 303, 319

P

parenteral 234, 243, 244–246, 250, 251
pH-responsive 343, 344
polyelectrolyte complexation 162, 180, 188
polymer matrices 141
polysaccharides 198–200, 205, 220, 223, 228
prodrugs 88–90, 92, 102
protein delivery 155, 156, 159, 165, 175, 177
pulmonary 327–329, 331, 338, 339, 342–347

R

release mechanism 167, 177, 184
responsive 234, 237–240, 243, 244, 246–248, 250–252

S

smart 234, 236–238, 251, 252
sodium alginate 200, 201, 226
stimuli 234, 237–240, 243, 244, 246–248, 250–252
stimuli-responsive 1–3, 7, 12, 15, 18, 343, 347

stimuli-responsive systems 25, 32, 45
sustained release 75, 76, 81, 83, 154, 158, 159, 165, 167, 174–176, 180, 183, 184, 186
swelling 116, 117, 128, 133, 138

V

vaginal therapy 279, 292, 295
vesicles 52, 54–56